THE SILENT CHILD

THE SILENT CHILD

Communication without Words

Editor
Jeanne Magagna

Assistant Editor
Michelle Scott

Routledge
Taylor & Francis Group
LONDON AND NEW YORK

First published 2012 by Karnac Books Ltd.

Published 2019 by Routledge
2 Park Square, Milton Park, Abingdon, Oxon OX14 4RN
52 Vanderbilt Avenue, New York, NY 10017

Routledge is an imprint of the Taylor & Francis Group, an informa business

British Library Cataloguing in Publication Data

A C.I.P. for this book is available from the British Library

ISBN-13: 978-1-85575-5185- (pbk)

Typeset by V Publishing Solutions Pvt. Ltd., Chennai, India

"The aim of art is .... to understand first of all."

and

"...if we listen attentively

we shall hear a faint flutter of wings,

the gentle stirring of life

and hope."

Camus (1960, p. 266 and p. 272)

This book is dedicated to Anne Alvarez, supervisor, Bryan Lask and David Wood, directors of inpatient units, as well as to all those parents and young people who help us to understand children's communication without words

CONTENTS

PART II: YOUNG CHILDREN

PART III: YOUNG PEOPLE

ACKNOWLEDGEMENTS

We would like to acknowledge the following people who have contributed to our work: Tara Pepper Goldsmith, Ellen Jaffe, Mel Perks, Yissca Schiff, Feroza Seervai, Erin Thompson. A particular thanks to Isabel Owen for her careful editing of some chapters.

Special thanks also to those at Karnac: Oliver Rathbone, Lucy Shirley, Kate Pearce, and Alyson Silverwood, who have facilitated the publication of this book.

We are grateful to the following publishers for permission to print previously published articles:

Chapter Two: Sage Publications has given permission to republish Milo's mother's article "Pervasive refusal syndrome: a parent's perspective", *Journal of Clinical Child Psychology and Psychiatry, 6*(3): 455–469.

Chapter Four: Taylor and Francis has given permission to republish Alex Dubinsky's (2010) article "The musings of babies: reflective thinking, emotion and the reintegration of the good object", *Infant Observation, 13(1)*: 5–13.

Chapter Twelve: Karnac has given permission to republish Jeanne Magagna's (2004) chapter "'I didn't want to die, but I had to'": the pervasive refusal syndrome". In: G. Williams, P. Williams, J. Desmarais, & K. Ravenscroft (Eds.), *Exploring Eating Disorders in Adolescents: The Generosity of Acceptance, Volume II* (pp. 107–138).

We are also grateful for the permissions to reprint the following:

Excerpt from Leunig, M. (1990). *A Common Prayer*. New Blackburn, Victoria, Australia: Collins Dove, reprinted with permission from HarperCollins Publishers Australia.

Excerpt from Greene, G. (2004). *The Quiet American*. London: Vintage, reprinted with permission.

Excerpt from "East Cocker" from *FOUR QUARTETS* by T. S. Eliot. Copyright 1940 by T. S. Eliot; Copyright © renewed 1968 by Esme Valerie Eliot. Reprinted by permission of Houghton Mifflin Harcourt Publishing Company. All rights reserved.

Excerpt from Camus, A.(1960) Albert Camus Notebooks, 1935–1942. New York: Knopf and Paris, France: Editions Guillimard.

Excerpt from Camus, A. (1960) Resistance, Rebellion, and Death (pp. 249–272) London: Vintage (Penguin).

Excerpt from Greene, G. (2004) The Quiet American. London: Vintage (Penguin).

Excerpt from MacNeice, L. (1940) Plurality. In: M. Longley (Ed.), Selected Poems (243). London: Faber and Faber, 1966. (Permission from David Higham).

Excerpt from Moreno, J. L. (1946a) Psychodrama Vol. 1. Permission obtained from Moreno's wife, Zerka Moreno.

Excerpt from Seervai, F. (2003) 26th January Mumbai, India: Spenta Print (privately published). Permission granted by Feroza Seervai.

Excerpt from Simon, P. The Sound of Silence. Columbia Records: Catalogue number 4–43396. New York: Permission obtained from Paul Simon Music: New York, New York.

Drawings in Chapters 8 and 17: Permission from Yessica Schiff.

ABOUT THE EDITORS AND CONTRIBUTORS

Nancy L. Bakalar, MD, is a psychoanalyst in private practice in Lone Tree, Colorado, just south of Denver. She completed her analytic training at the International Institute for Psychoanalytic Training (IIPT) in Chevy Chase, Maryland, where she is on the teaching faculty. She is also a faculty member of the International Psychotherapy Institute (IPI), where she teaches and supervises students, and coordinates and teaches distance-learning infant observation seminars by conference call, linking participants from across the United States. Dr Bakalar is on the faculty of the University of Colorado School of Medicine and the Denver Institute for Psychoanalysis. She is the chairman of the Scientific Program Committee of the Denver Psychoanalytic Society, and is a member of the Boulder Institute of Psychotherapy and Research. Dr Bakalar jointly edited and contributed chapters to *Intimate Transformations: Babies with Their Families* (2005).

Naomi Ben Simon, SRN, currently works privately as an individual and couple psychotherapist in London and provides a teaching/work discussion group to the psychiatric nurses of the Child Psychiatry Inpatient Unit of Hadassah Hospital in Israel. Previously, she qualified as a registered nurse and then as a marriage guidance counsellor. Subsequently, in 2005, she became a member of the Tavistock Society of Psychotherapists and Allied Professionals after doing trainings in observation and psychotherapy with children. For over twenty-five years, she has been evolving a method of using stories and life-discussions alongside creative group activities to facilitate communication between non-speaking and speaking children within the inpatient and outpatient psychiatric services in the Royal Free Hospital and then in Great Ormond Street Hospital for Children in London.

Melanie Bladen, MSc, is a clinical specialist physiotherapist at Great Ormond Street Hospital in London and has worked there since 1998. She graduated from Coventry University in 1993 with an Honours Degree in Physiotherapy. She previously worked at Birmingham Children's Hospital and has been in the field of paediatrics for fifteen years specialising in child psychiatry and chronic fatigue syndrome. She has been working with children suffering from a pervasive retreat from life and various other disorders. She received her MSc in Physiotherapy at the University of East London in 2007.

Sarah Dixon, BSc, worked at Ellern Mede School, which is part of the Ellern Mede Centre for Eating Disorders in London. She was a mathematics teacher for the first three years, and subsequently became the head teacher of the school. During this time, she developed her skills in reintegrating young people into their home school after a hospital admission. Before joining the Ellern Mede School, Sarah worked in diverse independent colleges. Several years ago, she then moved to Abu Dhabi, UAE, where she is employed by the Beaconhouse group who work for the Abu Dhabi Education Council to facilitate higher standards and interactional teaching in government-run mathematics departments.

Alex Dubinsky, PhD, is a child and adolescent psychotherapist in private practice. He teaches on the Observation Course at the Tavistock Clinic in London. He also teaches on the Observation Course and the Child Psychotherapy Training at the Martha Harris Centre in Larmor Plage, France. For many years, he has also been supervising infant observations and the clinical work of professionals in Moscow, Russia.

Jo Guiney, MSc, is currently completing doctoral training in Clinical Psychology at University College London, where she is carrying out research into the effects of developmental adversity on attachment style and social processing in adolescents. She studied Psychology, Philosophy and Physiology at the University of Oxford before working for over three years as a Therapeutic Care Worker at the Ellern Mede Centre for Eating Disorders. Following this, she completed an MSc in Psychodynamic Developmental Neuroscience at the Anna Freud Centre, University College London, and the Yale School of Medicine. Whilst at Yale, Jo researched the relationship between early adversity, brain structure, and mood disorders in adolescents using structural magnetic resonance imaging.

Bryan Lask, MB, BS, FRCPsych, MPhil, is Emeritus Professor of Child and Adolescent Psychiatry at the University of London; Honorary Consultant at Great Ormond Street Hospital NHS Trust; Research Director, Ellern Mede Centre, London; and Visiting Professor at the University of Oslo. He is also President of the Eating Disorders Research Society and recipient of a Lifetime Achievement Award from the Academy for Eating Disorders (2011). He has previously been a Consultant Child and Adolescent Psychiatrist at Great Ormond Street Hospital NHS Trust and Visiting Professor at the University of British Columbia, Vancouver, Canada. His research areas have included many aspects of child psychiatry, particularly the psychological aspects of childhood illness. More recently, his clinical work and research have focused on early-onset eating disorders. He has published ten books, nearly two hundred peer-reviewed papers, and numerous chapters in books edited by others. He has also been the Editor of the *Journal of Family Therapy* and *Clinical Child Psychology and Psychiatry.* He is well known as a leading expert in eating disorders, and he lectures internationally.

Natalie Le Clézio, BA, is currently completing a DPsych in Counselling Psychology at City University and works, at present, at the Maudsley Hospital in both the Adult ADHD unit and CASCAID, a specialist service for people affected by HIV who also have mental health difficulties. She has worked with narrative in a diverse array of community settings, including HIV-affected communities in southern Africa, immigrant communities in the UK, and among various online communities of young women. She studied both psychology and sociology at the University of Cape Town and the University of Cambridge, and is now returning to psychology after several years in the creative and strategic divisions of the advertising and marketing industry. She sits on the British Psychological Society's Division of Counselling Psychology Committee, as the representative for trainee counselling psychologists in the UK. In her spare time, Natalie is also involved in creative writing.

Jeanne Magagna, PhD, was Head of Psychotherapy Services at Great Ormond Street Hospital for Children, London, for twenty-two years. She currently works at the Ellern Mede Centre for Eating Disorders in London. She received professional qualifications as a child, adult, and family psychotherapist from the Tavistock Clinic in London. She also obtained a doctorate in psychotherapy from the University of East London and the Tavistock Clinic. Jeanne is the vice-president and joint coordinator of training for the Centro Studi Martha Harris Tavistock model trainings in Florence and Venice. She edited *Universals of Psychoanalysis* (1994) and jointly edited *Psychotherapy with Families* (1981), *Crises in Adolescence* (1994), and *Intimate Transformations: Babies with their Families* (2005). Her special interest is the application of infant observation to work with people in various educational and hospital settings, and she has been involved in long-term video-link seminars to pursue this interest. She has published and taught in Australia, Europe, India, South Africa, South America, and the United States.

Milo's mother wishes to remain anonymous. After writing her previously published classic chapter, which is already considered a source of consolation and support by many parents of ill children, she has continued to use her creativity to pursue an artistic career.

Tara Pepper Goldsmith, MA (Oxon), MSt (Oxon), teaches infant observation at the University of Roehampton, London. She was co-leader of a young people's group on the Mildred Creak Unit, an inpatient psychiatric unit at Great Ormond Street Hospital. Prior to this, she worked as a voluntary counsellor in London primary schools, and for six years she was *Newsweek* magazine's London arts correspondent.

Cynthia Rousso, MSW, MA, is a psychotherapist working with young people and families in both private practice and in the NHS, where she is part of the Child and Adolescent Mental Health Service specialising in eating disorders at the Royal Free Hospital. She completed her graduate degrees at New York University (MSW) and the Tavistock Centre/University of Essex (MA). Cynthia has lived and worked in various countries outside of the United States since 1998.

Ankur Sharma, MB, BS, MRCPsych, is an amateur artist and trainee child psychiatrist in London. His interest in art and child psychiatry is interrelated, for he finds that art is a very useful medium to form therapeutic relationships with young people. In his own artwork, he focuses on emotive elements, using colour to highlight these. He has contributed two abstract artworks that made the cover image of the *British Journal of Psychiatry* (February 2009) and the *American Journal of Psychiatry* (May 2010), and he has had a solo art exhibit in Italy.

Michelle Scott is currently working as a psychotherapist in private practice and on various book projects. She has a background in arts and media but retrained as a mental health nurse at Napier College, Edinburgh, in 1998. She has worked in the specialist field of eating disorders for ten years and completed her MSc in Psychodynamic Counselling at Birkbeck College, London, in 2005. Michelle has a particular interest in using the creative arts in therapy, and has done so both with children at the Ellern Mede Centre and with adults at the Maudsley Hospital in London.

David Wood, MB, BS, FRCPsych, MIGA, is a consultant child and adolescent psychiatrist, group analyst, and family therapist, and the Clinical Director of the Ellern Mede Centre in London, a specialist inpatient service for young people with eating disorders. He began his medical career as a general practitioner, but moved to specialise in psychiatry in 1982. Subsequently, he trained in child and adolescent psychiatry and family therapy at the Tavistock Clinic, London, and in group analysis at the Institute of Group Analysis in London. He has specialised in the treatment of eating disorders in young people since 1995. With others, he set up the Ellern Mede Centre in 2001 and has spent the last ten years developing that service. He has a special interest in the integration of systemic, psychoanalytic, and neuroscientific thinking, with special reference to the development of self-regulation and mentalization, and how these ideas can inform the development of treatment programmes. He focuses on the use of group methods and a total therapeutic milieu approach to help the young people with eating disorders and the staff who work with them.

Charlotte Wormald, MSc, is a trainee clinical psychologist on the Salomon's doctorate course at Christchurch Canterbury University. After completing a degree in English Literature at Trinity College Dublin, she worked as a journalist. Subsequently, she completed a conversion course to psychology and an MSc in child development. While completing her doctorate, Charlotte is also an honorary research associate at the Institute of Psychiatry, King's College London, and in the Great Ormond Street Hospital Feeding and Eating Disorders Service.

INTRODUCTION

Jeanne Magagna

A baby begins communicating with the mother in the first moments of life. If all goes well, the baby looks into the mother's eyes, notices the father, and sucks at the mother's nipple whilst cuddling into her body. The baby is born during a nine-month history of being connected to the mother's body rhythms and the sound of her voice. The baby is born with a need for the mother to hold him in mind and lend meaning to his experiences of comfort or distress, to hold and protect him securely so he feels safe, and to meet his other physical and emotional requirements. The mother is dependent on the baby's signals through gesture and sound to assist her in meeting his needs. If mother and baby are attuned to one another, the baby successfully beckons mother through cries, and subsequently uses gestures and words to tell mother and father what is happening to him. Sometimes, though, the baby stops vocally signalling to the mother when in distress, language fails to develop, or the young child who had begun speaking regresses to a non-speaking state. When these events occur, parents and professionals become alarmed, for they are aware that a difficulty has interfered with the attunement between the mother and child. The child has stopped using the mother and father as a secure base for emotional development.

This book, *The Silent Child: Communication without Words,* is intended to help parents and professionals compassionately comprehend the child's difficulties in depending on someone to receive their communication. This involves the child's difficulties in signalling to the mother and having the signals accepted, the child's difficulties in developing language as a separate person and creating a bridge with another, and the child's difficulties in continuing to use words as a way of communicating states of mind to *the other* once the capacity for speech has developed. Naturally, the child's difficulties in depending on others is influenced by the quality of caregivers and other family members who are influenced by current and trans-generational family relationships.

This book arose from our necessity to think about and describe some of our intuitions about how we might work with emotionally regressed children who entered hospital in full retreat from the external world. With their eyes shut and bodies immobile, they refused food and stopped talking. Underneath these regressive symptoms involving a pervasive retreat to not-talking and not-thinking about an emotionally disturbing inner and outer world that has felt unbearable and unmanageable, there were many varying degrees and types of psychogical problems. Initially, as parents and professionals, we felt very incapacitated in using some of our repertoire of learned skills in helping such a child who didn't talk to us. As a leader of a work discussion group with nurses, I realised that if I helped them learn to observe their own emotional experiences minute by minute and *see with the child's eyes*, a form of empathic identification with the child, and then *see with the parents' eyes*, the nurses and therapeutic careworkers would become effective in finding their own unique and creative ways of being emotionally present and therapeutic for both the non-talking child and his or her parents. Similarly, when I was using this same approach in my work with the parents in a parents' group, parents worked together to regain their confidence as caregivers to a very ill child who didn't speak to them.

Therapeutic work with a non-speaking child is best done if both the multidisciplinary team and the parents think of being on a journey in which all are required to develop and find words about their own experiences in working. As part of this philosophy, I encouraged professionals, parents, young people, and myself to write about our experiences, for ourselves. Eventually, one parent wrote for *The Times* (2002); another parent, whose chapter is in this book, wrote for *The Journal of Clinical Psychology and Psychiatry* (Chapter Two). Then we decided it would be useful to share our experiences in a book for you, the reader, in order that you might go on and further this approach to working with the child who is communicating without words.

Professor Bryan Lask was the Consultant Psychiatrist in the Mildred Creak Unit at Great Ormond Street Hospital at the beginning of this work with the children who had given up life. He encouraged us to work slowly, with patience, supporting one another, while not putting pressure on the child to speak. I encouraged him to allow me to offer a modified individual psychotherapy to the children. In Chapter One, Bryan Lask muses on the "The sound of silence". Although he has written many chapters on what he calls the "pervasive refusal syndrome" (Lask, 1991, 1996, 2004), Lask has chosen to focus on his way of thinking about and working therapeutically with a thirteen-year-old anorectic girl who refuses eye contact, food, or conversation with anyone. He describes how a sigh, a sob, a shriek, a groan, and a laugh are all very significant communications. His hypothesis is that a child may become "silenced" and our task is "to embrace the silence, for the sound it creates tells us so much". Lask is a very charismatic, therapeutic clinician who allows us to watch his patient, clear, not too wordy, step-by-step interaction with a child who is not using words to communicate.

In "Milo was a normal boy" (Chapter Two), a mother very movingly describes her agonising journey with her husband in trying to understand and help her eight-year-old son, Milo, who gave up talking, walking, and eating. Milo's mother and her husband participated in the parents' group connected with the children in hospital. This was difficult for them for they felt themselves to be "very different" from the parents whose children were less ill and making more rapid progress in recovery. However, many parents benefited from learning about their unique ways of being with their child. Milo's parents had to develop many creative skills as parents with a non-speaking child and at times the journey was overwhelming. As part of the recovery phase for the parents, I suggested that they share their work with other parents and professionals in order that others might learn from their thinking together and develop ways of *being emotionally present for Milo.* During the critical phase of Milo's illness, his mother felt that "to share the problem and admit the bewilderment and distress would have caused them to break down and cry and cry". Now, that Milo had recovered, writing "her story" seemed to be a cathartic way for Milo's mother to lend words to her unspoken painful experiences. Similarly, perhaps my own interest in writing about "communication without words" derives from a desire to create a narrative about my own unverbalised states of mind present in both my experience in my own bilingual Italian family and my sometimes painful and arduous experiences working as a psychoanalytic psychotherapist with non-speaking children. Chapter Three, "Communication without words", describes five of the states of mind underlying "silence". The infant observation vignettes are used to assist parents and professionals in their quest for understanding the infantile part of the non-speaking child who initially makes them feel terribly rejected. The five states of mind illustrated are: giving up, feelings of persecution, holding onto physical sensation in lieu of thinking and speaking, feeling hatred toward the other, and creating a loving communion.

Young children

Alex Dubinsky, in "The musings of babies" (Chapter Four), continues the exploration of children's capacity to communicate through using infant observations. His detailed vignettes assist us in understanding the child's initial attempts to form symbols and thoughts, and to communicate in words. In his chapter, we see beautiful moments in which the baby is imaginatively trying to discover symbolic representations of the loved and good internal mother. We also discover how the capacity for thinking and speaking evolves in normal infant development.

In Chapter Five, "A baby's 'broken bridge' to the parents", I describe how the development of thinking and speaking can be hindered by the nature of the family interactions. Lack of emotional containment of the distress in early infancy can prompt a child to resort to non-thinking and to the use of bodily sensations to "hold the self together emotionally and physically". This chapter presents a picture of the infantile states to which non-speaking children regress when their psychic structure is overwhelmed with experiences of emotional turmoil linked with rage, anger, misery, despair, fear, abuse, and other forms of trauma.

In Chapters Six and Seven, I describe ways of working with parents and young children using family psychotherapy and individual psychotherapy in the presence of the mother who helps me understand her child. Illustrated is my approach of using the parents as "colleagues" to foster a shared experience of observing sequences of interaction and sustaining one's own inner feelings and the child's feelings sufficiently long to lend thinking to them. I say to the parents, "I need your help, help me to observe and understand your child." I also involve the family in an exploration of internalised trans-generational trauma expressing itself in current parental interactions with the therapist and the child (Faimberg, 1988).

Older children and adolescents

Although a child is not speaking, that does not mean that his or her siblings can't facilitate understanding of *the unspoken* feelings present in family interactions. For this reason, when a child is not speaking, I feel it is important to undertake *extended family explorations* involving the whole family in using dreams, drawings, drama and play. Focusing simply on the symptomatic not-speaking child by providing speech therapy and/or individual psychotherapy does not do justice to *the unspoken issues* imbedded in transgenerational and current family interactions. In Chapter Eight, "Extended family explorations using dreams, drawings, and play when the referred child does not speak", I describe ten techniques for developing understanding of *unspoken aspects* of family relationships that require repair.

Those children whose relationships have become unbearably emotionally intense may feel pushed into complete withdrawal from the external world through shutting their minds, their eyes, and their mouths. Regulating their emotional experience through retreat may also involve regression to not-eating and not-walking. A young psychology graduate or nurse, but also any experienced clinician, confronted with such a retreating child can feel intense feelings of inadequacy, emotional tension, and hopeless despair. Once again, putting into writing the tedious and emotionally turbulent journey one has taken with such a child is an emotionally useful experience for every staff member.

I encouraged Jo Guiney, a young therapeutic careworker, to put her experiences "into a story". Her chapter, "Inpatient care of a child who does not talk, walk, or eat" (Chapter Nine) involves a helpful form of self-reflection. Writing helps staff members "put the pieces together inside" both during and after the emotionally wearing process of working with a very withdrawn, persecuted young person. This is true particularly because such a child makes a staff member feel rejected, and this in turn evokes all sorts of internalised experiences of rejection. Jo Guiney has spoken openly about how important it was to keep hold of her own emotional responses to the rejecting, non-speaking child in order to facilitate a dialogue with her. In particular, she highlights those emotional experiences which inpatient staff often feel they aren't supposed to have. These include feeling irritation, infuriation, a sense of being drained of life, or feeling inadequate and helpless. She makes us aware that a *work discussion seminar* for the staff group to explore the staff's emotional attitudes to a young person is particularly helpful to foster thinking about the non-speaking young person's state of mind that gets projected on to the staff and influences their relationships with the family and each other.

Many professionals may be called to intervene with children who are not talking. This is particularly true if the children have given up walking and eating as well. In my role as a consultant psychotherapist, it seemed important to work alongside a physiotherapist, in this case Melanie Bladen, to support and foster an integration of our therapeutic methods of approaching a non-speaking young person. In Chapter Ten, "Collaborating, containing, inspiring confidence: physiotherapy with a child who does not talk, walk, or eat", Melanie Bladen and I illustrate the therapeutic mind–body dialogue between child and physiotherapist through these six concepts: collaboration, curiosity, containment, confidence, creative imagination, and surprise. Melanie's physiotherapy insights are helpful to all staff members and parents, for they remind us to hold the child's bodily experiences in mind and to understand the experience of *the whole of the child.*

This requires that we give time and space to becoming aware of how our encounters with the child affect *both* our bodies and our minds (Dosamantes, 1997).

One way of giving time and space to holding the bodily and emotional experiences of the child within ourselves and lending thinking to this experience is through writing. In Chapter Eleven, "The silent child in school", a young teacher, Sarah Dixon, develops a creative way of elaborating on her relationship with a silent child: in the evenings, she writes letters to the child talking about her experience of the day. These letters are not given to the child, but they inform and modulate Sarah's way of being with the silent child on the subsequent day of school.

In Chapters Twelve and Thirteen, respectively, Dr Nancy L. Bakalar and I separately explore the question, "Can psychotherapy be therapeutic when a young person is not speaking?" These chapters are designed particularly to assist clinical teams who have rejected young people who attended psychotherapy sessions but *"did not show the motivation 'to work' through talking"*. One of the premises in these chapters is that some of the most important and difficult implicit memory experiences have not yet been symbolised and therefore *are not in a suitable form for speaking to take place.* Rejection of the non-speaking child feels particularly unfair, particularly since some children, like the child who created the "no entry" cover drawing, have been forbidden to speak. It is important for us to remember that a silent child can still think alongside a therapist thinking aloud.

Therapeutic work is essential to help the young person find a capacity and a wish to think alongside the therapist. The therapist's use of bodily and emotional countertransference experiences is a focal point for transformation and modulation of overwhelming emotion. This makes it possible for emotions to become symbolised, regulated, and suitable for verbal discourse. These chapters demonstrate the unfreezing of "encapsulated parts of the self' that are in a frozen state in the unconscious" (S. Klein, 1981). In the therapists' descriptions of the analytic process, it is possible to discover the way in which emotions are brought to consciousness, depicted in dreams, drawn, and discussed by the young person (Magagna, 1999). The reader also discovers therapeutic ways of working with what feels like "an impossible therapeutic impasse" (Rosenfeld, 1987). Likewise, Cynthia Rousso (Chapter Fourteen) is undaunted by the responsibility of working with a family of a non-speaking, non-eating, pervasively refusing young person. Rousso reveals how she grapples with "non-talking family patterns of interaction" which arise in response to too-intense and therefore overwhelming emotions. She also makes us aware of how words can be used as a necessary protection to evade the emotional impact of a critical emotional point. One is reminded of Winnie, in Beckett's *Happy Days* (1961). Winnie was an impulsive talker trapped in a wasteland of words. In her chapter, Rousso also describes therapeutic ways of relating to the family's use of evasion, projection, and containment of feelings.

For many years, Dr David Wood, in his role as clinical director of an inpatient unit for eating disorders, has also been embarking on what in the 1980s leading clinicians said was impossible: working in large and small therapeutic groups with young eating-disordered and pervasively refusing children who might sink into a deep, opaque silence that can feel like it will last forever. He describes how a barely adequately functioning protective ego boundary might leave a young person feeling an overwhelming anxiety of "losing oneself" if she or he talks to others. In his chapter "Opaque silence in groups" (Chapter Fifteen), Wood affirms his belief, and knowledge gained from his experience, that therapeutic groups provide "repeated, corrective, emotionally charged experiences which foster emotional maturation" (Foulkes, S. H. 1964, p. 82 and 129).

Of course, there is an even more difficult silence to bear: that is the silence of a young person in a coma. The problem for family and professionals surrounding a coma victim is that they can begin to relate to the young person *as though the young person is dead.* Imagine awakening from a coma and people are ignoring you because they feel you are dead. *There is no one to come alive to!* The young nurse in Almodóvar's film *Talk to Her* (2002) realises this as he is movingly and continuously present and sometimes talking to a young dancer while she lies in a coma for months before she "comes to life" again. With this film in mind, I provided Skype supervision for the work of Irith Barzel Raveh, who worked with families and multidisciplinary teams on several Israeli medical wards for coma victims.

Usually, a portion of coma patients, even those with some brain functioning, die; however, the eighteen coma patients in this small pilot study using the Bick infant observation method survived. The staff involved with the patients and their families had conducted *close, detailed observations* of the patients accompanied by staff *work discussions* thinking about their observations and countertransference experiences. Barzel Raveh's conclusion in "From being nobody to being somebody" is that "the quiet, non-intrusive containing presence of the observers who are fully available for the coma-patients and their families, can make the *seemingly dead* patients *come alive* in their own minds" (Barzel Raveh, 2009). This may lend confirmation to the notion of patients' mental consciousness, a notion that exists in the eyes of the families who desperately look for contact with their child overtaken by a coma. The coma victim may awaken, not with his/her full capacities, but with the awareness that he *has remained alive in the mind of a caring family and staff.* This seems to make all the difference when traversing the distance between an unconscious coma-state and consciousness. Reaching towards and grasping onto consciousness may be facilitated as one awakens if the surrounding people are holding you in mind. This work is mentioned here to illustrate the extent of our interest in helping professionals work therapeutically with families and their children, however ill they may be.

Creative activities for non-speaking children

People often repeatedly try to get *words* from withdrawn young people. It can feel very intrusive to these young people not ready to give words to their experiences, and they often retreat even further. When I worked in a creative group, I realised that young people often draw or sculpt their experiences a few weeks or months before they feel able to share their feelings in *verbal dialogues* with their individual psychotherapists. For this reason, it seems essential to provide group opportunities for non-speaking children to gather and transform their unspoken sensations and feelings in artistic or musical ways. Symbolisation of the non-speaking child's feelings is assisted by the presence of other children who are expressing their feelings through art and music as well as through conversation with others. Usually, the group leaders begin the creative group with stories, films, and themes connected with the group's current emotional experiences. In doing this, the leaders offer the group members an invitation to express their own feelings connected with the themes, or to choose to express something else. The non-speaking young people in a creative group can be safely guided to freely share symbols of what is inside themselves. Tara Pepper Goldsmith and Naomi Ben Simon in Chapter Sixteen state that the creative group can function as a container for the not-speaking young people's unconscious, unprocessed emotional states. By gently offering insight and interpretation to the group, the therapists began to help the young people to hold their emotions and think quietly about them to themselves. Silent thinking occurs while drawing and sculpting long before the young people opened their mouths to speak to anyone in the group.

This story of therapeutic work with non-speaking children ends with "Roar and rumpus: engaging non-speaking children through stories and songs" (Chapter Seventeen). Charlotte Wormald, who has written this chapter, was about to leave her job when I accidentally discovered her interest in children's literature and asked her to write this chapter. She was assisted by Natalie Le Clézio, who is interested in writing and music, and Ankur Sharma, a child psychiatrist who has been drawing and writing poems as part of his growing interest in creative communication with a child. Milo's mother and father (Chapter Two) had been encouraged by me to both create and to read children's stories linked with a particular themes in Milo's emotional journey towards recovery. For example, the parents created a story about courage which they told to Milo before and after his first journey away from the hospital. This chapter assists staff and parents in thinking about relevant story themes they might use to help a child feel understood during times when the child *shows* but *does not speak* about particular emotional states present in their mutual encounter. At times when children are particularly overwhelmed by emotions, they don't feel it is possible to think about their own feelings. The authors state, "Meta-narrative functions as a wedge," an "in-between story that is not about the young person in question and that is not even narrated by or interrogated by that young person". As the authors suggest, it is certainly "sometimes easier to approach oneself and easier to eventually communicate with an-other" using stories, poems, and song lyrics. Most importantly, the chapter suggests:

> "The child's silence should not function to silence the person with him."

In conclusion, I would like to mention that many of the chapters are written by parents or young staff, who had not yet completed their professional training and were working alongside older staff members. Almost as a necessity for therapeutic work to occur, everyone working within the hospital teams; staff, parents, and young people, were encouraged *to give words* creatively to their deeply moving emotional experiences. Understanding the countertransference experiences, both in working together and with the silent child, was an essential aspect of our staff *work discussion* groups, parents' groups, supervision, and/or personal psychotherapy. In presenting this book, I am suggesting that writing about one's experience can be part of the therapeutic work to answer the question, "How can I make more sense of my experience of my encounters with a child communicating without words?" I am very grateful to these writers for their thoughtful, sensitive, courageous, and creative endeavours to penetrate beyond what they already knew.

Jeanne Magagna, The Editor

NOTE: All descriptions of families and their children have been heavily disguised to preserve confidentiality. Each chapter uses either "he" or "she" to avoid referring to an individual with the pronoun "they". Obviously, a regressed child who is not walking, not eating and not speaking can be of either sex.

PART I

INTRODUCTION

CHAPTER ONE

"The sound of silence"

Bryan Lask

Hello darkness, my old friend
I've come to talk with you again
Because a vision softly creeping
Left its seeds while I was sleeping
And the vision that was planted in my brain
Still remains within the sound of silence.

—*The Sound of Silence* (Simon & Garfunkel, 1964)

Many clinicians in our field consider working with the persistently silent child to be one of the most challenging of all clinical situations. This brief essay attempts to refute that view and indeed to demonstrate that "silence" is neither silent nor challenging, but rather a very loud and meaningful communication.

Case vignette

Let us consider Sarah, thirteen, with an eight-month history of anorexia nervosa, who has been on a child psychiatry inpatient unit for six weeks. Sarah has consistently refused to eat or drink, sits alone, miserable and tearful, head bowed, shoulders stooped, and face invisible behind her long hair. She talks to neither the staff nor other inpatients. At meal times, she eats very little, and this extremely reluctantly, slowly, and sparsely, whilst avoiding all eye contact and crying silently. During the rest of the day, Sarah shuns all contact and spends as much time alone as she possibly can. In her therapy sessions, she repeats this behaviour and all attempts by her therapist, and all other clinicians, to engage with her are met with profound and persistent silence.

We will rejoin Sarah later.

Definitions and concepts

In the clinical setting, "silence" is generally taken to mean, literally, "a lack of verbal communication". As such, it challenges the clinician's skill and, often, patience. However, this definition is problematic. A lack of verbal communication implies an absence of words that can be understood and responded to. But non-verbal communications, such as a sigh, a sob, a shriek, a groan, a laugh, whilst lacking words, are each in turn very significant communications.

Let us therefore broaden the definition of silence to "a lack of audible communication". Thus we include a sigh, a sob, a shriek, a groan, a laugh. In so doing, we instantly broaden our conceptualisation of silence and therefore enhance our potential for understanding it.

Such a definition is still, however, problematic. How do we conceptualise the scenario described above in which Sarah sits silently, making no sounds, whether they be verbal or non-verbal? She is truly inaudible. But is she silent? From an auditory perspective, she is indeed silent. But is she "silent " from a metaphorical perspective?

Metaphorically, "silence" is used to mean "a lack of communication". Does this broadening of the definition help? Although seemingly nihilistic, it does indeed! Watzlawick (1967) made the point that "because behaviour does not have a counterpart, there is no anti-behaviour" (p. 48). To put this in another way, there can be no "non-behaviour". Returning to Watzlawick (1967), "it is impossible not to communicate," thus there can be no such thing as non-communication. Therefore, silence is not only a behaviour, it is a communication. Furthermore, it is a very clear, loud, and unambiguous communication. There can be no disputing such a behaviour; it is silence in the loudest possible way. And this is not simply pedantry, it has significant clinical implications.

Before turning to these clinical implications, there is another important construct to be considered, that of "volition". Volition means "the act of making a choice, selection, option, free will". When Sarah is "silent", is this volitional? Has she chosen to be silent? Was this but one option of many for her? Is her "silence" of her own free will?

To answer such questions, we need to know much more about Sarah than is in the information provided so far. In other words, the answers are likely to be determined by numerous, as yet unknown, circumstances. We need therefore to consider the question: "Why is Sarah silent?" To find out, we need to understand more about Sarah, but how can we do this in the context of her "silence"?

The dilemma of silence—a very simple conceptual framework

A dilemma is a state of uncertainty or perplexity, especially when requiring a choice between equally unfavourable or unpromising options. So where does this philology leave us when we ask, "What can we do about Sarah's silence?" When politicians are asked difficult questions, they tend to bluff their way through, or answer a totally different and unasked question, or respond: "With respect, that is the wrong question!"

So with respect, I contend that asking the question "what can we do about Sarah's silence?" is the wrong question. I believe a more constructive approach is to consider not a "*silent* Sarah", but a "*silenced* Sarah". So the question can be re-phrased as "How can we help a *silenced* Sarah?" And this opens up numerous possibilities, each based on the premise that Sarah is silenced by her dilemma.

So how can we help Sarah with her dilemma? That is *our* dilemma! In other words, what are our options, all seemingly unfavourable, in trying to understand and help Sarah resolve her dilemma? What has silenced her?

Children are silenced for many reasons: emotional turmoil such as rage, anger, misery, despair, fear; abuse, other forms of trauma, threats; lack of trust; shame; inability to find the right words and confusion. So what can we do to help Sarah and other silenced children?

Pictures speak louder than words

Let us revisit Sarah and consider here a few basic principles:

We recall that Sarah sits alone, miserable and tearful, head bowed, shoulders stooped, her face invisible behind her long hair. The maxim "A picture speaks a thousand words", first stated by an emperor of the Xia Dynasty in China about 4,000 years ago, remains just as pertinent today. We overestimate the verbal and underestimate the non-verbal. Once we acknowledge this, then the "problem" of silence is no longer a problem.

Sarah is "speaking" very loudly, she is "saying": "I am lonely, miserable, scared, unworthy". She does not need to say this with words because she shows it silently, and if we cannot "hear" this communication, then we increase her sense of loneliness. Thus, our mind-set needs to be one that embraces the silence, for the sound it creates (*The Sound of Silence*, Simon & Garfunkel, 1964) tells us so much.

Context

Is this conversation better held with Sarah alone, or with her parent(s) or other carers? All possibilities should be considered. It should not be a matter of either/or, as all scenarios can have value. Seeing Sarah alone provides a context that reduces any pressures or conflicts associated with her parent(s)' presence, ensures privacy and supports confidentiality.

In contrast, parental presence may have its own benefits. It could be reassuring and may feel safer. It does have the added advantages of parents observing how the clinician communicates with Sarah and learning what underlies her silence. The clinician might talk with a parent about what Sarah may be experiencing and in the meantime observe Sarah's responses to this conversation. The decision is best made in consultation with Sarah. She may offer no verbal reply but we have now established that it is impossible for her not to communicate on the matter.

I would proceed as follows, using as gentle a tone as possible:

BL: Sarah, I'd like to try to understand what is so troubling you. If it's okay with you I'm going to spend some time with you just trying to get to know you a little.
Sarah: [No verbal response, no movement]
BL: For some people, such conversations are easier held with just the two of us, but other people prefer to have a parent or someone else with them. It's entirely your choice.
Sarah: [No verbal response]
BL: It's perfectly okay not to reply, but I'll just give you a few moments to think about it, then I'll check with you.
BL: [Remains silent for half a minute or so and then assumes Sarah is not going to give either a yes or no verbal, or non-verbal response]
BL: I wonder whether you can indicate if you do have a view on this? Perhaps just a very little nod or shake of your head in reply to each question, but please don't worry if you can't or prefer not to respond, that's quite okay. So, I'll ask just a couple of very short questions; the first is: "Would you prefer to have someone with you?"
BL: [I then wait a few seconds, and if there is no response:]
BL: Okay I wonder if it would be okay for it just to be you and me?
BL: [I repeat the few seconds wait, and then:]
BL: Sarah, if I've understood correctly, you haven't expressed a preference?
BL: [Silently waiting]
BL: So, if it's okay with you, I'll decide?
BL: [Silently waiting]

Assuming no obvious choice by Sarah, I would then decide on her behalf. What I decide is based upon other factors, which will be specific to each "Sarah". Obviously, if Sarah somehow indicates her choice, then I would fully accept and respect it.

The principles in the above "conversation" include a soft tone of voice, a very gentle pace, clear explanations, plenty of time to consider and answer, and non-obtrusive observation of Sarah's non-verbal communication. This process may best be described as "tracking". There is no attempt to get responses from Sarah; rather the clinician stays with the moment, notes her "communications", considers them, and responds gently, empathically, and non-judgementally.

If Sarah had given any obvious response I would have checked this out to ensure I had understood correctly. Here is an example:

BL: I'm not sure if I got that correctly, Sarah, but I think you are indicating that…

Once the decision has been made with regard to who will be in the room, we can move onto the next step.

Musings with Sarah

In the absence of verbal conversation, I choose to use the concept of "musing" - the process of calm, quiet, curious contemplation. However, I do this aloud. In other words, I think aloud.

BL: Sarah, I have a somewhat strange way of doing things, and I do hope you won't mind too much. I like to think aloud about what might be happening for you. So I may just say a few things, then stop, think about them silently, then think aloud again. I hope that will be okay with you. Now I absolutely don't expect you to reply, though of course you can if you want to, but I am not expecting that, and that's fine with me. I hope that's okay?

From here on, I gently state what I am thinking may be happening for Sarah. What I say will be based on what knowledge I have of her and what knowledge I have regarding why children are "silenced", as discussed before. Possibly most importantly, I use my own "feelings", my gut instinct, and my "heart", in my attempt to understand what Sarah might be experiencing. A useful guideline is to track my "countertransference". Assuming that when we start the session I am feeling relatively emotionally neutral, I note my own feelings as the session proceeds. Awareness of a sense of sadness, fear, and despair suggests to me that this may be what Sarah might be experiencing.

The "conversation" may proceed as follows:

BL: I am sorry to see you so sad, and have been wondering why this might be..... [Pause]..... I know you have been very sad recently..... and worried..... and other things too..... I'm trying to think about what might have gone wrong to so upset you.....

It is essential to proceed very gently and slowly and, of course, to watch for any non-verbal communication such as a shake or a nod of the head, a tensing of muscles, a sigh, a groan, crying, fidgetiness, or further withdrawal. Any of these is an important communication and would modify the content of my musing. In the absence of any such response, I would continue:

BL: What I've learned from other people of your age, who have seemed as upset as you..... is that many different things can happen..... at school..... at home..... somewhere else..... sometimes there has been teasing..... bullying..... arguments..... even worse things..... violence..... other horrible things..... sometimes when things go wrong other girls have felt it's been their fault..... they wrongly think they have deserved it.....

I would pause for a bit longer here. Then I might ask:

BL: I wonder if any of these things make any sense..... mean anything to you?

Until this point, and this may well be fifteen to twenty minutes into the meeting, there may have been no signal of recognition, no verbal response. But in my experience, it is extremely rare for there to be no response to that last question. In fact, I cannot recall of any such time. Almost invariably, there is a nod of recognition or acceptance.

BL: It seems like something I said was important for you.
Sarah: [Sarah moves her head almost imperceptibly]

BL: I wonder which of the things I said was important….. maybe I could just very carefully check this out….. and of course you don't have to respond.
Sarah: [Sarah makes another very slight move]
BL: Teasing….. bullying..... arguments ….. fights…..
Sarah: [Sarah gives a very slight nod]
BL: So that seems like there are some fights going on…..?
Sarah: [Sarah nods]
BL: At home.....
Sarah: [Sarah nods]
BL: That's horrible for you…..?
Sarah: [Sarah sighs]
BL: I'm wondering who's fighting…..
Sarah: [Sarah does not respond verbally and doesn't change her posture]
BL: I'm guessing mum or dad may be involved…..
Sarah: [Sarah nods]
BL: Mum and Dad are fighting…..
Sarah: [Sarah softly cries]
BL: That sounds very scary…..
Sarah: [Sarah cries more intensely]
BL: And I am guessing you are worried about how it's going to end…..
Sarah: [Sarah nods]
BL: Worried that someone will get really badly hurt…..
Sarah: [Sarah cries and looks up]
BL: Maybe we can try to discuss this further if you are up to it…..?
Sarah: [Sarah nods]

Sarah has said nothing throughout; but she has communicated very powerfully and conveyed that she is willing to continue. The hardest part of the work has been done.

But what if she had shaken her head to convey that she did not wish to continue?

BL: Sarah, I can see how horrible this is for you….. I don't want to upset you more ….. If you would rather stop right now, that's fine.....

At this point, I would carefully *track* her response, and if she indicates she wants to stop, I would fully accept that:

BL: Sarah, I'm sorry things are so awful for you ….. I think you're right to want to stop….. I'll think about what I have learned….. and I would like to try and chat more about it next time….. I hope that's okay with you…..

When we next meet, I would recall our "conversation" and check with her that I had understood correctly. If so, then I would gently seek her permission to continue. If she conveys that I had got something wrong, then I would use the same approach to clarify. If she conveys that she does not wish to continue the conversation from last time (this has never happened to me), I would muse on where I had gone wrong.

Using such an approach requires tact, patience, curiosity, and a willingness to accept little or no apparent progress. It is essential to remember that Sarah has been "silenced" and that whatever has silenced her is far more powerful than she is. Acknowledgement and acceptance of the fear of speaking is reassuring for her. Sarah is in a dilemma and silence is her way of managing. It can be helpful to acknowledge this by saying something along the lines of:

BL: I've been thinking about you, Sarah, and what I know about you..... It sort of feels to me that not saying anything is for you the only way you can manage just now..... If that's right, you shouldn't try to change things for a while..... It's quite okay to hold onto something if it helps a bit.....

Throughout this "conversation", I would continue *to track* her responses:

BL: Sometimes it just seems so difficult to know what to do..... Sometimes people think that whatever has gone wrong, it's their fault, even when it's obviously not..... Sometimes people are told it's their fault, even when it's obviously not..... It can even happen that people are threatened that if they say anything, worse things will happen.....

I am making plenty of pauses and doing much tracking here. I try to stay with the moment, to understand the feelings present between us, to gather my thoughts, and to find the right words.

BL: I don't know if any of this applies to you, Sarah, but if it does then I think it's important for you to know that when adults are fighting, whatever they say to you about it, it is not your fault..... and whatever you may think, it is not your fault..... and you don't deserve it.....

There are more pauses in my speaking as I *keep track* of her expressions and body postures, noting their qualities and Sarah's mood.

BL: If adults say horrible things to you about you or about other people, then they are wrong to do so..... Adults must always take responsibility for their own behaviour. .....

This approach seems helpful regardless of Sarah's "diagnosis", background, length of illness, or intensity of silence. In fact, Sarah has anorexia nervosa and it might be useful to illustrate how this technique can be used for that illness in which children and adolescents quite commonly find it difficult to discuss their thoughts and feelings. This is hardly surprising in that anorexia nervosa is a confusing illness to all concerned, full of apparent paradox and contradictions.

For example, Sarah is very thin but feels very fat. She may feel well but look, and at times feel, very ill. She looks fragile but behaves with great strength. Her stomach feels full despite not eating and is therefore actually empty. Mostly, Sarah starves herself but sometimes cannot avoid bingeing. She is obsessed with food but does her best to avoid consuming any. Her self-esteem is very low despite her being a popular, talented, and successful child. Sarah feels as if she has no control, or is likely to lose it completely, but presents to others as very much in control. Having previously been a conscientious perfectionist, eager to please, she is now rebellious and uncaring of how others feel. At times, Sarah knows she is ill but at others has no sense of ill-health. She sometimes perceives the illness as a friend and comfort, but at other times she experiences it as an enemy and tormentor. Therefore, sometimes Sarah is more aware of its advantages and wants to stay with the illness, but at other times she is more aware of the disadvantages and wants to recover. What family and clinicians believe to be supportive and helpful, she experiences as coercive and persecuting.

It is hardly surprising that Sarah is confused, and perhaps overwhelmed, by powerful feelings.

Musing with the Sarah who has anorexia nervosa may go along the following lines:

BL: Sarah, from what I've heard from other girls with anorexia, it's really a very confusing and frightening situation….. They are told they're very thin when they feel very fat….. They feel full even though they've not eaten much at all..... They feel like they've eaten lots but are told they haven't….. They feel ashamed of eating….. They feel guilt about it….. Losing weight feels good but everyone else says it is not….. Thoughts nag you not to eat, tell you are greedy if you do, that you are bad….. but the thoughts can also sometimes seem supportive and comforting….. People get cross with you for not eating even though you feel it's the best thing for you…..

Throughout this musing, I watch carefully for any response, any sign of recognition. If there is, then I might acknowledge that "perhaps that bit meant something to you…..?" And I would continue with the musings along the same lines.

If there were no such sign of recognition that something I said resembled what Sarah felt, I would continue:

BL: I am not sure if any of that was of any relevance to you, Sarah….. I hope it will be okay if I just go through some of those things again…..

I then repeat each in turn, slowly, gently, and with pauses between. It is unusual for there to be no response. Should that be the case, then I might simply acknowledge that these things are really hard to think about and it's fine not to respond. I reiterate that I don't expect her to respond and that's fine.

An alternative approach is to muse more directly about the pros and cons of anorexia nervosa:

BL: Some girls have told me that the good things about having anorexia are much stronger than the bad things….. They say that there are lots of good things about it….. such as they feel proud of managing to avoid eating….. proud of losing weight….. They feel better….. They think they look better….. They feel in control….. They don't feel ashamed of themselves….. or disgusted with themselves..... They feel less anxious….. That's lots of good things..... It's not surprising you'd rather stay with how things are…..

The same principles as outlined above apply throughout this process.

Whatever the content and responses during such "discussions", I suggest that I will think about it all and that maybe we can meet again soon. Sometimes it can take a few sessions before Sarah feels safe enough to contribute, and patience is of the essence.

Conclusion

Hopefully the principles of this "musing" approach are clear. The aim is *not* to "get Sarah to speak". The aim is to *understand* Sarah's dilemma and *to help* her to tackle it. There are many variations to this approach and clinicians are encouraged to try them out. One will work. All we need to do is "listen"; listen not only with our ears..... but also with our eyes..... our knowledge..... our experience..... our instincts..... our hearts..... and, above all, we should listen to *the sound of silence*!

> And the vision that was planted in my brain
> Still remains within the sound of silence.
>
> (Simon & Garfunkel, 1964)

CHAPTER TWO

"Milo was a normal boy"

Milo's mother

Milo was a normal healthy eight-year-old boy. Until.....

The illness started as an apparently harmless 'flu bug', but within days had him writhing with pain, and calling out. He was admitted to hospital with suspected appendicitis, but not operated on. His illness was blamed on a "virus". After a few days, he moved to a more specialised children's hospital. He was in great distress, crying out, not eating and not taking interest in any activity. It was clear that the medical and surgical staff did not know what was the matter with him, although he had several physical tests. At this stage Milo was repeatedly calling out "I have a bad pain" and "It's getting worse". This was all he said, he could not converse, but clearly wanted us there to reiterate his distress, and to comfort him. I sensed irritation from everyone on the ward. Suddenly Milo whispered to us "It hurts to talk", and went silent. His silence gave a certain relief to others on the ward. However, he resumed calling out as before on the following day. We were told that Milo had a psychological problem, and he was seen by a psychiatrist.

Milo's illness was not given a name, nor was he offered any help. He was discharged shortly afterwards, in an extremely distressed state. He was calling out loudly in a non-stop manner. He could not walk or stand. He hardly ate and only drank with great encouragement. We were offered tranquillisers to calm him down, but no other support or help. He was having increasing difficulty with eating and drinking. We were anxious about his physical deterioration, and on our suggestion it was arranged that we would return with Milo to the hospital every week to have his weight monitored. The psychiatrist offered an appointment six weeks after discharge. For the next two weeks, Milo continued to call out all day at home, from the moment he woke until about midnight, until again one day it "hurt to talk". Suddenly he called me over, whispered a little, and told me about the pain, "It is still getting worse" and "It hurts to talk". Then he became agonisingly silent and passive. I can't explain how much I wanted to take up the screaming for him.

The only time Milo spoke a few words was in the darkness at bedtime. During the day, he kept his hands over his face, seeming absorbed in his world. In fact, he was aware of everything going on around him. He wanted to be close to us physically, to stay in the same room, or to lie in our arms. He kept his hands over his face when there were people around, and he peeped out a little if it was just family present. He would lie passively in our arms or lie on a sofa if it was only the family in the room, but would curl into a ball, as if to hide, if anyone else came in. Occasionally, if he couldn't bear what was going on, he would shout out "No". We could see that he was watching and noticing what was going on around him.

At night, and in the dark, he relaxed enough to uncover his face and whispered a few words. These were not conversations, more often they were to tell us, "Bad pain", and "Still getting worse". He wanted us to be very involved with his suffering. At night he could not relax to sleep unless one of us lay in bed beside him for about two hours. Also, he used to wake up sometimes during the night, and always very early in the morning.

As the weeks went by, and we returned to the hospital with a weaker and more ill child, the physician arranged brain scans, endless blood tests, and other "investigations". The results of the tests coming back as "all clear" was reassuring for us, but confusingly upsetting for Milo. It seemed he was distressed that, despite his very real pain, his pain was not being identified.

It was difficult to answer Milo's cries of pain. All we could do was to acknowledge them, and indicate to him that we were still trying to get to grips with them. We told him we knew how bad his pain was, and that we had told the doctors. We reassured him that we would continue to tell them. We understood that he was suffering. We told him we would not leave him. In our own minds, we were acutely aware of how helpless we were to relieve his suffering, even though we were doing everything imaginable to try to help him. We were seriously concerned that something might be being missed.

After Milo had been unwell for about two months, his care was transferred back to the original hospital where he had first been seen. An action plan was set up which involved hydrotherapy, sessions with an occupational therapist, and us seeing a psychiatrist without Milo present. They freely told us they had not seen a case like Milo before. Milo became dangerously thin and dehydrated, and we admitted him to hospital to have a naso-gastric tube put in place. We felt we were like Judas, betraying him by subjecting him to such a difficult procedure and hospitalisation, but the naso-gastric tube and hospital admission gave Milo the nutrition he needed to stay alive and fight on. The whole incident makes me shiver with disgust.

In passing, and almost by mistake, a junior doctor mumbled something about "pervasive refusal syndrome", a diagnosis that had not up until now been mentioned. He said Milo's condition seemed similar. Immediately when we arrived home, we researched what he had said and found articles by Professor Bryan Lask, a Consultant at Great Ormond Street Children's Hospital. We requested that our doctor make a referral to him, and telephoned Professor Lask. After various comings and goings and a lot of assertiveness on our part, we received an appointment to see the team of specialists in the Mildred Creak Unit at Great Ormond Street Hospital. Waiting for the appointment seemed like forever. Milo was assessed, as was the family. It was quite strange because, up until that moment, I had not really realised how we were under scrutiny.

The doctors in GOSH were very clear with us that it was by no means certain that Milo could be cured. They impressed on us that the hospital plan was a difficult one to follow and that it would take about a year of work with Milo as an inpatient. It was hard to embrace the fact that this meant Milo would be away from home, and the family, for such a long time. But it was imperative for us to agree and commit to it because it was Milo's best chance.

The practical difficulties of Milo being at best, 2 hours, away from home were stressful. It was very nerve racking to face the logistics of living with a plan that meant we should visit Milo three times a week, and attend GOSH one day a week for therapeutic meetings including individual therapy for Milo, family therapy and a parents' group. There didn't seem to be enough of us as parents to spread around.

Milo has four siblings, then aged between two and thirteen. They were stopped in their tracks by his illness. At the beginning, when he was in hospitals near home, their outlook was that Milo was in hospital for a short emergency. The upheaval at home was alright for a few days. Perhaps the children even quite enjoyed the excitement of going to friends' houses and things being unpredictable for a little while.

However, when the local hospitals initally sent Milo home, his siblings became slightly detached from him. I noticed they would talk to him, but would immediately look to me for the answer. They knew he could not answer them. Milo's two-year-old brother was slightly afraid of him; Milo, the brother who had been such fun, was now totally different. The younger child worried he had or would hurt Milo. Perhaps he felt rejected by the way Milo seemingly ignored him.

Time went on, Milo went to hospital, and things got no better; in fact, they felt worse. Milo's siblings seemed to be putting on a brave face for their friends. They didn't complain and tried to help. Milo's sister did caring things at home, and took over mothering roles. They didn't ask us about Milo, and soon started to reassure us that he "looked better". I discovered later that the children had actually asked their grandparents if Milo was ever going to get better.

One joy of Milo's illness was that his sense of humour remained almost wholly intact. This was a real bridging lifeline for all of us. We did not hear his voice, but when he laughed as he always had, we knew we were on the same "wavelength". Milo's siblings appreciated his sense of humour, because when they were funny, he laughed at them. This helped them not to feel so rejected.

My husband and I spent a great deal of time at GOSH, and we had to spend the weekends apart. There were times when this was very difficult, and after several months of this happening, the children complained that they never saw us together. They felt rather like children caught up in a divorce. Caught up in their sibling's illness, they began soul-searching about whether or not they could be partly to blame. Our children needed reassurance that they too were special, and that Milo's illness was not anyone's "fault". They felt less anxious and more involved through our telling them about much of what was going on for Milo. I noticed they also listened very carefully to everything I said to other people in case they had missed something.

The notion of exclusive family space was something I had enjoyed but not seen as a necessity before Milo was unwell. We had often commented on how good it was to be all together, with no extras, but since Milo's illness, we have consciously sought time alone as a family. As parents, we have also been aware of giving each child more individual time. During Milo's illness, the children needed it as time to feel safe, to be themselves, however they felt. Most noticeably, Milo's youngest brother regressed to wanting baby comforts and suffered quite difficult separation anxiety when we were not with him.

Communicating with the outside world

The outside world was anyone outside of the immediate family. Friends had to learn how we wanted to be treated, and we had to learn how to handle our new circumstances. Previously, we had usually been open and talked honestly, but we wanted to say nothing about Milo's illness, except to the professionals. With the professionals, we had to speak openly about every aspect about Milo and the family. Talking to professionals felt much easier than side-stepping friends.

People have a natural curiosity, and understandably our friends were concerned about how we were all coping. At the early stages of the illness, we had no answers, and later on, when we did, we didn't want to share the information. This was not out of any shame; it was simply all too "raw" to be able to discuss with people who might not know how to respond. Enquiries made out of good will didn't need hard facts; it was almost as if people making such enquiries were the ones most needing reassurance. However, as parents of a very unwell child, we felt ill-equipped to deal with the questions. We were struggling to come to terms with the situation ourselves. It seemed as though the better people knew us, the better they knew not to press questions and knew that we would answer when we felt able to.

Very early on, I noticed that Milo's illness was inviting a wave of questions that I didn't want and couldn't answer. I felt bombarded. We all tried to discuss Milo as little as possible outside of the family. We never mentioned any details of Milo's symptoms, so only close friends realised that he was not able to speak, walk, or eat. It was too personal. Outsiders' questions went from the simple "How is he?" which it was relatively easy to deal with, to the more searching type, involving questions such as, "What's the matter with him?" and "Will he get better?" All of the inquiries were difficult. I actually wished people wouldn't ask anything! There were days when I consciously avoided people in order to avoid talking to them. I felt such a confusion of emotions. I felt defensive for the family; I didn't want to share my distress and overwhelming feelings with other people. To answer their questions truthfully would have meant sharing something that I wasn't fully in control of, or fully understanding myself. I felt an outward composure gave me strength, no matter how I felt inside. I did this not just for the family and myself but also for Milo. It would have been too frightening for him to see his parents crumble when we were, after all, taking up his cry to be heard. No matter how we felt inside, we had to appear strong!

Maybe we were brittle and off-hand towards some people who were trying to help. Perhaps unintentionally we were, but in the "eye of the storm" survival that is what it's all about. In order for us to survive, we had to make certain boundaries within which we could cope. Then it became possible to carry on. By making boundaries, we were able to deal with people.

The way our boundaries worked was that we told everyone who asked the same thing about Milo (and still do). We worked out a verbal "news bulletin" strategy. It worked very effectively. As a couple and as a family, we worked out a "party line", and stuck to it vigorously. The party line was that "Milo had a bad virus, and was now in GOSH, and was getting better slowly". It parcelled a version of truth and gave an acceptable answer. By using the GOSH name, we were giving confidence, and by saying "getting better slowly", we were buying time. It also shifted the emphasis off the family. Inevitably, there were people who went on to ask more about "the virus", but it became easy, as we said it again and again, to reassure that GOSH had it under control. We kept to this story no matter what people said. I found that so many people were bombarding me that to tell everyone the exact same thing was important, or I would have got very muddled with my story! It was all quite rehearsed, but we had to hold ourselves together. I noticed Milo's siblings found it reassuring that I said the same thing to all enquirers. They were anxious in case they did not know everything. They liked to know what to say to their friends about Milo being unwell. I suggested they always said "getting better slowly".

One of the hardest things about answering people's questions was that it meant a type of sharing of a problem. At the time, we were trying so hard to keep ourselves together that the outside intrusion felt like too much pressure. To share the problem and admit the bewilderment and distress we felt would have caused us to break down and cry relentlessly. In the "eye of the storm" of Milo's illness, it was so important that we did not let go completely and sink into our distressing emotions too much. We needed every appearance of strength and optimism to tackle it. It was important for Milo that he knew we were in control, and that we were strong for him. Beneath the strong shell, a real tell-tale sign of how we felt was that we had to fight back tears whenever even the smallest good thing happened and when we met genuine kindness. Together as a very united couple, we were not able to talk about how it felt, because we knew completely how each other felt. We talked instead about how we could make things better.

People often remarked that they wondered how we kept up a jolly façade, when we had such a sick child. Little did they know; the reason was that we were trying to divert people's attention from what was actually going on, because we were incapable of sharing it with them.

Annoyingly, acquaintances started to offer help. The help ranged from faith healers, to advice to tell Milo to "pull himself together". The most welcome help came from kind people who gave support that was non-intrusive to the experience of being together as a family. Wonderful help came in the form of child-friendly meals; this meant I had more time to concentrate on the family instead of shopping and cooking. It was also great if friends offered to take the children on outings. If we knew they were happy, it made it easier to spend long periods of time away from home at Great Ormond Street Hospital. Most of all, we did not want extra people around the house. Home was our haven.

When Milo had been unwell for some time at home, before he went to GOSH, two close friends, who were doctors, offered to read stories to Milo and to look after him so I could do essential jobs. I gladly accepted their offers because Milo was happy to be with them and I could keep things "running" as well as I could at home.

All this time, we felt like marooned people, on a floating raft, not sure where we were headed and not sure how long we would be there. We were desperately frightened. Nobody appeared to know what Milo's problem was. It was very scary that because we appeared outwardly in control, people assumed we were. Before we brought Milo to GOSH, we received practically no help from medical professionals. In fact, our composure was to reassure Milo that we were struggling to get his cry heard. Inside my head, I felt like that Munch painting of *The Scream*, silent from crying, and contorted by despair.

The telephone was a nuisance. It never stopped ringing. Of course, we were pleased and reassured that people cared enough to ring us, but speaking to them was so difficult. Close friends seemed to understand, but it was with the kind people whom we knew less well that it was very hard. We still told everyone that he was "getting better slowly", but it was not always as convincing as it might have been, especially on our low days, and we dared not really tell the world how we felt or we might not have surfaced. Also, I wanted time I had at home to be spent with the family. The children understandably did not want me endlessly discussing their brother on the phone; their needs were just as viable. They wanted their turn of my attention. Time at home was time together as family!

When Milo was with us in places like waiting rooms, we tried to make sure no one noticed that he couldn't talk; whichever parent was with him chatted or read to him. We all felt very sensitive to the unintentional comments people make. There is no doubt that some people felt frightened by Milo's illness, even though we never gave it a name and they knew only that he was unwell. Illness and uncertainty stopped some people from speaking to us at all.

Communicating with Milo

We love Milo very much. His illness made it seem that he was in a terrible free fall and that keeping communication going with him, despite his not speaking, was our only lifeline. We were terrified by his sudden illness and its severity. Happily, Milo wanted us with him all of the time. We knew this because he was so upset when one of us was not with him.

Even when he was at his most withdrawn, we made all efforts to keep contact with him going by talking with him, reading to him, noticing how he felt, and staying silently with him at times. We used all sorts of ways to communicate, not all verbal. It was not difficult because we felt so passionately that communication was essential for both him and us. We lost any inhibitions with our efforts because of the intensity of our feeling. We knew we had to keep him emotionally alive and with us.

Our communication with Milo changed as time passed, and his illness went on. There were days when some ways of communicating worked better than others, depending on how we felt, and where we were. We continued to talk to Milo, as we would normally have done, but without expecting a response. We were careful as to what we talked about, but tried to talk about normal sorts of things. We talked about whatever was happening around us, always doing our best to see the moment-to-moment experiences from his perspective. We frequently acknowledged his pain. We made sure that what we were talking about was not going to cause him upset. It required a fine-tuned sensitivity to see what was best in the circumstances; sometimes he just wanted to be held and soothed, other times he wanted to be talked to. Understanding what Milo wanted at a particular time became easier with practice.

All that mattered was that we kept mentally "in touch". I don't pretend to understand the torture that must have filled Milo's thoughts, but by communicating with him in all sorts of ways, he knew we cared deeply, and were trying to reach him. We needed to remind him that his lifeline was with us. Besides communicating with Milo, we felt very strongly that we must communicate with the world on Milo's behalf. We felt ourselves to be ambassadors for "the well Milo".

Holding Milo and understanding his bodily expressions of comfort or distress was important, especially at the start of the illness. His facial expressions and body language were signals of how he felt. He was comforted by close physical contact. Initially, he did not walk and barely moved his limbs, and so we held and carried him rather like a small child. He relaxed when he was cuddled, and he liked being gently stroked. When upset, Milo's whole body became tense as he curled up into a ball and hid his face. However, when he was relaxed, he spread his fingers so they slightly parted over his eyes, so he could observe us, almost secretly.

When Milo was unhappy, writhing around in discomfort and calling out, he wanted reassurance that we were beside him. He didn't hear much of what was said to him. He cried out louder if one of us was not constantly with him, but was reassured by our presence. He liked the reassurance of our voices. We read him stories, spoke soothingly to him, and told him how sorry we were about his pain. We told him that we were explaining his pain to the doctors. It was better if we were with him singly, because he seemed more comforted by the attention of one person speaking to him. His interests were focused solely upon himself, he didn't want to hear any news of his siblings or school friends. He didn't like it when we were both beside him, and talking together. He did not want the presence of a couple, but rather wanted to be coupled with one of us.

Before being admitted to GOSH, while Milo was not moving, not speaking, and barely eating, and later when he finally began to come home at weekends, non-verbal communication between us seemed quite easy. In the familiar surroundings of home, we all felt more relaxed among ourselves. We used to talk as normal in the family: we included Milo in the conversation while not expecting a verbal response from him or, at times, not expecting any acknowledgement that we had spoken at all. His siblings tried to include him too. They would ask whichever parent was there for his answer. When we were answering for Milo, we always prefaced any answer with, "I think Milo wants, likes ...". We sat next to Milo when we were answering for him and looked to see his response. We deflected attention away from his lack of speech by adding in expressions like, "Milo usually likes/wants/thinks.... And I expect that is what he wants/thinks today." When things didn't please Milo or when we answered the wrong thing for him, such as agreeing for someone to come to the house, he made it very clear that we were wrong, by tensing up or writhing with anguish. Then we would comment that, "Milo is letting us know that we were wrong with what Milo wants," etc. While we were trying to accommodate Milo, we did our best to make things fair for his siblings so that they did not feel he took precedence over them.

Physically, Milo was lying on a sofa or deckchair, unable to walk or talk, and was being tube-fed. He was able to move his limbs if he wanted but would not move on request. He liked to be with the family, but did not want any involvement beyond being near us. He would recoil if asked to do anything such as hold something for a sibling. We always knew when he wanted to go to the lavatory because he indicated this through some bodily movement, but other than that, he did nothing at all for himself!

We ensured that the one of us looking after the children during the day did not spend the whole time concentrating on Milo. Although we were usually within sight of him, we carried on with whatever had to be done, and we also spent time with the other siblings. We moved Milo to the garden if we went outside. He was content to observe normal goings on, as long as we had no visitors and no demands were made on him. We would make comments to him, like, "can you see what x is doing, look he is in the tree", and then carry on, making no comment about whether Milo had looked or not.

There were times in each day when it was possible to be alone with Milo. Whichever parent was around would sit beside Milo, and spend "special time" together. He would relax completely and we would spend however long was available in a companionable "muse". Like any conversation, this one-sided talking with "one side non-verbal", used to begin on a mundane level, musing on the day, goings on with family, and progress on to a deeper level of how we both felt. I would tell Milo all the things about what I would like to happen, or about how I felt about people we knew, or how I felt about things going on. I would tell him interesting things from the news. Then I would muse out loud with Milo about how I thought he might be feeling. I used to speak about the obvious mundane things, "I suppose you get fed up watching x being silly", or things like, "Isn't it hot?" I felt I could ask questions, as long as I spoke without too much of a question in my voice and almost answered them my self, "Do you get uncomfy sitting here? [Short pause].... I know I certainly would."

I tried to guess what he might have been thinking, and then said it out loud, so that he would know I was really trying *to feel his thoughts*. I would muse sometimes, but not often, that I was sorry I couldn't hear what he was telling me. I very occasionally said in a very quiet, undemanding way, as though I was just sharing a thought, "I wish you could talk to me." I tried to follow these rather desperate remarks with, "Never mind, I think I know a lot of what you want to tell me." Using words like, "explain to me", "tell me", "show me", "want me to know", were key to communicating. We certainly didn't want Milo to feel under pressure to talk, and therefore consciously avoided using the word "talk".

We assumed that Milo was at the same intellectual level as he had been, and had the same interests. Even though he appeared to have regressed to a "baby-like" state and was at times afraid and not thinking coherently, we were adamant that mentally he was still a bright, enquiring, if unwell, eight-year-old. Our talking with Milo was not unnatural or forced. If we were too stressed and it was difficult to relax and talk spontaneously, we might just stroke Milo. Occasionally, we would sit still with him in silence. There was an occasion when Milo and I were musing, Milo in my arms, and I felt totally bogged down with the situation. Suddenly, I couldn't stop myself and I burst into tears. Milo said nothing but "looked" me the most amazing answer. At that moment, I realised fully that Milo DID want to come back to the world, and it didn't matter how long it took, but it would happen!

Communicating with Milo in hospital

The plan the hospital set up for Milo was that he was to be a full-time inpatient. We had set visiting times as his parents. Our visits were Saturday and Sunday from late morning to mid afternoon, and Wednesday mid to late afternoon. We also saw Milo for an hour or two for family meetings on Monday. We telephoned the unit each evening for a bulletin on the day, and then spoke for ten minutes to Milo while he remained with his ear to the phone. No one else visited or phoned Milo.

When Milo finally arrived at the GOSH inpatient unit, he had been unwell for four months, and not talking for the last two of those months. Our time with Milo in hospital was slightly "unreal" at first. Initially, we felt that our conversations were slightly forced, because everything was so unfamiliar, and we felt observed by everyone on the ward. However, because thinking about and speaking to Milo was our primary link to Milo, we quickly overcame our inhibitions in order to feel fully attuned to him through our words and gestures.

We were deeply sad that he had to be in hospital, being tube-fed, in a wheelchair, and away from home, yet enormously relieved that his illness was being addressed. Milo was withdrawn and depressed, and it was difficult to feel his feedback because everything and everyone was new to us. The first few weekends we spent in the hospital, we felt obliged to speak to the other children, and Milo deeply resented this. Understandably, he wanted us exclusively. We spent time in his room, and "mused" about how it felt to be in hospital. We talked in much the same way as we had at home. I would first spend time telling him about things happening at home. When I spoke about people, I always said, "x sends you their love", or, "x is sorry you aren't well", rather than, "x was enquiring about you". Milo would have been disgusted by the idea that he was being discussed. The "musing" conversations with him were not forced; I talked about whatever was on my mind. We sympathised with Milo, told him we missed him, and told him stories from home, particularly the ones we felt might seem amusing.

We did not tell Milo about the diagnosis of his illness, or about how long he would be in hospital. It would have caused him more pain to discuss his situation of being away from home for so long, or his cure. At that time, he was not able or did not want to think about being part of the world. Once Milo accepted that he was going to be in hospital, he accepted being away from the family. He didn't cry when we left, but was sad.

We decorated the space in the room he shared with another child with photographs of the family and places we had all enjoyed together. We talked to Milo about himself and these many times together with us as a family, and we sensed that this often gave him pleasure. After a period of "trial and error" we worked out how to handle the hospital visits best. We usually visited Milo singly, one parent each day during the weekend, both parents on Mondays, and we tried to visit together on the mid-week evening visit.

The time in hospital worked best for Milo if we had done a certain amount of preparation beforehand. Whichever of us was going next to the hospital spent time thinking how to make the five-hour visit satisfying and interesting, with a bit of fun involved. We had a hospital visiting basket that we kept for putting things in to bring to show Milo. There needed to be stimulating times with him as well as time to relax together. The hospital care plan was that we stayed on the ward all day, with a break while the children had lunch. My way of handling the visits was that I brought a storybook, a detailed factual book, some photos, letters, a notebook, and felt-tip pens. There were plenty of games on the ward. In my mind, I had a plan for the day.

When Milo was first in hospital and very withdrawn, we spent most the time in his room and about a quarter of the time in the communal area. I tried to make communal time towards the end of the visit. This integrated Milo physically back into the group of children before the separation. During the communal time, we would all watch videos together. Room time with Milo was spent going through the things I had brought, and talking to Milo about each of them. At first, Milo used to be very withdrawn and showed little reaction, except displeasure or boredom! As he became less depressed and physically slightly healthier, he became more interested in factual illustrated books, and these were great to discuss. We looked at all sorts of books, including many cross-section diagrams of buildings, animals, and ships. Looking at books seemed to absorb his imagination, and it gave lots of "hooks" for conversation. We made up stories for him relevant to the current issues that he was facing, such as stories of fear or courage. When we were looking at books together, I used to point out things, for instance, places to which we had been or to which we might like to go. At the beginning, he didn't like to even think about the future and about making progress to exist outside of the hospital, but gradually this attitude diminished. We also used to look at photos. I liked to have photos of home near Milo because it made talking about home more real. There were photos of the "well" Milo among all the others. "Well" photos were treasures because it subtly reminded Milo that he was part of another world besides the world of illness. I used to know when Milo had had enough because he used to look away when he became distressed or had become bored.

During the hospital visits, we also worked on a "Milo's life" scrapbook. This was a large album we made to show Milo his life events, in as much detail as we could muster. The book had lots of photos of Milo from when he was a small baby. We discussed how we had planned for his birth, the days leading up to it, the event itself, and all the excitement regarding his being a newly born baby. We also included lots of stories about his growing up. We used to make about three pages during each visit. Milo watched and got pleasure from this. He used to look at the book when we were not there. Initially, he was not able to turn the pages, but ward staff would spend time looking at the book and, through talking about the pictures, reinforce his sense of self. While we were making the life-story scrapbook, we talked a great deal about him. Making the book also underlined that there was another life waiting for Milo when he was ready.

On the three days when we were not in the hospital, we used to phone Milo in the evening. We started with one parent being with Milo, and phoning the other parent at home. The parent who was with Milo set the scene by telling the other parent what had been happening that day with Milo, and then held the phone to his ear while the other spoke to him and told him news from home and about his siblings. Once we had established this, the staff arranged for Milo to be by the phone each evening at a special time, and we would call from home. Milo found it annoying to be asked what he had done that day because he was actively "not doing", so we substituted with phrases like, "has anything interesting been happening today?" We used such phrases as, "Dad mentioned such and such a match was on, so and so hit an amazing shot". Initially, Milo used to recoil if an expression implying his involvement was used. It seemed appropriate to acknowledge when Milo felt very unhappy, depressed, and wanting to retreat from us. We used expressions such as, "I expect you are unhappy about such and such. I know I would be." When we were speaking on the phone, we always allowed short answering pauses, but only short ones. Sometimes, there was very little news to tell him during the course of a day, but he was content with even the smallest details. Until we got used to the one-sided phone calls, we used to make a list of things to tell him before we got on the phone. The calls were a way of helping Milo to feel we loved him and were thinking of him. They also became a reminder to him that he had a family and that life was going on outside the hospital.

Communicating ... the next six months

After about three months in hospital, Milo no longer kept his face covered and he sat up unsupported. Physically, everything else was the same: he still had the naso-gastric tube because he would not eat, he did not speak, and he was virtually immobile. We communicated in all the ways we had before, but the longer time went on, the more fine-tuned our communication became.

We had our first happy breakthrough when Milo smiled at one of us when we arrived on the ward and gave a wave of sorts when we left. As this progress had taken six months from the start of his illness, we were naturally overjoyed. The problem was that it would have been counter-productive to acknowledge our pleasure at his step forward towards us. As Milo did not feel well enough, and did not seem to want to join the well world yet, it would have been alarming for him if he felt he was progressing, even very slightly, towards life.

As very small glimmers of improvement became apparent, we slightly altered our ways of communicating so that we could further facilitate Milo's movement towards a life outside hospital. We had to retreat very slightly from doing as much as we could possibly do, to doing almost but not everything. For instance, I began by placing his hand on mine while I was brushing his teeth, and I handed him the towel to dry his face, instead of doing it all for him. We made no comment about whether he did an activity or not.

Milo was slowly emerging from his engulfing illness. It was imperative that we communicated without speaking the words, that there were ways to rejoin the world. It was also important that he moved forward because he felt ready to, rather than feeling "pushed" by us or our needs to have him better. After six months of being almost continually inside the hospital, Milo was allowed home for short weekend visits. It felt like a milestone, for it was a big adjustment for Milo. Such a step forward communicated to him that he was not the acutely sick child he had been some months previously. This was a metaphoric "hard pill to swallow" because, by accepting that he was well enough to come home for short periods, he had to accept that he was slightly improved. By being improved, albeit with still a very long way to go to being well, he had to relinquish some attention. He would no longer have one parent all to himself for two full days and two half days a week. He felt both very frightened and angry as he made the first few trips home. His fears and anger were further aggravated because at first he came home by car, but after a few weeks we had to make the trip by train. He clearly expressed his displeasure towards train journeys by being obstructive and unhelpful when we were moving him.

We continued to make our mid-week hospital visits. In order to help Milo move on, it became apparent that it was better to spend time with him in a different and more active way. We were able to take him in his wheelchair to the park or hospital café. At first, he was frightened by the newness of the situations and all the change moving outside the hospital ward implied. The idea that we would shift our attention onto anything but him was resented. For example, he was angry even if we ate anything when we were with him! Gradually, during time away from the unit, he was able to accommodate all the changes to his situation and he became more accepting.

We did still spend quiet time together but the emphasis was less on his being passive. We still read to Milo and made his life-story book, but we made subtle adjustments to what we expected from him. For example, when I was doing the book I would not pick up the pen or glue stick if it fell. I would leave it, making no comment if he picked it up and handed it back. Gradually he did assist by doing that kind of thing. Once he did something once, we assumed we could expect him to continue to do it, but we were always wary not to overstretch him by making too many expectations too quickly upon his emotional resources. We began to include Milo in playing board games, moving his piece as we took turns in the activities. Milo would observe and slowly over time he began to get quite animated over certain games. Milo needed to know that he was still entitled to lots of "special Milo time" and that by moving forward he would not lose the special time, just spend it doing different things.

It would not have been helpful, in fact it would have been counterproductive, to tell Milo what we were slowly trying to achieve. Our aim was to make the world seem an attractive alternative to a hospital ward. We wanted to communicate to him that by letting go of "illness" and all the more intensely given benefits that go with it (attention, sympathy, caring, protection), he could rejoin his life, still filled with attention, sympathy, caring, and protection, albeit offered in an age-appropriate way. We offered Milo life as it had been, or a life a little bit different. We wanted Milo to know that there was a family and a life outside waiting for him. Milo's not speaking, eating or walking did not involve a decision on his part to be unhappy and "sick", but the alternative to "sick" had to be attractive so that Milo would want to embrace it. Presenting this to Milo became a major but subtle undertaking.

As Milo became used to going out when we visited him, and playing games with us, we were gradually able to introduce more challenges. We were working very closely with the ward staff and told each other privately about every nuance of achievement. For instance, one day when the staff were taking Milo to the hospital shop in his wheelchair, he used his feet to push open the heavy swing doors opening out to the next corridor. Once we were told of this, we assumed he would do the same for us and never allowed him the opportunity to backtrack. Again in the wheelchair, I put my purse on his lap and said, "mind that for me". (Not "hold", rather "mind".) He did not let it drop and I realised that slowly, very slowly he was letting go of his illness and finding his eight-year-old self again.

We spent more and more time outdoors in the ward roof-garden. We also spent time reading and talking, and gradually we began playing increasingly more physical games. I say reading and talking, it was one of us who was with Milo who read the story or talked, but we had honestly virtually not noticed Milo's lack of words. He did communicate, *on his terms*, perfectly.

By now, Milo had been ill for one year and in hospital for seven months

As Milo was getting physically stronger, he also showed more enthusiasm for things that pleased him. The staff took him on several hospital school outings to museums, parks, and galleries. While there was still no verbal response from Milo, clearly he was responding to all that he saw. He began to use his hands to make simple models and to turn pages of books. If the children around him were playing, he wanted to join in, watching, but on his terms. He began to enjoy their jokes. He also began to grunt to attract attention and he would then mime what he wanted to convey. He didn't want to be left out of the group now!

Remember, this all took many months, but it was PROGRESS

Something that was very hard to understand was that Milo made his first bursts of progress with the children on the ward, then in the hospital school, then with the ward staff, and only quite a long time later with us. We were very confused as to why it wasn't with us first.

Could he not see how much we cared? The key to why his progress was like that IS just that. He was testing the results of his actions with the people who weren't so important first. He was worried that by showing us aspects of his "well-self" too soon that he would lose the special things that he received from us through being ill. In particular, if he was ill, he did not have to share us with the rest of the family for so much of the time. Also, there was a certain safety in practising being well with the children, because children practise all sorts of things with each other.

By being taken to the hospital roof-garden regularly, Milo began to get involved in the children's games. They used to play a game similar to hockey. From being a spectator, Milo was put sitting in goal, as goalie. He began to move his legs along the ground to stop the balls. A few weeks later, he was still enjoying the game, and had started to shout, "No", and say, "Hurray", when he stopped the ball. The next progression was table football. He would start by sitting on a chair at one side of the table and one of us would play against him. This involved him in lots of movement which he was happy to do, always with no comment from adults. When he got involved in the game, he would kneel up on the chair to get better control and shout, "Yes, no, hurray!". He was keen, but the secret of success with all the activities was to stop them while he was still very much enjoying them and not too tired.

Almost spontaneously, Milo was beginning to get more and more involved in physical activities. In the ward, he would catch and throw a ball with the other children, and he knelt in his chair to get a good view of interesting things. He began to do jigsaws, make models, and join in school activities. He was still naso-gastrically tube fed, but he was no longer revolted by people eating near him. Also Milo was obviously much more interested in everything. On the telephone he would occasionally say little words like, "Why" when we were telling him news from home. Increasingly, he didn't like female staff to dress him or take him to the bathroom.

When we were with him, we gently nurtured his speech by not explaining things in great detail so he would want to know more. After a few weeks, he began to say a few words like, "How".

During weekends at home, he was making bumper progress. From the first six months in hospital when we saw agonisingly little progress, we were now seeing almost daily progress. Granted, Milo did not or could not talk, walk, or eat, but he almost could. His attitude towards everything had changed. He was no longer totally introverted and depressed. Milo had been unwell for a very long fifteen months, and in hospital for ten months, but we were very heartened.

Up until now, we had almost not dared to push Milo. We had taken the lead from the hospital staff to do as they instructed, which is to be patient so that he could choose his own steps forward. Suddenly from observing Milo's progress we felt empowered to lever him on slowly but surely. We were able to gently insist on certain things happening. For instance, one day while we were visiting him, we brought him to the hospital café at lunch time. We were very clear that he was not having anything to eat or drink but that we were, and that we would like him to stay with us because we had come to see him. He found it annoying to have his wishes dismissed, but he was able to cope with sharing the space for us to have our lunch.

Physically, Milo was now strong and had lots of energy. He was moving around on his knees, semi-crawling, and clearly had the physical strength to walk, but he did not have the emotional strength or confidence or will to do so. The crux came when his already battered wheelchair was sent to be repaired and never came back. Milo was led around by two members of staff, holding him under his arms. Some days later, Milo made a sign that he wanted to be moved. The nurse, feeling that he was emotionally strong enough, said to Milo that there was only her around, not another staff member to help out and that if he wanted to move, they would have to work together. He rather grumpily accepted, and from then on only one member of staff helped him to walk. We took the opportunity some days later to singly bring him to the bathroom door, and suggested he might go in himself, which he did.

We never commented, we just tried to maintain the progress which Milo made on one occasion and pressed on with very minute expectations of him. As each stage was consolidated it was appropriate to say things to him such as, "It's easier without the wheelchair". We continued to speak to him on the phone each evening. The weekend visits home became longer, so Milo spent three nights at home each week, and four in hospital. We were confident at home with him and felt we could gently nurture his progress there while he was outside the hospital ward of ill children. We were able to insist on certain things such as sitting at the table during family meals. Milo enjoyed being part of the family and took an interest in that in which the family was involved. At this stage he could just about walk unaided. He showed all the usual feelings of happiness, anger, boredom and pleasure shown through laughter. He only spoke key words like, "How", "When", "Yes", and "No". It was as if he had regressed to having only a very basic knowledge of the language for his own use, but we felt almost certain that he understood everything.

While having Milo home on the weekends, we made sure we allowed Milo plenty of special time with one of us, so we could muse on the new experience of being at home. We told him occasionally how brave he was to be trying so hard. We made it clear that we were all very happy to have him around. We reinforced the idea of bravery by reading him stories about brave people, so that he could identify with their strength.

It was clear that Milo was progressing fast. He was saying one or two key words to make a statement and he secretly used more words when he was with his siblings. He wanted to be included in everything and was very clear about what he wanted. Milo's one major bugbear was his naso-gastric tube. He disliked everything about it, particularly having it stuck to his cheek, having it changed and all the attention it attracted. The ward staff began to talk to Milo about his leaving hospital. This was quite something for Milo to think about. Once he acknowledged that he enjoyed home and family, he embraced the idea of home rather than hospital. Any apprehension he had was about leaving hospital rather than about coming home.

Milo had been in hospital for a whole year. It was coming towards half-term time, and Milo was going to spend the week at home. We were planning a family weekend away by the sea. Before the trip Milo needed to have a new naso-gastric tube. This was a necessary routine that occurred at regular intervals. The old tube was removed but Milo could not bear the idea of a new one. His special staff member was with him and saw the opportunity to say to Milo that he could be brave and try to have drinks instead. This was a very momentous step for Milo. He was ready to do it. This signified a grand farewell to so much of illness. By being prepared to drink, he was taking a very positive step towards being a well-person. In choosing to drink/ eat, he was saying, "Yes" to us. In choosing to lift up the drink, he was saying, "I'm back". Everyone could see how much courage he had to draw on to actually lift the drink to his mouth. He drank special milkshakes and it was only a matter of days before he wanted to mix in other flavours. He began experimenting, adding ice cream to his drink, and he also started to drink orange juice and water. Milo appeared pleased by his courageous step. We didn't congratulate him explicitly, that was too direct. Instead we acknowledged how brave he was being and how nice it was to see his face properly.

All this time he was just saying one or two words in each sentence. We made sure not to interrupt what he said. It was faltering speech like a person speaking a foreign language. He continued to make hand gestures as he spoke. While he was home for half term, we felt he wanted and was ready for another "push". Without discussing it beforehand, we put some stewed apple at his place beside his milkshake drink. No one commented and the rest of us ate our meal. Without comment, Milo rather hesitantly picked up the spoon and ate the stewed apple. We could hardly believe our eyes! The same thing happened at the next meal. Once we felt we had consolidated this process of eating a little, a few days later we varied the small portions we gave him to be as similar as possible to what the family was eating. He was ready to be congratulated on the "brave steps" he'd taken. We were able to remind him that a little more food meant a little less hospital milkshake. He became interested, but not obsessive about watching me prepare food. He was not calorie conscious but was keen for "proper food". He had never liked processed food so this was not a change. He was happy to eat the things he had helped cook, and later all food, regardless of who prepared it.

When he returned to hospital after the ten-day break, we were worried that Milo might revert to "sick" ways, because he appeared to have virtually abandoned them. He did not want to go back to the unit, and this pleased us too. It said to us that he wanted to abandon sickness. However, he went back and continued to move on rapidly towards recovery. He talked more and more fluently, began to run about, ate more and more, abandoned his special drink, and was virtually his old self.

He continued to come home for long weekends. As he was spending longer at home now, the hospital staff helped him integrate into a new school. Together we worked out that it would be better for Milo to start a new school, which the hospital teacher visited. The hospital teachers explained to the new teachers that they must praise the work Milo did and not over exert him. It was explained to his new class that Milo had been unwell but that he was now better. We began introducing school into the time when Milo was at home. At first he went just for one afternoon a week and as the weeks went by we built on this. Suddenly we reached a point when he wanted to be at home and never return to hospital. Wow!

When Milo had reached this point, he was discharged within a few weeks, returning to the unit every week for the first few weeks. We were reassured that we could call the unit anytime but there was no need. Outpatient appointments continued. Milo spoke, ate, ran around and did everything much as any other nine-and-a-half-year-old, but he did have a limp, as if to remind everyone of his "scar". He was quite pale, but quickly integrated with his new classmates and got on with school.

At long last, Milo was well again!

Afterwards … the conclusion

As soon as Milo began to make strides back into the world, we became supercharged with huge energy. Nothing seemed impossible and everything was worth a try. We could hardly believe that Milo was well again. We had never allowed ourselves to contemplate that he might not be, yet at the same time had not dared to think how he might be after the illness.

I still remember that when he was unwell, one of the most painful things was seeing his friends. Their wellness, his sickness; the contrast was unbearable. Now of course, he is like his friends, they all look wonderful and healthy and full of vitality. He is achieving great things at a top university, startlingly fit and he's always sensitive to supporting "the underdog". It is hard to believe he went through so much suffering himself. I still find myself wondering what on earth went wrong. Did something go wrong? Will we ever know?

As a family, and as a husband and wife I feel we achieved something enormous too. It was the worst eighteen months of my life. Undoubtedly, we are a strong couple, but having gone through this crisis, the family unit is extra strong and loyal, and we have deep family ties. We never discuss Milo's illness with other people, and people we have met subsequently do not know the history. As time passes, the experience of Milo being so very ill is often still in my mind yet gradually getting buried in my "annual rings". It will never really vanish. I am so thankful that we found the right specialist care and that we were able to do the work necessary for such a good outcome.

Postscript: Milo has now completed his university studies.

CHAPTER THREE

Communicating without words

Jeanne Magagna

A little about me

I was born in America residing in my Italian grandmother's home. Everyone spoke Italian to each other and spoke to me in broken American words. During the endless hours I spent with Nona, my grandmother, I watched the look on her face, the gestures of her hands, the way she laughed, frowned, and walked around with her hunchback protruding. I loved her dearly and yet I only learned one word of Italian from her, "*zitte*", which means "be quiet!" I did not speak then, but I felt the feelings of the speakers, observed their gestures, listened to the intonations of their voices, and even joined in their laughs. Their personalities entered me in this way and became part of me.

Infant observation

Later, I did weekly infant observations under the supervision of Mrs Esther Bick, who was encouraged to initiate this pioneering work in 1948 by Dr John Bowlby at the Tavistock Clinic. I became utterly convinced of the therapeutic value of the observer who does not speak much, but simply observes and compassionately empathises with the child, through getting in touch with the flow of the child's gestures, the sound of her cry, the look of her eyes. Through the observer's compassionate observation of the infant-mother relationship there seemed to be a transformation of the child and mother's interactions. The observer's silent understanding was being offered to both the mother and the baby. It could only be experienced through empathic attunement between observer, mother and baby.

The application of infant observation to work with the silent child

As I did in my grandmother's home and in infant observation, I use this experience of understanding through observing as I work as a child and family psychotherapist with the eating disordered children who do not communicate with words, but only through gestures and projections of states of mind into me. After many years of working with non-speaking children, I have come to understand how essential it is to patiently hold hope and trust that a compassionate understanding rapport with the child will enable the child to reach out to grapple with life and try to understand his or her own emotional experiences.

As a result of this experience I can say, as you meet a mother/father/baby or a child, a question is being asked of you: "Can you understand me?" To understand you must reach into the depths of your own emotional experience at that moment to understand that which cannot yet be communicated in words. As you do this, I believe that both you and "the other" can repair some broken connections between the verbal self and the as yet unsymbolised self.

Exploring five states of mind of the child

I shall now describe *five states of mind* in babies, which might help you in your therapeutic encounters when working with a non-speaking child. My aim is to show you how infant observation will help you move beyond the symptom of the young person's not-speaking to understanding the child's *communication without words*. As Bryan Lask suggested in Chapter One, the child is not silent, he is simply not speaking!

I shall proceed by sharing brief observations of five different states of minds in babies relating to members in their families. I shall then link the discussion of each baby's different infantile experiences with five different states of mind, which may be present in the non-speaking young person. There are many more feelings present in a personal encounter and I am illustrating only some states of mind commonly experienced by the non-speaking child in psychotherapy.

The first state of mind: giving up

The following observation of a five-month-old baby described in *Intimate Transformations: Babies with Their Families* (Magagna, Bakalar, Cooper, Norman, & Shank, 2005, p. 25) shows how unnoticed sibling relationships affect a "sense of self".

Infant observation one: "Anna", five months; "James", twenty-three months

Anna, five months, is sitting in mother's lap, facing out, having her bottle. She has both hands around the top of it while mother holds the end of the bottle. Her brother James comes near with Anna's dummy. Mother tells James, "Don't do that!" but James continues to push the dummy into Anna's mouth until the bottle is forced out. Anna whimpers. James climbs into mother's lap. Mother faces Anna away from her body. Anna looks stupefied with her eyes glazed over and unfocused. Her fists are tightly closed, but the rest of her body is limp. Anna remains motionless and when mother puts the bottle into Anna's mouth again, Anna doesn't suck. Milk dribbles out of her mouth. Anna rocks herself. Her eyes are still blank and unfocused as she leans back onto mother.

> There are repeated sequences of James doing such things as pushing Anna off her chair, taking her toys, taking the space on mother's lap, often leaving Anna excluded from mother's care and attention. As time progresses with this going on, when Anna's mother comes to her, Anna's body becomes rigid, rather than cuddling into mother's body. Anna is hostile to mother for not protecting her from James repeated physical intrusions into her personal space and her rapport with her mother. Now her relationship with her mother is an intensely ambivalent one.

Thinking about infant observation one

In trying to understand the meaning of a non-verbal gesture, it is important to do a process recording in order to find answers to the following questions:

1. What is the sequence of interaction?
2. What do you think baby is feeling over time and how is that shown?
3. What do you think mother is feeling over time and how is that shown?
4. How do you feel witnessing this? Does it resonate with any experiences you have in your therapeutic work with a non-speaking child?

1. *Let us look at the sequence of interaction:*
James pushes the dummy into Anna's mouth and repeatedly intrudes. Mother uses verbal remonstrations, but she does not protect Anna physically from James' physical intrusions.

2. *What is Anna feeling?*
Anna is feeling unprotected and misunderstood by mother. She looks stupefied, her eyes are glazed over, and she is not focused on anything particular. Her body has lost its resilience and hangs limp. Anna moves into "blanking it out", dissociation, a kind of not thinking. She does this for *she feels helpless* to change the situation. The only thing that Anna is able to use to keep herself feeling safe is the tightness of her fingers clenching into the safety of her palms. When she goes into these dissociated states, she seems to feel: "I am not experiencing this bad experience, I am not here." Physiologically, she is developing acute hypervigilant anxiety responses which will continue later in life.

3. *What do you observe in mother's actions and how do you think mother is feeling over time?*
Mother seems slow to protect Anna physically from the intrusion of James. It may be that mother experiences the presence of Anna as a disturbance to mother's very intimate relationship with James, her older child. Mother has difficulty identifying with Anna. Often, mother ignores Anna as mother plays and talks with James. Mother seems to lack the capacity to meet the emotional needs of two very young children *simultaneously*. One wonders how mother's internalised sibling relationships might interfere with an empathic identification with Anna.

4. *How do you feel witnessing this scene? What is your countertransference as you identify with each of the three family members?*
You might feel sorry for all three parties as well as angry with James for intruding, angry with mother for not protecting and understanding Anna's experience, and worried about Anna. Anna's passivity also involves letting go of "her fight", and all her aggression gets projected

into James. He becomes "the bully" and Anna becomes "the victim". Anna is only five months old, but she is getting cast into a "helpless victim role".

Now let us link this infant observation with therapeutic work:

The first example of a clinical encounter: the silence of "giving up"

How might this state of mind present in an older child? Often, a young person with an eating disorder starts out by fighting against medical staff and parents who are threatening their omnipotent control of anorexia nervosa. The young person starts obsessionally counting calories, not eating, being extremely controlling. At a certain point, if he becomes physically ill, or he is feeling no one really understands what he is experiencing internally, or if he is separated from his parents when he lacks the inner resources of good internalised parents, which allow him to be separate from them, the young person collapses into dissociation, bodily limpness, feeling helpless to make any change in the situation, giving up, not talking, not eating, and maybe not moving at all.

A child gives up and retreats into not-speaking in the context of family relationships. For this reason, it is essential to offer family therapy to understand what is not being acknowledged emotionally and spoken about in the family. The child's non-speaking might be linked with his own or the family's *denied* feelings which can not be spoken about and have just been sensed by the young person, with no inner freedom to speak about what is being sensed. There may also be physical, sexual, or emotional abuse, but not always!

"Giving-up", non-speaking Russian "Marina", eleven years old

Here is Marina, eleven, in a family session with two younger brothers and an older sister, Josephina, fourteen, and her parents. Marina is hunched over with her long, curly black hair completely draping over her face. She has not spoken to anyone for months, nor has she eaten. She is naso-gastrically fed. Marina sits immobile in a wheelchair for she also does not walk. No one in the family answers my question: "I wonder what you are feeling being here together in hospital today?" It is clear that Marina is in "not-speaking" mode. There is silence in the family. I position a little chair right beside Marina and I ask Josephina, the older sister to sit in it. I ask Josephina to speak as Marina in the first person, and I ask her, "What might be the matter?" Josephina says, "I am frightened. I don't want to be in hospital away from my family. I want more time together with my mother. I am worried about her."

I then ask mother to "be Marina" by sitting next to her in the little chair. I ask, mother, "being Marina, what else are you worried about?" Mother replies, as Marina, "My brothers are rough. They hit me sometimes when they are cross with me. It hurts." Mother looks very sad as she speaks for her eleven-year-old daughter Marina. I ask mother, who is still speaking "in the role of Marina", "Does your mother know any other reasons for your hiding away?" Mother, being Marina, says, "I am frightened."

Mother starts crying and wiping away her tears. I gently say to her, "Your tears are saying something to me." Mother says, now in her own identity as mother, "I cannot cope any longer. I miss my family in Russia." Father joins in and says to me, "The family has been very sad

> since the paternal grandmother has died six months ago. That is when we moved here from Russia. Everyone is missing Russia. We have to speak English here. We miss our language, our family, and our life there."
>
> As the sessions go on for a few months, the older sister, Josephina, bravely describes how her father drinks, gets furious with mother for not disciplining the children, shouts, hits when he loses his temper, and throws plates around.
>
> Father defiantly says, "They need some rules. The children are all running wild, they are spoiled by mother who buys them a lot of things and doesn't discipline them." Mother is twenty years younger than her husband. She treats him like the parent and feels bullied by him, aligning herself with the children against the "bullying father". Father feels responsible for everyone in the family as though he is "the only parent".
>
> What is unspoken is that the family is angry, terrified, feeling out of control, unsafe, and unhappy. The family's fear and unspoken shared sadness has been projected into the identified non-speaking child Marina. Marina is helpless and overwhelmed by the family's terror and sadness.

As I reflect on the pervasively retreating, not eating, walking, speaking children who have given up hope, I become aware of intergenerational silences, family silences, the child's denial and the child's dissociation, withdrawal from unbearable pain, and retreat from "family secrets". Here are just a few of the family relationships which seem to be present when a child retreats from thinking. These family situations, if they are not accompanied by thinking, talking and dealing with what is going on, can drive a child into a retreat from the spoken word:

1. The grandfather has witnessed his Lithuanian Jewish family being murdered in front of his eyes, but has never spoken about it. The family style is to be strong, not speak about pain, and not talk about difficulties, for discussions regarding psychological or physical pain and/or difficulties might upset family members.
2. The mother in an Arabic family is being beaten by the father's mates, but the family can't talk about it because they are afraid of what father will do to them and afraid of losing any financial support to have a roof over their head. The non-speaking child finally lets me know.
3. There is severe bullying by the older boys and also by the American father in the family, but the mother and her non-speaking, anorectic daughter at times deny it. At times they are simply too afraid to speak about it, for fear dad will return to the United States and leave the family completely.
4. More commonly, there is depression in the parents accompanied by severe denial and fear of the painful emotional issues that the non-speaking child may be facing. The parents' transgenerational conflicts have led to weakened internal psychic structures, and it feels "just too much" for the parents to acknowledge how they are not understanding their non-speaking child's emotional needs. Denial and/or lack of resolution of intense conflictual feelings is often the family context in which a child stops speaking.
5. The identified patient knows about the homosexual or heterosexual affairs of the father and/or mother and does not speak, not just about this, but about all sorts of aspects of his family's

conflicts and unhappiness. Hiding painful issues from awareness, "not thinking about them" and using "distraction" gradually become a forceful eradicating mechanism, through which the child can lose parts of his capacity to be mindful and ability to speak about emotional experiences.

When the family has no system of interaction which involves holding feelings of family members, trying to make sense of them and speaking together about them, there develops an overload of overwhelming feelings, which drown the identified non-speaking child. One non-speaking anorectic young person living in a family in which all members relied on manic denial of feelings to cope said finally, "Inside I felt like the toilet pipes were bursting. I felt I was going crazy. Then I stopped eating, I turned away from others, my family, my friends." For her, there was a sense of accumulating traumatic, destructive experiences with no inner psychic structure, but also no family mentalizing structure to facilitate bearing, understanding, and putting a stop to destructive emotional interactions in her shouting, quarrelling family.

When they were young adults, some formerly not speaking, not eating, not walking (pervasively retreating) children contacted me. They made me aware that we were required to find a way of gaining a much deeper understanding of the family dynamics, involving the child in a retreat into helplessness and not speaking, walking, or eating. This was always so difficult when no one seemed able to speak about "the issues", which sometimes weren't fully apparent to anyone in the family.

In particular, the young people who came to talk to me as adults let me know that when they had been inpatients the parents' and siblings' mental health involving emotional neglect, abuse and violence seemed to be underemphasised. Often, we had been aware of these issues, but not aware of how ongoing and severe they were because all family members were "not speaking" to avoid family break-up, the prospect of which felt even worse than what they were currently experiencing. Some families of non-speaking children did break up, and some of these children went to boarding school, which was felt to better meet their best interests, even though the full details of their family situation had not been revealed.

Some children who originally did not talk, walk, or eat after they recovered from their illness went on to live quite happy, productive, normal lives. Not *all* the families of these non-speaking children had severe difficulties, and it remains a mystery as to why these particular children found it so difficult to stay connected to life. Perhaps "not talking" about things, because of a difficulty in bearing psychic pain and conflict, simply left them overwhelmed and drowned by unbearable feelings.

However, the child who "gives up" and feels "dead-alive" has *sometimes* experienced trauma from projections from the family or external people as well as having the internal trauma of being overwhelmed with feelings. Such a child has inadequate inner psychic apparatus (mentalizing, internalised parents) to think about the feelings and work out solutions to the difficulties which the child is facing. The non-speaking child often has feelings that cannot be symbolised, verbalised, described to others, or mastered.

There are major limitations to what can be achieved relying solely on ordinary verbal communication with such a child. The first therapeutic work involves receiving projections of the child's states of mind; holding the feelings inside oneself, trying to puzzle over the feelings and bodily experiences one has, giving the feelings some words or a drawing, and then thinking about what the child is feeling. Sometimes the clinician, as well as the child, might find it helpful to use drawings, sculptures, sand-tray representations, music, and later writing stories and poetry to process experiences in a therapeutic encounter.

The second state of mind: the silence of "I am afraid of being here - keep away!"

Showing a negative reaction rather than being passive and not emotionally present to external life is a sign of a self remaining emotionally intact. A fearful or angry flinch away from a therapist is progress from unfocused dissociation, for there is still hope that both the child and the therapist can notice and change something in the fearful situation.

Here is an example of a negative reaction, which is a sign of a mind facing a persecutory experience rather than denying it:

> *Infant observation two: "Tom", three and a half months*
>
> Mother anxiously holds the baby. Immediately, each time mother shows baby the bottle, he looks at it as though he doesn't recognise it. He then becomes serious as he looks at his hand and rotates it in front of his eyes. Then, with his left hand, he grasps his right wrist and brings his fist to his mouth. Saliva bubbles are coming out of his mouth. Baby then sucks his tightly closed fist. For six or seven times, mother takes baby's hand from his mouth to try to insert the bottle. Baby immediately puts his hand back in his mouth. Mother pushes the baby's hand away and inserts the teat of the bottle. Baby sucks once and spits out the teat. Each time this sequence is repeated, mother becomes increasingly insistent as she firmly presses the bottle hard into baby's mouth.
>
> Baby grasps the bottle with both hands, pushes it away, and spits out all the milk from his mouth. Mother becomes more nervy, forceful, and angry as baby becomes increasingly strong-willed in rejecting both the bottle and mother. Baby vomits the milk, returns to sucking his thumb, looking away from mother, with his other fingers tightly clenched, near his chest.
>
> (Magagna, 2002, p. 137)

What is important in processing this infant observation is to observe the specific sequence of interaction and put oneself in the shoes of each person in the interaction. Asking questions about one's emotional experience while observing deepens and more fully elucidates the observational process.

Thinking about infant observation two

1. What is the sequence of interaction?
2. What do you think baby is feeling over time and how is that shown?
3. What do you think mother is feeling over time, and how is that shown?
4. How do you feel witnessing this; does it resonate with any experiences in your work with a non-speaking child?

1. *Let us look at the sequence of interaction:*

The bottle is threatening. The baby retreats to the blockading thumb as a primitive protection against the anxiety. Mother takes away baby's self-protecting thumb used to armour himself against the persecutory bottle / mother.

2. *Can we now empathically identify with the baby?*

The baby is persecuted. He is frightened of the bottle's entry into his mouth. It has become bad through circumstances which we don't understand. He is turning to his own system of defence, putting his thumb in his mouth, clenching his fist, tightly closing his eyes. This is his armour to protect him from the anxiety of the horrible bottle.

3. *Can we understand now how it feels to be baby's mother?*

Mother is panicked because of her need to keep the baby alive through food.

She is not able to identify with the baby's persecution because she is so worried about what she is not doing; feeding him.

Mother becomes angry and frustrated because of her sense of impotence.

Mother then becomes controlling and intrusive. She is not able to think, not able to talk to the baby, not able to experience how threatened the baby feels if she takes away his thumb or inserts the bottle into his mouth.

Mother ultimately is feeling terribly persecuted by the baby who is refusing what she is giving him for him to remain alive!

4. *What is your experience in witnessing this, and does it remind you of any experiences in your therapeutic work with a non-speaking child?*

The experience of observing mother and child interacting like this is very upsetting.

If you are identified with the baby, you can get angry with the mother for being so intrusive.

If you are identified with the mother who is feeling so impotent, you can also get "fed up" with the baby. The anger can interfere with understanding the sense of persecution in both an impotent mother and a frightened baby who has lost a sense of the goodness in his relationship with the food / the mother.

The second example of a clinical encounter: "Keep away!"

A similar kind of scenario often occurs when parents first bring a non-speaking, non-eating child to an inpatient unit. Terror can also occur when a pervasively retreating child begins to again *be mindfully present* to his own feelings, from which he has previously been dissociated.

Our task with the non-speaking child recoiling her body and glancing away, suggesting that we should "keep away", is to understand the experience *both* in oneself and in the young person. We must understand the young person's transference to the therapist, and therapist's countertransference to the young person, just as we did in the previous uncomfortable baby–mother feeding interaction.

Then we have to think of:

1. Identifying with the young person's transference.
2. Understanding our countertransference; how we feel at that moment.
3. Thinking about how we speak.
4. Thinking about where we should locate the feeling: *in us* or *in the young person*?
5. Thinking about the feelings that are existing in each person in the encounter.

"Keep away" gestures of silent "Jane", fourteen years old

Jane wasn't told that she was being admitted into the inpatient unit. Her parents were afraid of what she would do if she knew beforehand. When Jane came with a strong, defiant stride into the therapy room, she averted her gaze and went to the window, where she stood with her back firmly positioned to keep me out. Her face, covered with long, blond hair, was invisible throughout the session as she looked out of the window.

"We need to find some quiet space within ourselves to understand the child, before we 'do' anything verbally. If we speak before we feel, the child becomes disturbed". (Dosamantes, 1992, p. 362).

1. *What is Jane saying?*

"Keep out! I don't want you to get in! I want to be out of here!" Her firm stride, her back to me, looking out of the window, indicate: "get out!"

2. *What is the therapist supposed to feel?*

I am to feel the rejected one, the pushed-out one. Jane is projecting into me "the bad unwanted feelings".

3. *Where should the therapist locate the feeling; in Jane or in the therapist?*

Like the baby who didn't want the bottle in his mouth, Jane is not wanting me to talk about the feelings *inside her*. She doesn't want me to come closer, she wants to push me out. For this reason, the interpretation has to be about feelings outside her, what John Steiner (1993) calls, "therapist-centred interpretations", which *locate feelings first in the therapist* and only later within child when the child has the capacity to think about feelings inside her.

What could we say? "I am not wanted here. I should leave her alone and not offer this time to think with me." Could I say, "I should 'let you out' of this place that feels like a prison, keeping you here for 50 minutes?"

4. *How should the therapist speak?*

Jane is being firm, with her hard back pushing me away. When I speak, I need to keep attuned to the strength of her emotions as she "shuts the door" on this unwanted me.

5. Jane is feeling persecuted and rejecting my overtures, and I am feeling "no good" and that nothing I say will feel good to her at this moment. I can just understand that is how she feels.

Jane's protective, blockading thumb consisting of not speaking, not eating; keeping her hard back facing me represents her way of keeping away what she experiences as intrusive: a therapist trying to understand how she feels. Understanding threatens Jane's own protective armour of denial, of not-thinking about difficult emotions.

Jane had difficulty in sleeping, but had no access to her dreams. Jane was lonely underneath, but had no access to words for her emotions. Jane's body was cold, tired, but she seemed to have no sensation of heat, cold, or tiredness. She was in an armour, which was firm in relation to me, but also the armour separated her from her own vulnerable, emotional self underneath. She was using *primitive omnipotence* (Bick, 1968) as her protection, for she was insecurely attached to her mother and lacked internal mentalizing parents. For this reason, she was terrified that therapeutic understanding was going to "crack" her self-protective armour—all that she had to keep safe!

This understanding is all based on *countertransference:* the feelings I listen to silently within myself until I know what I feel inside while with her. I then need to consider what feelings I am holding in projected form for Jane and what feelings belong to me. I need to be firm in my voice because she is in her "soldier self" armoured against me. Work with the non-speaking child isn't about asking a lot of questions, for an unwilling child will feel that questions are intrusive. The task is to ask questions about what *you as a therapist* feel. The task is also to ask what is projected into you as the therapist at this moment. Therapy involves listening to the music of your soul.

What is healthy about this situation? Jane is struggling against that which persecutes her. She is putting up a fight. She *hasn't given up* trying to protect herself! Believe it or not, that is a strength. She still has some hope that she might get things working with people the way she thinks they should work, or she wouldn't be fighting. Passivity, when the child feels limp and helpless, is much more worrying!

This is what one can typically receive from frightened people newly admitted to an inpatient unit. They have had some difficult experiences or they wouldn't have stopped eating and wouldn't stop speaking in the session at this point. "I shouldn't be here..... my parents are the ones who have a problem. They think I have anorexia nervosa. They are just trying to make me fat." This would be what Jane might be saying if she were speaking rather than not-speaking to me. She said this later in the therapy. Jane was experiencing what a motivational therapist would call *a phase of denial*.

But wait a minute! If you take these statements metaphorically, perhaps it is true that the child's psyche is being saturated with undigested intergenerational conflicts, and conflicts of the immediate external family and her own internalised family. This is partly what is responsible for making her feel fat and visually perceive herself to be fat.

The third state of mind: silently using adhesive identification which can involve holding onto physical sensation, muscular rigidity, or the sameness of an object in lieu of having an internal space to contain emotions

Third infant observation: Baby Eric, four months

"Baby Eric is lying on mother's lap. She isn't holding him firmly and in response to this lack of holding baby stiffens his body and back with his head pushing back. His back and neck are stiffly arched over mother's legs... Stiffening of musculature is baby's way of trying to make a stiff, holding container for himself with all the energy he can mobilize... At other times a colourful, striped, jump-suit, which always hangs nearby, is often used when baby is not 'emotionally held' by mother. He stares at it intently, 'holding on to it' with his eyes" (Magagna, 2002, p. 85).

These behaviours are described as using adhesive identification measures in lieu of a secure internal or external mother being present at that moment.

Holding the lips together and tightening of the stomach and body musculature are required when the infant is terrified and cannot trust the mother to attend to him. Spitz (1965) noted that babies in hospital who were nourished but did not have a primary caregiver attending to their psychological needs stopped crying and later died. Tightening of the lips, muscular rigidity, holding onto a physical sensation or an object is thought of as *adhesive identification* (Bick, 1968), which is used in lieu of both physical holding and psychological containment by the mother and/or an internal mental structure to contain emotions. Sometimes parts of the body get frozen in an extended period of muscular tightness and physical pain. The muscular contractions can cause both a feeling of paralysis and actual physical impairment to mobility.

The mouth is the bridge between internal experience and the outside world represented by mother. When the link with the mother is broken, the bridge to her, the mouth, stops opening to let out cries, sounds, or words for her (Rhode, 1997, p. 17). The mouth may remain closed with the lips adhesively stuck together, for to open the mouth can bring fear of everything, all of the self, falling out. Opening the mouth may bring the fear of crying and never stopping. Opening the mouth may also bring the fear of becoming trapped in emotional overload without any internal psychic structure for reflective functioning.

A mother who often fails to respond to a baby's cries can contribute to a child having an insecure attachment to her. The child will then stop crying for mother when in need of her. When a child expects to be understood, words can feel like a way of getting through emotionally and eliciting a response. When the expectation of mother's understanding is weak, words can feel like something that is concretely lost from the mouth, like losing a part of the self into the void. The lips adhere to one another as a protection, as a means of control to survive psychologically without falling apart.

The third example of a clinical encounter: using adhesive identification

Silent "Lara", aged fifteen, using adhesive identification to hold herself together emotionally

For several months, Lara, who was suffering from anorexia nervosa, was silent. Later on in her sessions, she cried out in pain. She had been suffering for two years from an abdominal pain for which the doctors could find no cause. She no longer walked because the pain was so

> severe. Upon admission, she whispered to her mother that she did not want to talk to anyone because in her year-long previous hospitalisation, everyone kept saying her physical pain was not real. Feeling terribly disappointed that no one understood her, Lara stopped talking completely.
>
> In the sessions when she started crying, she paused in her crying only sometimes, in order to hear my words. I stayed with Lara's crying about her pain rather than trying to explain it was nothing. Sitting alongside her, rather than facing her, I echoed her cries, taking care to pace and attune my cries in a way that matched her cries. Subsequently, I spoke in the first person, "No one understands me. Jeanne doesn't understand me. I am in too much pain to talk. The pain hurts so much it takes over my mind. Please understand how much it hurts inside."
>
> As the sessions went on, I would create stories about "the pain" using made-up characters, talking about the hatred of the non-understanding therapist, the non-understanding doctors. I accepted the physical pain and how it felt to be overwhelmed by it. I was aware of a shared family system of denial of psychic pain. It was particularly obvious that Lara's mother would deny pain or get too upset if she acknowledged problems. I was also aware that I needed to accept the *pain as physical*, regardless of any medical diagnosis. Lara's soul was breathing through her body. Her body was reflecting the pain.
>
> Gradually Lara used eye-blinking to signal to me. Later, she began moving her head to signal yes or no to my aspects of my conversation with her. She was like a strict teacher firmly signalling to me if I "got it right" or "got it wrong". Much later, when she found words again, Lara described her hallucination of a man's voice coming through a door and her nightmare of being stolen by a man and taken away from her home.

In a series of instances of non-speaking young people, holding onto a physical pain of an earache, a headache, a sore leg, seem to be unconscious protections against becoming conscious again of anxieties of a terrifying psychotic nature. Adhering to a physical pain can be a protection against losing one's mind!

Through my work with Lara, I have thought more about the infant left alone in her bedroom while the parental couple share a night together. The baby cries with the anguish of being separate from mother or separate from father and is jealous of the couple's togetherness. Also, the baby's body, if the baby is left to cry for some time, suffers the pain of physiological responses to prolonged panic and crying. This pain at a physiological level seemed to be re-experienced in the session and requires therapeutic containment through feeling the young person's terror prior to transformation from physical pain held onto adhesively in lieu of an inner psychic structure for mentalization to take place. Later, the physical pain became transformed into symbols of psychological issues. Much later, it was possible to talk to Lara about her psychic pain that had contributed to her unconscious retreat into illness.

In the hours spent with the non-speaking Lara, I continue exploring what is happening inside her and inside me. I imagine that somewhere there is a wish for a regeneration of a silent, encrusted part of my infantile self and of Lara, that has never been spoken to, never been heard. Somehow Lara, myself, and every human being probably entertains a wish for a dialogue with the encapsulated part of the personality, a part of the personality deeply buried in the unconscious that is isolated, lonely, and out of communication with both the conscious self and the unconscious dreaming self.

The fourth state of mind: the silence filled with hatred and subsequent persecution

Bowlby's book *Attachment and Loss* (1969) is essential reading to carefully distinguish the non-speaking child's sense of being persecuted by the therapist from the non-speaking child's hatred and rage towards the therapist. A therapist new to a child may be experienced as threatening to his defensive armour. The two phenomenon hatred and persecution are often confused because the child's hatred to the therapist creates a "bad therapist" who is then persecutory to the child. Hatred and persecution require disentangling through observation of gestures and body postures as well as through noting one's countertransference experiences. First, though, let us look at an infant observation where the child begins to experience anger, rage, hatred towards the mother, followed by a sense of persecution.

Infant observation four: "John", eighteen months old

> This is an observation made by the Robertsons (1971): John, whose caring parents were having another baby, placed him for nine days in a residential unit. The nurses were young and friendly, but the system of group care does not allow any one of them to substitute for the absent mother. John tries hard to make a relationship with the matron to get the comfort he needs, but he is defeated in getting her attention, and he becomes increasingly distressed. The nursery nurse's work pattern prevents John's individual needs for substitute mothering from being met. He becomes upset and tearful. Then for a few days, he begins crying in a very strong, protesting way. The staff are used to crying children and don't respond to his cries. Their philosophy is that John will cry less if they respond in this way. He is angry with his absent mother, for she has left him and he is not protected from the attacks by the other children. Gradually, he becomes hopeless, listless, and depressed. When the mother returns, she feels a stranger to John. Mother has turned into a persecutory figure for she has been filled with all John's projections of panic, rage, and hostility towards her for leaving him in this unknown place, with unknown caregivers, in an unprotected situation. When mother says hello to John for the first time, he hostilely turns away from her. She feels rejected, for she has become John's persecutory mother, now perceived as a "bad object" filled with his bad projections of hostility.

Hostility to mother turns mother into a dead mother filled with bad 'stuff' of hostility. The mother has not been kept alive as a good mother inside. A child has to have a good and strong mother present, internally and / or externally capable of bearing hostility. When the internalised mother and external mother is uncaring, weak, or filled with too many projections of hostility, she is no longer a good mother; instead, she is a bad object. It will take some time for John to return his mother-in-his-mind into being a good mother who can accept his anger and hatred for leaving him alone and unprotected in the strange situation.

The fourth clinical encounter: The silence filled with hatred and subsequent persecution

Hatred and rage usually occur in therapy after the young person is less dependent on primitive protections against anxiety, such as omnipotently controlling intake through vomiting or starving or self-harming. Pseudo-independence is reflected in states of mind suggesting, "I can take care of myself, I don't need anyone else." Hatred and rage emerge when there is a growing dependence on the therapist and the therapist's reflective functioning offered to the young person.

> *Sixteen-year-old "Hanna"*
>
> Hanna came to the UK with her American family while her father was on a university sabbatical. She has long, dark, unruly hair. After six months of virtual silence accompanied by crying in therapy, Hanna is beginning to depend on me. Just before my frequently discussed two-week holiday, she says, "If I were really courageous I would really bloody myself." She adds, "How can I make anyone take care of me if I am not ill?"
>
> When I return from holiday, Hanna is furious with me. She walks into the first session with her head down and hands clenched; she immediately walks out of the therapy room and does not return. She refuses to come to the second session. When Hanna arrived on the third session after my break, she does not meet my glance when I greet her, nor does she respond to my hello. She is silent for a very long time.

What can I do? I can interpret the need for safe space, a bodily position to hold herself together. With her body and her fingers tightly curled up, she feels better. I can acknowledge Hanna's sense that there is a split between her body felt as safe and the outside world, represented by me, felt as bad. On the other hand, I could create a story, sometimes with dolls or animal families, not speaking to her directly but rather to myself, so she won't feel intruded upon. She can feel free to be curious about what I say. She can choose to listen or not listen. She can think or not think with me. Creating a story to the side of her allows her to feel she has "to search me out" rather than feeling I am pushing my thoughts into her mind.

Despite Hanna's persecution, hatred and rage, a question is again being asked of me. She is asking, "Can you understand me?" Compassionately comprehending Hanna means that I must meet at least these six requirements:

First, I must pay rapt attention to the bodily experiences of both the young person and myself. This involves the following:

- Rapt attention to what I observe concretely, such as asking myself about the direction and feel of her eyes looking: Hanna's eyes are turned away from my gaze.
- Rapt attention to what Hanna's hands are telling me. For example, they may be tightly clenched, extended in tight musculature, spread out like spider legs, hurting each other, picking on nails, fidgeting on a mole, spot or pulling on the hair. In fact, Hanna's hands were tightly clenched.
- Rapt attention to what her feet are telling me. They may be tightly intertwined with one another, tapping the floor, kicking quietly outwards, holding toes clenched, while pressing them tightly onto the floor. Hanna's feet were pressing tightly against the floor, as though she were holding herself together psychologically by sticking to the floor in an adhesive way (Bick, 1968).

- Rapt attention to her breathing. For example, there could be relaxed breathing linked with sadistic phantasies of attacking someone, there could be constrained breathing trying to hold the rage in. Both Hanna and I were experiencing a shallow kind of breathing reflecting anxiety.
- Rapt attention to the tightened musculature used to hold Hanna's body firmly. I noticed that Hanna's muscular rigidity created an impression of an ice sculpture. There could also be aching pain in her body due to the muscular rigidity.
- Rapt attention to fluctuation of her bodily states and to the moments in our non-verbal/verbal dialogue when the fluctuation occurred.

Second, I must tolerate the frustration of not-knowing and not understanding. I must bear the frustration of feeling ineffective.

Third, despite the aggression in the room I must strive to be compassionately present, empathic and non-critical towards the feelings emanating from myself and Hanna in that present moment. That is the only way that I will lessen the cruelty of the harsh superego punishing Hanna by creating symptoms and guilt.

Fourth, I must make a decision to speak or not speak about the gradually forming thoughts about the present moment with Hanna.

Fifth, it is important that I accept that unprocessed anguish and suffering have contributed to a broken symbolisation and a broken verbal bridge to me. Hanna's missing the sessions is a form of *acting out* what couldn't be put into symbolic thought.

Sixth, and most importantly, Hanna has a right to be alone with her feelings. Only when Hanna feels sufficiently held together internally and trusts me will there be a sharing of the encrusted hidden parts of Hanna's self which require understanding, regardless of whether or not there is verbal conversation.

> *What could I do and what did I do in this situation?*
>
> I tentatively told Hanna a story of our time together before the break. I mentioned how she had felt she could count on me a little. I also described how she had also told me that she wanted to bloody herself before I left for holiday. I wonder if she was in a rage with me for leaving her just when she had thought I might understand and help her.
>
> Hanna remains silent and immobile as though she hasn't heard a single word.
>
> I then say it has been difficult for her to come back to see me. I suggest that she has struggling with the temptation to run away from me, but she came to the session. I add, "Even though you are here, you and I are confronted with these feelings, whatever they may be."
>
> You may notice, I am not asking questions. I am making a tentative running commentary which implies curiosity and allows the possibility for Hanna entering the conversation through listening, thinking, feeling or words.
>
> Near the end of the session Hanna haltingly decides to speak with me in a voice which is aggressively chopped up so that it is virtually mute. Hanna mumbles, "I feel really bad about myself. I have a very angry, nasty side." She, her parents and two brothers

> have all been involved in hitting one another. "I am worried everyone will reject me for having it."
>
> Hanna adds, "You feel different to me now you have come back. I don't like you. I don't like feeling I dislike you so much. You have become a stranger to me. Before I thought you liked me, but now I feel you don't like me."
>
> I wait briefly and then suggest, "Maybe you have been very angry with me. You hated me for leaving you". I tentatively wonder, "It could be that now I am filled with your hostility. It feels to me that the hostility now in me is boomeranging back at you."
>
> Hanna replies, "I felt like slapping you. I can't imagine that you can feel me disliking you and not dislike me." (Dislike is a mild word for her hostility!)

As I reflect upon this session, I realise that not coming for therapy, not speaking with me may have been Hanna's only way of modulating her out-of-control, violent feelings.

I discover subsequently that Hanna had filled the holiday by watching violent and sadistic films; one safe outlet for her aggression. Over time I realise that a very uncomfortable silence accompanies Hanna's hatred and rage when she feels completely misunderstood by me, or criticised by me. On these occasions, I again puzzle over my countertransference and talk about what has happened in these moments between us just before Hanna abandoned a verbal interchange with me. I mull over possibilities aloud to myself, wondering if I have understood anything about the hostile silence.

Alan Schore (2002a) suggests that the therapist's own bodily sensations in the therapeutic encounter are needed to provide a deepening of empathic connection with the child. The therapist's body is especially involved in the reception of transferential projections of split-off parts of the self. Schore agrees that in order to transform the child's distress, the therapist must go beyond mirroring. More than the clinician's verbalisations it is his/her non-verbal activity, the bodily and emotional containment by the therapist of the child's projected and disavowed experience that needs to precede verbal processing (Dosamantes, 1992, p. 362). It could be argued that these spontaneous, emotional pre-attunements constitute a conversation between the limbic systems of child and therapist. The pre-attunement experiences create a safe holding environment promoting transformation of the personality (Hadiks, 1994).

I shall now describe another experience that has happened with several young people, including this time with Hanna.

> Hanna is sitting with her head in her hands at the beginning of the session. I feel physically drained of life and then gradually become aware of a pervasive pain in my face. It is as though I have been and am still being battered. I use this experience to describe how there is something that seems to be battering the life out of this experience. Using third-person descriptions of an experience present in the room, I go on to describe how there is some pain, some lifelessness here.
>
> After a very long silence, Hanna describes being assailed by inner thoughts saying, "You shouldn't talk to her, it's all useless, nothing will change. You shouldn't eat, you can't gain weight, you are horrible, you are just fat, that is all!" She reports this event factually with no

flicker of desire to challenge these thoughts. She is flattened. It is I who has to struggle to come to life, to release life from deadness, to feel her aggression against her life in therapy, against my work.

At times, I wonder if part of what is also essential for transformation through projective identification is my seeing Hanna's facial expressions of hopelessness, despair, terror, disgust, shame, excitement and rage, and her seeing my facial responses to her. I recognise Hanna's emotional state by seeing and experiencing her bodily and facially expressed, non-verbalised affective expressions. It is this seeing, receiving and responding to Hanna's non-symbolised emotional state, which is a central therapeutic component of the non-verbal communication in therapy.

The fifth state of mind: the silent loving communion between the child and the therapist

> The therapist should enable the child who arrives to the session disgruntled like a lion to depart like a contented lamb.
>
> (Meltzer, 1984)

Infant observation five: "Eric", one month old

I observe Baby Eric, one month old, sucking mother's nipple calmly while looking first into mother's face and then more directly at her eyes. The rest of his body is very still, with his arm resting against his waist. He moves his hand along mother's blouse, holding on it momentarily. He glides along mother's breast with his fingers. After a while, he stops sucking and he looks up at mother's eyes in a more intimate, attentive way than before. Then he smiles, and mother says he enjoys staying awake for much longer periods now.

By four months, you can see that the pleasure of being deeply understood fosters an ordinary dialogue as part of the mother–baby relationship. I observed Baby Eric when mother was talking with him. He takes his fingers out of his mouth, breaks into a smile and then a laugh, with a kind of "goo-aah-hi" series of sounds. He becomes more excited as he waves his hand in a flopping motion. As mother talks to him, he makes more sounds (Magagna, 2002, p. 86).

The fifth example of a clinical encounter: the silence in a more loving communion

Once the protective defences against intimacy have been lessened, the pleasure of being deeply understood creates in the young person in therapy the possibility of a similar psychological growth and happiness to what was experienced by baby Eric in his loving relationship with his mother.

Sixteen-year-old "Hanna"

Hanna had not spoken to staff, family, or me for several months of her admission to the inpatient unit. She had lived a kind of masochistic experience of life without any point. She didn't

> talk for, in her words, "There was no point". When she did talk, she said she just wanted to run away from her life, but there was nowhere to run. Her family situation was very difficult indeed, and she spent a lot of time crying and saying she had had too much, she was worn out, she couldn't live.
>
> At the end of her inpatient admission, Hanna said, "I hate to admit this, but this has been the best experience of my life." It seemed most appropriate to sit quietly together while meditating on Hanna's experience of the pleasure of being understood.

The psychotherapeutic experience requires some silence—silence for meaning to emerge and silence for meaningful insights to seep profoundly into the psyche.

T. S. Eliot in his *Four Quartets* (1940) helps us to understand when he says:

> I said to my soul, be still, and wait without hope.
> For hope would be hope for the wrong thing: there is yet faith
> But the faith and the love and the hope are all in the waiting
> Wait without thought, for you are not ready for thought:
> So the darkness shall become the light …
>
> We must be still and still moving
> Into another intensity
> For a further union, a deeper communion.
>
> (T. S. Eliott, 1940, pp. 123–129)

Conclusion

I have drawn the links between observing an infant with a mother, and therapeutic work with the infantile and mature parts of the non-speaking young person.

Five of the states of mind which may underlie silence have been illustrated: first, giving up; second, being afraid; third, silently using adhesive identification; fourth, feeling hatred and rage; and fifth, experiencing a loving, understanding and deep resonance with the other.

Most importantly, I have emphasised the importance of linking the internalised family relationships of the young person with the external context: the inpatient dynamics, the unspoken issues in the family, and the family's system of communication, as well as sibling, school, and peer dynamics.

Lastly, I have described how the therapeutic person's task is to be fully present to one's deep emotional and bodily experiences, one's countertransferences. Being with the child involves rapt attention to every nuance of the communication between child and therapist.

In each moment of your therapeutic encounter, a question is being asked of you. When the child is not speaking to you, *even more* is being asked of you. You are being asked to transform non-symbolised, inchoate experiences into thoughts suitable for shared understanding to emerge.

PART II

YOUNG CHILDREN

CHAPTER FOUR

The musings of babies: reflective thinking, emotion, and the re-integration of the good object

Alex Dubinsky

Bion's work, *Learning from Experience* (1962) in particular, demonstrates that one can speak in a coherent manner of the baby's thoughts and thinking. We will consider here a particular situation which shows how the baby's thinking contributes to the deepening of the relationship with the mother, and thus to the child's development.

When babies feel they cannot or should not turn for comfort to their mothers, they may instead direct their unconscious thoughts towards the good mother in their internal world. Thinking these thoughts helps restore their relationship with that good internal object. The baby can then turn back to the mother in external reality. The relationship with both the good internal mother and with the mother in external reality is consolidated while the store of unconscious thoughts increases. This is conducive to growth, provided the avoidance or splitting off of angry or painful feelings does not become a predominant feature of the child's personality.

These considerations emerged from observation material reported by students in infant observation seminars. Some of this material will be discussed in detail below. Indeed, the succession of observed gestures, expressions, and utterances allows us to understand something of the baby's thoughts and feelings, whether conscious or unconscious, through a process of interpretation. The plausibility of such interpretations depends in part on their providing a coherent description of these thoughts and feelings over a period of time as they prompt each other and replace previous thoughts and feelings. The interpretations must also be consistent with the emotional quality of the observed situation. Some of these interpretations are based on psychoanalytic understanding of the infantile clinical material of children, adolescents, and adults.

A representation is considered to be symbolic, or a symbol, when the thought, and what the thought refers to, and what represents that thought in the external world, remain distinct in the baby's mind. When this distinction is blurred, the phenomenon of "concretisation", studied by Segal (1957) and Bion (1962), occurs. The symbolic representation of unconscious thoughts provides the means to communicate with the internal world (Segal, 1957). In this way, symbolic play and gestures allow the baby to think about emotional relationships as they occur in the internal world in the way that a dream allows us to think our unconscious thoughts (Meltzer, 1983).

Baby "Phoebe"

Baby Phoebe is a passionate and forceful little girl.

> *"Phoebe", six weeks and five days old: an intense feed*
>
> Phoebe is first feeding with a hand on each breast. There is a brief interruption and both hands are again in fists, but this time her hands seem to be resting on the breast from which she is feeding. The index finger on her right hand starts to move up and down almost in synchronisation with the feeding. Her mother comments that Phoebe likes to have her eye against her hand as she is feeding, so much so that she gets a little red mark under the eye. Her eye rests on her left fist which his resting on the breast.

The fists Phoebe puts on both breasts indicate that in her mind there are two breasts from which she can feed and which she wants to possess. The eye pressed against her fist suggests that she has a thought of penetrating into the breast like the nipple entering her mouth.

The finger marking the rhythm shows that Phoebe takes part in the feeding with her whole being. The urge to identify with the flow of milk, through projective identification, probably induces a confusion between the rhythm of the flow of milk, the thought of it, and its representation by the beat of her finger. If this is the case, the representation is not symbolic and is an instance of "concretisation" of a thought. The thought of penetrating into the breast is probably similarly "concretised", so that the breast is experienced as being actually entered into. This is in contrast with the fragment of an observation that now follows in which the gestures are symbolic.

> *"Phoebe", thirteen weeks and four days old*
>
> After feeding Phoebe, mother sits her up for a moment on her knee so that Phoebe is facing the observer. She has a drunk, dreamy look on her face. Then mother lays her down across her lap. Phoebe puts her finger and thumb in her mouth. Mother comments that she does this as soon as she finishes feeding. She adds that sometimes the baby makes herself gag by putting

> her hand in too deeply. After a moment, Phoebe's hand comes out of her mouth and she puts one hand into the other. Her feet are also crossed at the ankles.

In this observation, Phoebe is not overwhelmed by the urge to swallow the nipple and the breast. She does not perceive the finger and thumb in her mouth as a breast and nipple which have to be swallowed and thus, she does not make herself gag. Finger and thumb provide a symbolic representation of the thought of the nipple and breast. The thought and its representation become the object of further elaboration as Phoebe puts one hand inside the other and crosses her legs. The thought is now that of her being physically and emotionally close to her mother and holding something, in the manner of the mouth closing on the nipple.

In contemplating this observation we see that 'in the manner of' suggests that the gesture of putting one hand inside the other is a symbolic representation. It corresponds to the notion of the paired mother-baby. This notion of a couple is a significant elaboration of the baby's initial experience of the existence of the mother. The emotion permeating the relationship between mother and child is the very stuff from which this notion is constructed. The representation of this notion, in turn, sustains the existence of this link in the way that language sustains both our emotional involvement and our thinking. Phoebe is more than satiated and she does not want to suck again at the breast. Her gestures represent symbolically the very intimate relationship with her internal mother which she is preserving in the alcove of her unconscious thoughts. She is ready for a different kind of interaction in external reality. Indeed later in the observation, Phoebe is happily gurgling in response to her mother's playful words.

Baby "Joey"

Joey is a little boy who wants more emotional interaction with his mother, who loves him dearly but is very busy,

> *"Joey", one year, two and a half months*
>
> Mother chuckles whilst sitting down on the sofa in front of him. She kneels, getting close to him. "Hello Joey", she says fondly. He looks at her with big eyes. His sister comes in. Within half a minute, Joey crawls quite quickly to the corner of the room, then turns round so that he is facing mother and his sister again, though he is looking at neither of them. His action has stopped somewhat abruptly. Perhaps he looks a little subdued. Now, as he stands himself up against the armrest of the sofa where the observer is sitting, his eyes light up again, and they rove the room quickly. Mother is watching him intently, sitting a few feet away on another sofa. She is looking at him, though she seems very tired.

When his sister comes into the room at the very moment he is marvelling at his mother's fond attention, Joey turns away from mental pain. His mother is now perceived as a bad object, and he splits off his interest and his love, as well as his jealousy and anger. Joey now seems subdued. Although he probably feels lonely, Joey does not turn to the observer while standing up close to him. He is able to tolerate mental pain, and this allows him to feel and think. The proximity of the observer evokes the thought of a good presence which would alleviate his misery, an experience that has its source in the good maternal object in his internal world. As the observer is made to represent that object and to confirm its presence, Joey's eyes light up again and rove the room. He is probably searching for new representations of this internal object.

> Eventually mother leaves the room. After a few moments, Joey crawls very quickly towards the piano. "You want to play the piano?" asks his sister, and she lifts the lid. Joey rests the forefinger of his left hand on one key, and the forefinger of his right hand on another key. He repeatedly presses the key with his right forefinger. It sounds like a broken record, he is looking at the wall with a glazed, slightly lifeless expression as he presses the key.
>
> After a few seconds, he abruptly moves off the piano and crawls quickly towards the closed cupboard underneath the television set. He stands up and manages to open this cupboard which is full of equipment and, under the supervision of his sister, rummages in it with his hands, appearing to the observer to be "investigating". He then gets down on all fours and crawls to a music box, which plays different tunes as he presses the keys. He then crawls back to the piano, stands up again, and presses a key with his right hand.

Joey gives an impression of restlessness as he gives up each activity so quickly and moves from one to another. It is striking. He seems to be in search of something. He gets down again and crawls quite quickly out of the room, traverses the hall, and goes to the kitchen where his parents are talking. Brought back by his sister, Joey rolled a ball towards the observer. Soon he enjoys being changed by his mother.

When his mother leaves the room, Joey unconsciously fears to lose his good internal object as well and again he feels lonely. The thought of losing that internal object makes him go to the piano and try to evoke its distant voice. Now that this thought has found its representation, Joey wants more than to hear a voice. This evokes in him the unconscious thought of getting access to the internal object's mind, which he represents by the enclosed space inside the cupboard. He then wants to make the voice of his internal object talk or sing to him. As these thoughts succeed each other, the emotional relationship with that object is re-established. Only then, Joe goes to the kitchen to seek his mother in external reality.

The depressive anxiety of losing his good internal object has sent Joey to the piano where with lifeless eyes he repeatedly presses the same key. A part of him, which contains this internal object has been split off but is still within reach. Like Perceval in the Legend of the Grail (Chrétien de Troyes, 1183), Joey has embarked on a quest for symbolic representations of the loved good internal mother which ends in his seeking his mother in the external world. As in the Legend of the Grail, the purpose of the quest, that of regaining the good internal object, and the meaning of the particular representations, remain unconscious. Each symbol captures a particular aspect of the internal object.

Thinking can be sustained because Joey finds symbolic representations for his unconscious thoughts about the internal object. These representations in the external world momentarily give constancy to evanescent thoughts, until a new unconscious thought emerges, together with a new emotional experience, in the relationship with the good internal object.

As time unfolds, the emergence of new thoughts, conscious and unconscious, makes it possible for the baby to build, element by element, the apparatus required for thinking.

Baby "Roland"

Roland is a little boy who does not want to upset his caring mother. In the material discussed here, mother arrives late, which is most unusual for her. Also, mother would normally stay with him at the start of an observation.

> *"Roland", eleven months and two weeks*
>
> Mother arrives a few minutes late. She explains that Roland's brother is sulking. Roland is still in the car, in his baby seat. The observer sees him through the car window. He smiles at her and then turns his head away. He puts his hand on the soft furnishings of the car. Mother opens the car door to take him out. Roland looks at her and then turns to the observer to give her another smile. Mother is in a rush. She takes Roland inside the house, puts him on his play mat, takes his coat off, and goes to fetch the shopping.
>
> He smiles shyly at the observer and then delicately puts his hand flat on the carpet and looks at it. He turns, looks at the observer and smiles before turning to look carefully and smile at his hand caressing the carpet with a slow movement. He seems embarrassed by the observer's presence.

As his mother is upset and emotionally unavailable, Roland turns to evoking the softness of the breast. A tactile image is used as a symbol of their mutual tenderness. When observing his hand on the carpet, he is consciously aware of something most precious being the ultimate object of his gesture. This object belongs to another world not accessible to consciousness. That other world is the internal world which can only be reached by unconscious thoughts.

Great religious art puts us in a similar position. Both a believer and a non-believer touched by the art of the great Russian icons know these are representations of the deity. The particular experience is that of seeing a painting that points to another world. This pointing at is done through systematic stylisation, and the use of shapes and colours and harmonies that are not met in our everyday world. ("Ever since the earliest times, and increasingly after the Council of 787, the icon has tended towards a stylisation that is meant to make it a symbol of an un-depictable dimension" (Felmy, 1998, p. 4)). Sometimes, as in a haunting painting by Andrei Rublev of Christ the Saviour, the Archangel Michael, and St Paul, the figures appear to look at us from that other world. The emotional content of the icons is transmitted to us through our senses by the artistry of the painter. The conscious emotions that are evoked put the non-believer in touch with objects in the internal world. It also seems to me that the deeply religious icon painters were seeking through the intercession of the internal objects to bring the believer to sense the presence of the deity. Roland is not an artist at work. He is using a simple, tactile image to have a sense of the presence of a good internal object, and he does not want to be distracted by the presence of the observer.

> His mother comes back to the house with the food she has bought. His gaze follows her. He then takes a little brown stick made of plastic and applies himself to make it stand on his mat. Repeatedly, the stick falls down, but Roland continues to try and make it stand, alone, upright on the mat. His gestures are slow and precise. He is not interested in the observer.

Disappointment that his mother has not stopped to talk evokes the unconscious thought and wish to stand up, like a boy who can already walk, and stand up for himself and attract his mother's attention. The rest of the observation will suggest that the stick was also a symbol of virility.

> Mother says she will prepare some soup for supper. She puts what she needs on the living room table close to us. Roland's brother comes down with a black pencil and a colouring book. He is wearing the new boots mother just bought for him. He lies down close to mother and observer and talks about completing his colouring. Roland is looking at the observer for quite a long time while she gives attention to his brother. As soon as the observer turns back to him, he engages in a new pursuit. He is pushing the stick through the round hole in a box. It is the usual toy with a lid where there are openings in different shapes. He just gets the end of the stick in the round opening and then pulls it out. He repeats this a few times. Then he puts at the end of the stick a small container, maybe it's a cap used to close a bottle, and tries to introduce this assembly into the box. The little cap makes a noise as it falls into the round opening in the box. Roland opens the side door into the box and takes the cap back. He puts it again on the stick and tries again. He looks serious and seems far away.
>
> Roland watches carefully as his brother attracts the observer's attention.

Roland then uses the stick and the box to represent the internal mother's mind as an enclosed space and he would like to master how to get access to it. It then comes to his mind that the observer is now giving him support, like the stick, which also stands for the father's penis, and gives support to the little container in its endeavours to get inside the box. (This is symbolic play since Roland represents access to the mind as something to seek and not as something that has been achieved, although the stick really penetrates the box.)

> At this point in the observation, Roland's brother asks his mother to help peeling the vegetables. Mother replies that this is too difficult for him and that he can help her by playing with Roland. Roland is more present during this exchange. He is looking at each person in turn. Every time his eyes meet the observer's, he smiles. He takes a wooden half-sphere and puts it into his mouth, licking the round side. Holding it in his hand, he moves towards his brother and lets out sounds which express his excitement: "Ba, Ba!". His brother turns round and then restarts his colouring. Roland enjoys himself patting his brother's boots and then comes near him and tries to take away his black pencil.

After having sought first a tender closeness to the good mother in the internal world and then access to her mind, Roland wants to enter into a relationship with the observer similar to that of his brother with his mother. It seems that he still does not believe that he can attract the attention of his mother, who is talking to his brother. Instead, Roland chooses to establish a loving relationship with the observer. She now represents a mother whom he can reach emotionally, like the good breast symbolised by the wooden half-sphere that he licks.

At last, he feels strong enough to allow himself to experience both the admiration of his brother and the rivalry which he had split off. Roland even enjoys a sense of triumph as he approaches his brother while holding the little half-sphere in his hand: he is the one who has got the breast! With conquering assertiveness, Roland admires his brother's boots and tries to take away his pencil. By attempting to steal his brother's virility, Roland tries to possess himself of what in his unconscious thoughts made up his brother's capability to relate to their mother.

> Roland's brother resists, he does not want to give up. He settles on the play mat with his colouring book, taking over Roland's place. When Roland asserts himself and comes to play close to him, his brother leaves the room. Roland watches him go. He looks at the observer and then, with a big cry of admiration "ah", stretches his hand towards the halogen lamp which is switched on. He looks again at the observer and then turns to the bookshelf and, with the same enthusiasm, points at the books.

As soon as there is no competition from his brother, Roland feels again triumphant. He shares with the observer his admiration for the beauty and wisdom of the good internal mother whom, in his elation, he now believes is there for him to enjoy.

Roland's brother returns with some small toy cars, which he rolls on the back of the sofa. Roland extends both hands towards the cars. He opens and closes his hands and expresses displeasure by moaning and frowning. He imitates the noise cars make, "Brr", and remains in contemplation as he looks at his brother's game. He returns to the play mat and finds a red plastic ring. He pats it against the observer's arm and observes her face. She smiles at him and says, "It looks as if you want to play with me." He goes to the shopping bags and puts the red ring on a carton of milk and takes it back. He comes back to his play mat carrying his red ring. He places the red ring on a pole standing up on a base, takes it off, and puts it back a few times. Quickly, he now moves towards his mother's legs. He raises his head, stretches his arms, while opening and closing his hand, and says nicely to her, "Mummy".

As he covets the little cars, Roland is more integrated and can thus experience distress, anger, and rivalry. He then recognises that his brother is older and stronger and goes back to the play mat which is his "baby territory". Without collapsing, he has given up trying to equal or even surpass him. Instead, Roland becomes a competent baby who wants to have a close relationship with the good mother of his internal world. The red ring is used to represent his lips seeking her. Then, after resting these lips on the good breast, that is, the milk carton, Roland shows to himself that he can put his mouth around the nipple represented by the pole on its base. Like Joey, now that he feels close to his mother, Roland can at last turn to his mother in the external world. The word "Mummy" condenses all that he knows he will find in her.

Mother kneels to kiss Roland and says "What kind of a Mummy is this? She is always busy." Followed by his mother, Roland goes to the play mat. She kneels behind him as he is busy putting three rings around the pole. His mother congratulates him and Roland clasps his hands.

For a little while, he keeps removing the rings, putting them back around the pole, and clapping his hands. He then takes a little book and sits against his mother. She sits him on her lap and asks him to show her the duck. He delicately turns the pages and finds the duck. He produces an approximation of the word "duck". He turns the page, puts his hand on a balloon, and says "ba, ba".

Roland is now delicately turning the pages while his mother guides him in the discovery of his first words. A mother who opens up the world for you is so precious.

Conclusion

Babies may turn away from their mother in the external world in order to avoid feelings such as anger, jealousy, disappointment, or feeling satiated to the point of being emotionally overwhelmed. As a consequence, they may fear to lose also their relationship with the good internal mother and may embark on a quest whereby each new step is prompted by emotion and unconscious thinking. These babies follow a path marked by unconscious thoughts of restoring the relationship with the internal mother. When the mind's work is done, the baby has a sense of having regained the good internal object and turns back to the mother in external reality.

In terms of the emotional links of Love, Hate, and Knowing used by Bion (1965) to describe emotional relationships, what the baby may hate are the feelings that are perceived as too intense or dangerous. Together, Love and Knowing may restore the relationship with the internal mother, and then with the mother in the external world. Love for the internal object and the anxiety that it may be lost bring to the baby's mind thoughts upon which he or she reflects, protected by the relative isolation which the Unconscious provides. Knowing the good internal mother makes it possible for the baby to restore feelings of loving and being loved.

Acknowledgements

The observations in this chapter were made by students of the Tavistock Clinic in London and of the Centre Martha Harris in Larmor Plage, France. I was greatly encouraged by the enthusiasm for thinking shown by a baby girl I discussed in a previous paper (Dubinsky, 2007). The observer was bringing her observations of that baby to seminars held in Moscow.

CHAPTER FIVE

A baby's "broken bridge" to the parents

Jeanne Magagna

When a baby–mother/father relationship works, the baby keeps alive the desire to communicate with the parents through eyes, mouth, hands, body, and mind. The desire to be perceived and fully understood by his parents becomes a passionate one as the baby falls more deeply in love with his parents. He moves from crying to pointing to speaking and symbolically playing out his experiences as part of an intense wish to share emotional experiences and interests with them.

Unfortunately, pre-verbal relationships with the parents do not work for every baby, and the *emotional bridge* connecting the baby to his parents is sometimes broken. When this happens, a *basic fault* (Balint, 1968) occurs in the development of his personality. When faced with an emotional crisis at a later point in his life, the child will then be at risk of *regression* to not-talking, not-eating, and not being open to anything the parents have to offer him.

In infancy, when the *emotional bridge* to the parents is damaged or broken, the infant is desperate and tries to find a way of coping with the fear of dying, the anxieties regarding emotional disintegration, and the pain of being left alone. In early infancy, the baby lacks the inner capacities to bear such emotional experiences. Deprived of parents who are sufficiently responsive to his own particular needs, the baby turns to self-protection for safety. *Not-thinking* (Emanuel, 2001), often referred to as *dissociation*, becomes frequently resorted to as a primitive protection. Other primitive protections also develop as ways to keep the baby away from the risk of being vulnerable through needing parents who are not available to help him.

In order to facilitate the therapist's and parents' verbal *greeting of gestures* (Magagna, Chapter Seven) of a non-speaking young person in family or individual psychotherapy, I am going to describe the first year in the life of an infant whose *emotional bridge* to the mother is being broken in the pre-verbal stages of his development. This baby's broken *bridge to the mother* contributed to his lack of desire to reach out to his mother through vocalising, gesturing, forming words, and speaking. His personality was thus at risk of *regression to the basic fault* in his personality structure at times of developmental crises (Balint, 1968). I will also look at the possible origins of the problem in mother's or father's past, and see how a series of weekly infant observation sessions, and later participant observation sessions, were able to help the family towards a healthier, happier future.

I am grateful to the infant observer of the baby. Her observations depict the way in which Jon initially experienced a "broken bridge" to his parents. Weekly infant observation seminars are part of every child psychotherapist's training in the Tavistock Clinic and elsewhere internationally. Infant observation provides a crucial base for understanding of the baby's communication of his state of mind through gestures and facial expressions (Briggs, 2002). The observer visited Jon's home one hour a week for twenty-nine months. She had hoped to observe both the father and mother with the baby, but this rarely proved possible because of the father's long working hours.

Hopes and frustrations in "building a bridge" to the parents

Jon was an unexpected baby, born to a tall, stylish, red-haired, Irish-immigrant mother, aged twenty-three, working as a telephone operator, and a black-haired, stocky, jovial, Irish-immigrant father, also twenty-three, working as a computer shop salesman. The couple were married. Jon was delivered normally in hospital, and his young mother subsequently had several months of maternity leave. The observer began her work with the family when Jon was only a few weeks old.

In the first observation, there is a sense that mother is becoming aware of how very weighty a task it is to become a mother to a baby who is dependent upon her twenty-four hours a day:

Observation: Jon, five weeks

Mother tells the observer, "Jon seems to be so calm now you are here, but he was screaming before you arrived!" She adds, "Sometimes he gets so mad that he holds his breath. I think he really has a temper. He is better off 'hanging out' on his swing. Then he doesn't need me to hold him."

Jon is being jostled in his vibrating swinging seat. As the conversation between mother and the observer continues, he begins to cry, frantically waving his arms in the air and pushing his feet against the seat. Mother removes his blanket as he screams even louder. The baby wrinkles up his reddened face and tightly clenches his fists as mother moves her attention away from him and looks towards the observer. She explains, "I don't want to be mean to him but I want you to see what he does when he is angry!" Jon's cries escalate. Mother responds by saying to the observer, "He doesn't sound angry like he usually gets."

Jon begins to snort from nasal congestion and mother mimics him by snorting herself and then saying, "He sounds like a little pig!" She then begins to laugh mockingly at him. Subsequently mother pushes her baby a little distance away from her and bends down to check his nappy to see if it is soiled. It is dry. Gradually Jon's eyes begin to close

> and he eventually falls into a deep sleep. Mother feels visibly relieved and smiles at the observer.

Jon is becoming increasingly distressed, as shown when he wrinkles up his face, tightly clenches his fists "to hold himself together", and pushes his feet into the surface of the swinging seat (Bick, 1968). Mother appears to be uncaring to her baby when she does not respond to his unhappiness. Her making fun of Jon's uncomfortable breathing by saying, "He sounds like a little pig", feels hostile to his discomfort. Why is mother distancing herself from her painfully unhappy baby? Certainly, this must be occurring for a reason. It seemed that mother could not bear to be intimate with her distressed child, Jon, for his anguished crying evoked the mother's own unresolved conflicts, her sadness, her anger, her hurt, and her loneliness in relation to her own *internalised mother*.

Becoming a mother (or indeed a father) is a developmental process that starts with the mother's own experience of being mothered. The growth of the mother's capacity to mother "is rooted in the *introjective identifications* with parental objects which form the unconscious substrates of the self. Taking up a maternal role involves adding new dimensions to one's sense of self..... At the birth of a baby the mother has to sort out a new relationship to the internal parents which involves both identification with them and differentiation from them" (Rustin, 2002, p. 19). The mother's deeper containment of her own infantile feelings, in identification with her own internalised parents, strengthens the baby's *emotional bridge* to the mother. Michael Leunig explores this notion in his (untitled) poem:

> ... As she carried her child may she carry her soul.
> As her child was born, may she give birth and life
> and form to her own, higher truth. As she
> nourished and protected her child, may she
> nourish and protect her inner life and her
> independence. For her soul shall be her
> most painful birth, her most difficult child
> and the dearest sister to her other children.
>
> (Leunig, 1990, p. 41)

This poem describes how it is essential for the mother to give birth to her own inner child, how important it is for her to find the space to discover the truth of her emotional experience. It implies the need to form a picture of how one feels inside and to find nourishment in the form of emotional support, thoughtfulness, and protection for one's inner child, as well as for the actual child. This is true not only for the mother, but also for the father, and in fact for all of us, whether or not we have biological children.

The free associations that the mother makes during the course of the weekly observations express the mother's relationship not only with the external baby but also with her own *inner child,* and her relationships with internalised parental figures. The baby's feelings evoke the mother's own repressed infantile feelings.

Perhaps the mother was identifying with an uncaring internalised mother and running away from her own abandoned *inner child* living alone with grief. This results in Jon being left to suffer. Simultaneously, as his cries escalate, mother seems more persecuted by his crying: it makes her feel she is not a good mother. This *re-enactment* of an internalised mother, hostile to the vulnerable baby, is similar to unconscious *re-enactments* described by Fraiberg (1980) in, "Ghosts in the nursery: a psychoanalytic approach to the problems of impaired infant-mother relationships".

Jon's pain frequently receives *flat parental containment* (Magagna, Chapter Six) through distraction by inanimate objects, as seen here:

Observation: Jon, five weeks

> Jon is in a front pack next to his father's body. He squirms a little while burping and raising his arms into the air. Dad immediately turns on the kitchen sink faucet saying, "Jon seems calmed by the running water. He is also quietened by our fan's whirling sounds." However, neither Jon nor dad remain content with inanimate objects as distractions for Jon's distress. Father now places Jon on his knees, about six inches from his own face and begins creating a song. Jon has become very still and transfixed by his father's singing and compassionate, thoughtful attention. Jon also seems enraptured by dad's whispering, "I'm a cute baby", and "I've just had a bath and I'm all clean." This is such a beautiful intimate interlude between baby and his father!
>
> At the end of the session, as the observer was walking out the door, mother whispered, "My husband doesn't really know what to do with Jon yet. He treats him like he treats the cat."

For a little while, the father's relationship with his young son seemed thoughtful and loving. The baby needs to be accompanied by an adult mind which he can get to know, and which can get to know him. Just as the newborn focuses on the nipple, and very soon on the mother's gaze or the sound of her voice, so his attention and interest are held by the parents' interest focusing upon him (Miller, 2002). Why was mother denigrating the intimacy between baby and dad? Could it be that she felt jealous and angry as the left-out bystander? Perhaps the mother felt that her baby was receiving something good from the father which she herself wasn't at the moment able to give and which perhaps she was not currently receiving herself? Also, possibly the mother had not received such sensitive loving care, or at least had not been able to keep intact an internalised, good experience of being parented. The following excerpt suggests there is some maternal anxiety regarding emotional intimacy:

Observation: Jon, seven weeks

> Jon is sleeping on mother's chest with his mouth wide open as he smiles broadly. This is another lovely moment of intimacy which is suddenly interrupted by mother coldly saying, "I think his ears are big. Mine are smaller. I wonder where he got his big ears?"
>
> Baby remains peacefully sleeping against mother's breast. He smiles again, then opens his eyes part-way and looks up into his mother's eyes. Mother responds saying, "I can see there's nobody there when I look into his eyes."

This is such a very painful moment, for it is clear that baby is there, looking at his mother, wanting her, communicating his love to her, but mother is denying his very existence! Baby is partly conscious of the beauty of having a mother holding him, feeding him, and comforting him. "He is not completely conscious, but partly, and that is much" (MacNeice, 1940, p. 243). But why is the mother so fiercely protecting herself from the beauty and intimacy she could have with her baby? What leads her to point out the "bigness of his ears" and to blank him out, indicating "nobody is there" when her baby is smiling in her arms? Is it just too painful for the mother to come close to her vulnerable, dependent, loving baby because he evokes her acute awareness of her own unfulfilled longings? Something disturbing is happening within the mother, as seen in this next observation:

Observation: Jon, two months, one week

> It is just at this time that mother decides to leave the baby and begin to work part-time for twelve-hour shifts. When he is being left for long periods with the baby-sitter, Jon becomes more fretful. Simultaneously, and conceivably both because of her work and his crying, mother finds Jon to be an overwhelming burden. It is at this point that mother begins to regularly leave him to cry himself to sleep and to comfort himself when awake and crying during the night.
>
> At one point, Jon is left in his room in distress, struggling as if he wants to get out of the bed and crying so loudly and for so long that he begins to choke and gasp for air. Mother arrives to check on her son saying, "I don't want Jon to cry too long." But it has already been "too long" for Jon and the experience of being left in distress for "too long" is terrifying for him (Tustin, 1981). This is shown as he clenches his fists and tries to use his legs to push himself up from the bed. He is trying to get out of this terrible position of lying helpless on the bed, a miserable baby left without his mother, externally and also internally. Jon is relying on the clenching of his fingers to hold his "falling-to-pieces" self together. Then Jon's precocious agility becomes a necessity as he attempts to use his legs to push himself out of the position of being a "helpless, wretched left-alone baby".

There is a sense that mother's twelve-hour work shifts has disrupted an already *fragile bridge* between Jon and his mother. Jon's increased distress seems to result in his more frequently resorting to his own primitive protections against anxiety, rather than retaining his dependency on his mother to relieve his distress. A vicious cycle seems to be initiated: mother leaves for longer periods; Jon becomes more distressed; as a result, mother becomes more persecuted; mother detaches herself from Jon even more, and Jon is left crying for even longer periods of time. Jon turn's away from his mother to primitive adhesive protections (Meltzer, 1975). *Baby's bridge to mother* is being gradually broken and replaced by Jon alienating himself from mother. He is replacing her with his own body and sticking to objects as protections against overwhelming terrors. Perhaps it is worth explaining that the problem is linked not only with mother's way of responding to Jon, but also it is fostered by his helplessness, culminating in his being angry with mother for being absent. Jon's anger with his mother leads to his internal good mother becoming damaged. This internal situation of having only a frightening, damaged internal mother creates in Jon a terrifying anxiety. He experiences nightmarish images instead of a *good internal mother* (O'Shaughnessy, 1964).

Observation: Jon, three months

> Mother asks Jon if he is okay. His hands are more open now, but when he brings them together he places his thumb between his forefinger and middle finger. As mother walks past Jon to go into the kitchen mother tells him, "just a couple more minutes". Jon listlessly watches her go by. Sadness emanates from Jon's face and body. His arms are no longer being raised into the air with beckoning, waving, excited and agitated "pick me up" movements characteristic of his earlier weeks. Now Jon does not often seem to be signalling for his mother's help or attention when it would be helpful for him to do so. When he appears less demanding, mother describes how she has been taking anti-depressants for a year and is thinking of stopping them.

The combination of mother's depression, which required medication when mother became pregnant with Jon, Jon's birth, and the demands of work initially seemed to have swamped mother. There is a question as to whether or not during this time the anti-depressant had somehow led mother to feel distanced from psychic pain, not only in herself, but also in her baby, leading her to be less responsive to his needs. As a response to being left to cry for too long, Jon has become somewhat listless and is resignedly putting his thumb between his fingers rather than beckoning and crying for his mother. It feels like his thumb is used to plug up and banish his longing for his mother rather than being used to represent an *internal bridge* to a good mother in his mind.

The observer began to worry in earnest when Jon was seven months old and she saw on the mother's open computer screen a picture of dirty-faced baby Jon eating grass. Mother explained, "He did something worrying this week. I was weeding. First, he was just sitting there eating the grass, then he got a stiff weed and I thought, 'well that's ok', but the next thing I knew he had a big chunk of grass with dirt on it in his mouth. It was pretty funny! He was so cute! I took a picture of it." Mother then recounted how the computer picture depicted Jon with dirt all over his face and in his mouth. At first, mother and father had found this situation "funny", and this is why mother had photographed the baby, but now in the presence of a thoughtful observer, mother seemed to give a description of Jon which in its vividness projected worry into the observer.

This picture suggests that, symbolically, Jon is to hold "the rubbish", "the emotional baggage" that is too much to tolerate within the parental couple. It was very concerning to hear mother say, "Last weekend I installed a baby-cry-monitor system in Jon's bedroom, but then I decided to turn it off because he cried so long at night." Mother asserted, "I am not going to pick him up at night, because then he will certainly cry more." It appears that the baby's crying so distresses mother that she "turns herself off" like she turned off the baby-cry-monitor. Then she doesn't respond to baby at all! This is a scary metaphor that mother uses to show how she "turns off" Jon's cries, for they feel threatening to her precarious emotional wellbeing.

Mother seems to defend herself through keeping busy with household tasks. These allow her to distance herself from the demands of a very needy and dependent baby, who needs to be perpetually protected and *held in mind* by her. However, she asks the observer, "When are you coming next week? I will stop my chores for that hour", thus showing her own infantile needs and growing dependency on the observer's thoughtful, empathic presence.

Mother always seems to welcome the observer's visits. Sometimes, though, when the observer arrived and father was home, the observer would knock on the glass door and father would not get up: he expected the observer to fend for herself by opening the door to the house. His action seemed to reflect the couple's unconscious assumption that, "people should look after themselves, not be too dependent on others". Since there was as yet no family history available, it was unclear how the couple's shared philosophy of "you should look after yourself" had developed.

Fraiberg (1975) says that parents may have the determination to want something better for their child than they themselves had; however, conscious determination seems to fall far short of what is required. Fraiberg questions how we can know if the parenting will bring grief and injuries or become a time of renewal. The answer to this question must lie in the parents' use of defences to cope with a difficult past, but also in the parents' capacity to feel deeply and acknowledge the truth of their experiences. *Denial* of feelings that have accompanied painful experiences and the parents' *identification with the aggressor* are two common defences. Parents who use these defences of denial and identification may be unable to withstand the need to inflict their own pain upon their child, and will require some therapeutic understanding to respond satisfactorily to their child's needs (Fraiberg, Adelson, & Shapiro, 1980).

A potentially more attuned, healthy relationship between mother and Jon became further disrupted when mother went back to work and Jon became more distressed. By the age of five months, he began to avoid the gaze of his mother. At this time, she also complained that he frequently bit her breast and was less willing to eat the food she gave him. In some observations, Jon could be seen giving himself a sense of security by tightly clutching a set of metal keys. Jon felt desperate to hold onto the keys and, when mother wanted to dress him, she was required to struggle to prise them out of his fingers. The parents increasingly encouraged Jon to put things in his mouth, such as a pacifier or his thumb. This suggested their endorsement of dependency on an object other than the parents as a source of soothing.

Jon's avoidant attachment to the parents, his *broken bridge to the mother*, was becoming worryingly consolidated in his way of being: he consciously expected little from his parents, and he was clinging tenaciously to physical objects as a way to emotionally self-regulate and self-soothe. Jon gradually *dissociated* himself from his "vulnerable, helpless, crying self". When he was distressed, in the absence of a mother externally to come to his rescue and in the presence of a *persecutory internal mother*, Jon seemed to begin a retreat into his own psychic world, away from the unsafe external world (Meltzer, 1992). The only way to bear his experiences of distress throughout the long crying nights of infancy was to lose awareness of them. Jon's emotions and cries of distress and protest were frozen because there was no mother to respond to him and mitigate his distress through the night. The absence of Jon's cries of distress exacerbated the difficulty in a downward spiral of worrying interactions: Jon did not elicit mother's containment of his psychic disintegration, she did not respond to him when he needed her, mother felt even less responsive to him for he was not seeking her and then Jon felt doubly deprived of a mother (Williams, 1997a).

The repeated use of primitive protective mechanisms, such as keeping his mouth closed, holding onto hard objects like keys, a block and a screwdriver, the use of massive denial and dissociation, led Jon to an almost impenetrable cystic encapsulation of "the hidden tears of grief" (S. Klein, 1980). The tears are not only hidden from the mother, they are also hidden from Jon himself. Jon was beginning to use precocious motor skills and tenaciously hold onto hard objects not to facilitate the containment of emotional states but, instead, to bind his personality together. Thus, *adhesive identification* is used by Jon's personality rather than *introjective identification* with emotionally containing parental figures (Tustin, 1980). By seven months, Jon is more frequently locating the distress within his body. He has allergies, a hint of asthma, and frequent colds. Mother's anxiety is further provoked by her baby's illnesses. She feels something isn't right; she doesn't know what it is, but she feels persecuted by the experience of mothering her baby and finding that things are not going well in their relationship.

A manic defence

As time goes on, the baby's avoidant attachment to mother which hides his distress creates an even more uncomfortable phenomena permeating the family's psychic system: manic denial in Jon. Jon's "transformation of affect" from pain to excitement mirrors his mother's response to his eating the grass in an earlier observation. This form of manic denial is described by Melanie Klein (1935). Manic denial through laughter is best captured by a common American phrase, "Laugh, I thought I'd die". Manic denial, involving an aggressive act or painful experience which is greeted with excitement and laughter, is seen below:

Observation: Jon, seven months

Mother moans, "Jon is biting my breast when he nurses. When I say 'ouch', he laughs."

Jon is repeating his internalised parents' manic defence of laughing at an emotionally painful experience. He also has a fear of falling endlessly without being contained emotionally. This is played out through a game, as shown below.

Observation: Jon, seven months

> Jon pulls a basket toward himself, leans backwards until he almost loses his balance, and then he releases his grip. He repeats this falling action four or five times, following it with an excited laugh. Then he stares intently at the empty bottom of the basket.

Jon is terrified, particularly at night, but also generally when he feels like "a dropped baby". Through play, he is trying to *re-enact* this scary experience and work it through emotionally, but perhaps it becomes *a repetition,* rather than *a working through* of a frightening experience, for he also laughs as he nearly falls over. Perhaps this is a re-creation of the way Jon has experienced his mother and father laughing at his suffering on a variety of occasions. In laughing, Jon denies his terror of being "dropped emotionally" by his parents. His experience sometimes augments his terror as seen below:

> The couple mention that mother had accidentally let Jon roll off the bed, and the dad commented to his wife, apparently teasing her, "You wanted to try doing that again!" Mother responded to him, "If you had had done that, I would have killed you!" The parents are laughing and joking with one another.

The laughter of the parents is an attempt to move away from Jon's suffering and his vulnerable, helpless, dependent state of mind. The parents are using an omnipotent self to triumph over the infantile self, lending laughter to an emotionally frightening issue, linked with potential harm of their baby, Jon. Their laughter represents contempt for the plight of the distressed infantile self. This belittling is intended to diminish, as if by magic, contact with the baby's severe anguish, helplessness, and terror. Mother's comment that her own family has, "a lot of fun when they get together, they just play each other off, laughing at each other", makes one wonder just exactly what defences her family of origin employed in relation to psychic pain. Perhaps manic denial is what mother is using at this very moment in relation to her own psychic pain as well as finding it emotionally necessary to stay defended against her baby's suffering (M. Klein, 1935).

But why let their baby suffer? Is there some wish for the baby to suffer, some sadism toward the "little baby"? Possibly representing siblings towards whom they each felt rivalry, or is it just a sense of emotional inadequacy and persecution about the couple's own infantile helplessness and dependency that has never been properly understood and contained by their own internalised parents? It is this lack of *concavely containing internal parents* with whom the couple could identify which could promote their manic defence as a protection against psychic pain?

Inflicting self-harm rather than expressing aggression to the mother

Another concern is Jon's identification with an internalised intrusive and hurtful object when he repeatedly hurt himself on this occasion:

Observation: Jon, seven months

> Jon takes some keys and one by one he puts them in his mouth. He puts the long keys so far back in his throat that they occasionally make him gag. He makes an expression of distaste as he samples each key. After five minutes of this play, he pokes the key hard into the back of his throat and breaks into a sob. Mom responds with, "Ohhhh", picks Jon up, and places him on her lap, whereupon he immediately stops crying. Mother notes, "Already forgotten". Mother has momentarily responded to Jon, but both he and she quickly brush over the incident. When mother says, "Already forgotten", does this make it easier for her, too, to forget and put Jon's hurtful action and physical pain 'out of mind'?

Mother is increasingly aware of some ambivalence in her relationship with Jon. This evokes mother's memories of feeling "sad and glad" when her mother isn't visiting her. In this next observation, in "making the ball glow for him", mother is distracting Jon but also enabling him to find a way of expressing his assertive, aggressive self.

> *Observation: Jon, eight months, three weeks*
>
> Jon has a cold. He is watching mainly the observer, but also mother as the two of them talk. Then he crawls to mother's chair, pulls himself up to a standing position, and puts his mouth against the arm of the chair. Then he notices father's shoes and sits down to grab the shoelaces and put them in his mouth. Mother worries that the shoelaces may not be clean so she gets a ball and bounces it on the ground. This makes the special ball glow and mother offers it to Jon. He takes the ball and with both hands pushes it into his mouth. He subsequently tries to hit the ball against the arm of the chair. This game gets repeated as mother takes the ball, hits it on the arm of her chair, and returns it to Jon who reproduces mother's action by hitting the ball against the chair again. When the ball hits a surface it lights up.

Jon's aggressively hitting the ball against the chair seems to elicit mother's awareness of her own hostility. She tells the observer, "I am really angry with my mother, she left an electric heater turned on in the bathroom and that could have been really dangerous to all of us!"

By ten months, Jon is precociously walking unaided and carrying around a hard red Lego piece as a form of security. Jon has managed to prematurely develop physical maturity to move away from the vulnerable position of depending on mother to come to him to relieve his distress. He can walk where he wants to go! It is worrying that he is using "his red block", reminiscent of Tustin's (1981) *autistic objects*, for emotional safety in lieu of a secure attachment to mother.

Fonagy tell us that:

> The reactions of children under stress have their origins in the parents' defensive strategies. Many of the shortcomings in the mother's responsiveness to her child's needs derive from her own defences against acknowledging and understanding similar negative affect in herself. The mother's defences have their origin in her own developmental history and in turn make it

> difficult for her to respond empathically to affective signals from her infant. Because the infant cannot rely on his mother sufficiently to respond to his signals of negative affective states and thereby to reduce them, he must find alternative ways to diminish them. With an immature and as yet unstructured psychic apparatus, the infant will have to resort to some behavioural strategies.
>
> (Fonagy, 1993, p. 8)

It is important to note that, when the infant is regularly forced to rely on defensive strategies for mediating his emotional experiences, he can appear superficially calm. Although Jon spent many nights as an infant crying alone without eliciting a response from his parents, now Jon rarely cries. Instead, he has precociously learned to walk so he won't be helplessly stuck in a room while in distress. By the time he is two years old, despite the instigation of *therapeutic participant observations*, Jon is showing worrying signs of *"a broken bridge to the parents"*. He tunes out others frequently, has only a few intelligible words, often avoids eye contact with others including mother, and does not readily seek her out, even when in need of her (Hamaguchi, 1995). Instead, Jon uses his red Lego block, his screwdriver, his truck, his interest in doing mechanical things using tools from the toolbox. He can efficiently turn on the television, change channels, and look at various images on the computer, although he is not yet two-years old! There is a sense that some of Jon's anguish is encrusted under "his big boy self" *intrusively identified* with his grown-up, competent father.

Jon frequently averts his gaze when mother or the observer greet him or say goodbye. He appears similar to a child who has experienced the trauma of separation from his mother. Acquarone (2004) suggests that a baby should be able to establish eye contact within a relationship and maintain this contact for some time. Keeping the eyes averted seems to be a physical way of avoiding emotional contact and separation from important adults in his life (Fraiberg, 1982). Fonagy (1993) would suggest that Jon's defensive style of relating to his emotional experiences, including by laughing, reflects an *internalisation* of the defensive quality of parental reactions to his own affective signals.

This chapter has thus far demonstrated a baby's "*broken bridge to the parents*" which when intact would allow the baby to look towards the parents, smile, vocalise, and display emotional states such as sadness, worry, anxiety, and happiness. As mentioned before, when the early preverbal bridge to the parents is broken, a *basic fault* in the baby's personality develops which can promote *regression* during subsequent developmental crises (Balint, 1968).

What is the observer's role?

A child with early developmental difficulties such as Jon's can be therapeutically helped through "the adults appropriately sensing and responding to the child's rudimentary attempts to formulate and express his current mental state, his intentions and wishes" (Fonagy, 1993, p. 10). Bearing this in mind, as time passed the observer began to more actively make comments to mother or Jon about what Jon was experiencing. For the entire twenty-nine months, the observer was fully and regularly present for mother's mind, silently reflecting on her emotional states and those of her baby.

Over time, something more sensitive developed in the mother as she used the observer to think her thoughts aloud. She was beginning to unpeel her "thick skin" in relation to the pain of her baby and perhaps her own infantile self. Mother did this through re-enacting situations, for example, through letting the baby cry loudly for the observer to witness. She also used the observer to project a lot of anxiety into her through sharing free associations about the baby falling, eating grass, and crying unattended all night. Perhaps this was the only way, at that moment, that mother could communicate her anxiety about being a mother to the baby, and about feeling herself to be "an inadequate mother".

The observer experienced the projections of mother's anxiety with which mother didn't seem able to remain in contact. It was as though the mother internally had only a flat containment with an internal, unreceptive mother with whom she was identified to receive her own emotional concerns (S. Briggs, 1997b). We feel the mother desperately needs the observer to receive her words, feel their emotional significance, and then experience alarm and anxiety for Jon. The observer is also required to be aware of mother's denial of her own and her baby's needs for maternal care, protection and understanding.

The question is, should the observer's role be solely *feeling* very worried about Jon's emotional and physical safety, or does she need *to intervene, to act?* Should she intervene, for example, when Jon pushes the keys hard down his throat, eats grass, and crawls off out of his mother's eyesight? Our international video-link infant observation seminar strenuously debated, "What would be helpful to mother? How could the observer help the mother find her mothering role?" (Magagna, Bakalar, Cooper, Levy, & Shank, 2005). The seminar's first suggestion to the observer was to mirror the baby's experience, commenting aloud on baby's distress, helping mother think about her baby. They suggested exploring with mother what might be going on in baby's mind, empathising with baby's possible asthma when mother speaks with detachment about his breathing problems. Initially, the observer was reluctant to be more than an observer compassionately comprehending mother and her baby's experience. There was felt to be a risk that if the observer always accepted Jon's gaze and overtures then there would be a competition about who was the best mother in the room. Mother didn't seem to be inviting the observer to be more responsive to Jon. The observer felt she was walking on eggshells; she felt constrained. She seemed worried that she might put even more pressure on mother's fragile psychic structure if she remarked on Jon's possible feelings of pleasure and distress, noticing his gaze and the times when he smiled and liked receiving mother's care. We realised that the observer was establishing a therapeutic observational role, for mother looked forward to her visits. So we decided that it was important to be respectful to the observer's countertransference intuition that it was better to remain, for the time being, in the traditional observation role.

It is important here to emphasise that in any observation when the observer perceived an immediate and definite maternal lack of care in "being mindful" of Jon in dangerous situations, the observer felt compelled to intervene. Usually, however, an observer doesn't intervene directly; rather her weekly presence enables mother to focus on her baby and attempt to join the observer in discussing the baby's state of mind. Mother's increasing mindful attention to her baby can help her to keep her baby safe. I will now give some examples of the role played by the infant observer during her observations of baby Jon.

Observation: Jon, seven and a half months

Mum changes Jon's nappy and then walks out of the room. Jon looks as she leaves and aimlessly curls and uncurls his fingers. After a couple of minutes he starts crawling down the hallway after mother, crying. The observer says, "Mummy will come back." When mother returns, the observer says, "Jon was crying because he misses you." Mum says, "He almost never misses me. I leave him and he goes right on playing."

The observer has begun to take a more active role through talking about Jon's experiences to Jon himself and also to mother; mother is then able to talk about his confusing responses to separation. Mother is implying to the observer, that when the observer is not present Jon acts as if he doesn't miss his mother or need her. He just takes care of himself through playing with hard inanimate objects or his toys. Perhaps both mother and Jon have a different relationship in the presence of an observer offering "*compassionate comprehension*" of mother, of Jon and of Jon's need for his mother (Sorenson, 2004). Mother seemed to have *introjected* the observer's compassionate containment during the first twenty-two months of weekly observations. This was most apparent when mother began to think about the birth of her second baby saying, "I am not going to let her cry at night!" This excerpt demonstrates how much she changed into a much more containing, sensitive mother:

Observation: Jess, two and a half months, and Jon, twenty-five months

The observer arrives to find mother, with dark circles under her eyes, looking rumpled and exhausted. Mother lamented, "I have been awake all night because Jess was awake. I decided to go to her when she was crying. I don't know why she remained awake, could it be that she wasn't getting enough to eat because my milk supply was low? My milk supply is probably low because I have been so stressed!"

Mother subsequently goes into the bedroom to take off Jon's nappies and pyjamas and dress him for the day. As she does this, she is talking to Jon about what they are going to do during the day. As they go into the sitting room, the cat follows Jon. Mother continues conversing, telling Jon about the snow falling heavily and lifting him onto the window seat to see it. The cat jumps onto the window seat with Jon and this prompts Jon to begin chattering to the cat and mother. The words "kitty" and "snow" are partly intelligible in his flow of undecipherable words.

Meanwhile, Jess has been sleepily moving around in her cot trying to pull her arms up out of her blanket which is tightly swaddled around her. The minute her eyes open fully mother comes over to her saying, "Well, hello sunshine, how are you?" Mother lifts Jess out of the crib while asking, "Are you a happy girl?" Mother bends her face close to Jess while continuing to talk with her and then she kisses her several times. Later when she is being breast-fed, Jess loses the nipple, cries forcefully and angrily until mother replaces the nipple in her mouth.

In this observation, the mother shows how she is able to be more openly affectionate, putting her face close to Jess and kissing her. Mother seems to find it possible to reflect with Jess on her inner experiences, and by crying forcefully Jess ensures that mother attends to her displeasure when mother is not fully attentive during the breast-feeding. In this way, Jess facilitates mother being able to greet her distress and think about how a baby needs to be emotionally intimate with her mother, not just close to her nurturing breast. It is striking that mother can also bear to feel curious about Jess's distress and discomfort during the night. Likewise, when mother is dressing Jon, she feels as though he is her little friend with whom she is able to have a dialogue about the snow coming and later to share with him the pleasure of seeing the snow falling and covering everything in the garden.

Mother's behaviour with both Jess and Jon is now in marked contrast to when Jon was two and a half months, the same age as Jess is currently. When he was two and a half months, mother was leaving Jon to cry at night and talking about Jon in the third person rather than affectionately talking with him as a little baby with a mind and personality as she is now doing with Jess. Mother shows more attuned interactions and conversations with Jess, fostering Jess's belief that, when she cries to signal her need for her mother, her cries will be met. These seem to have resulted in Jess being a more emotionally engaging and responsive baby than Jon was at the same age. Also, the parents routinely laughed at Jon when he was suffering, but they no longer laugh at the children when they are distressed. It is obvious that the mother's capacity for *concave containment* has been enhanced by the emotionally supportive and thoughtful presence of the regularly visiting observer (S. Briggs, 1997b).

Nevertheless, Jon's emotional development remains a concern. He frequently switches on the television and glues himself to it. While he often "switches off his connections to the family", the family also worryingly forget about their connections to him. Jon's "being alone with grief" is hidden by his way of remaining isolated with his toy drill and toolbox and "living inside the television" in a sort of dissociative state. It is hard to comprehend how Jon feels about his baby sister Jess having a much more emotionally responsive mother than he had as an infant. Mother would shut off the baby-monitor for the whole night when he was crying. Perhaps Jon feels the benefit of mother's change to being a more communicative, friendly mother to him now. Certainly, Jon does not ever appear aggressive towards his baby sister, but one wonders if he has repressed jealous feelings brooding underneath his "big daddy pseudo-independent self".

As time progresses, mother is increasingly able to share with the observer her worries about Jon's emotional development and language delay. Because she is able to trust the receptivity of the observer, mother is also able to reflect more fully on the children and on her own difficult experiences as a child. In a wistful tone, mother describes, "My parents just let me cry at night. My mother wanted me to 'grow up' and took away my 'precious blanket' too early!" As mother becomes more reflective and open with the observer about her own emotional states and hostility to her own parents, she seems more able to access her love and to feel more affectionately attuned both to Jess and to Jon. As a direct result of mother's reflective responsiveness to Jess in her early infancy, Jess's psychological and language development continues to follow a very different trajectory from that of her brother.

Observation: Jess, three months, and Jon, twenty-six months

Mother is changing Jess's nappy on the couch. Jess is smiling at mother and sucking her own index finger. Mother is delighted with Jess, talking to her excitedly as she "gobbles her up", kisses her stomach, and comments on what a happy kind of personality Jess has. Mother also comments, "Jess is able to sleep much better during the night."

When mother goes to the door to greet a pizza delivery man, Jess looks anxious and afraid. She shortly begins to cry. Jess is comforted when mother returns. Mother says, "I try to calm Jess rather than letting her get too upset during the day since this allows her to settle down and sleep more easily at night."

Much of this time, Jon has been engrossed in watching a television programme and rolling a large metallic bulldozer toy around the living room. However, when mother starts feeding Jess, Jon goes to the cat and starts animatedly talking to him undecipherable words.

The observer is trying to be responsive to all three members of the family present and at a certain point she goes to Jon and talks with him about the cat while mother is breast-feeding Jess.

Mother is opening up and beginning to share her hostility regarding her own mother's misattunement to her during her own childhood. Mother is growing more responsive both to her own infantile feelings and also to her children's, but it is worrying that mother cannot become sufficiently intimate with the depth of Jon's emotional experiences and his need for her. This seems linked with Jon's emotions being hidden under his omnipotent attitude of, "I can take care of myself, I don't need you, mum". The observer tries to converse with Jon, although she can understand only a few of his responses to her. She is trying to both relate to Jon's present emotions and to demonstrate to mother Jon's need for a verbal, mind-to-mind interaction. During his conversation with the observer, Jon seems troubled by the dreary, rainy weather outside, which probably matches his own hidden tears.

Meanwhile, Jess seems securely attached to her mother and is thus more able to depend upon her mother's capacity to reflect upon her mental state, contain her otherwise overwhelming affects, and anticipate her psychological needs for reassurance, comfort, and support. Feeling consciously in touch with one's hurt and crying, when distressed, occurs when there is a secure attachment to a *concavely containing* caregiver. Trust in a caregiver occurs when the caregiver, usually the mother, will receive the baby's cries and mitigate their intensity through mindfulness (S. Briggs, 1997b). Jess has begun to *internalise* mother's increased emotional capacity for reflecting upon mental states. This means that Jess does not *massively deny* her distress, as Jon did, rather she cries and approaches her mother with her arms, hands, mouth, and eyes. This allows the crying infantile self to be consciously heard by the self and the parents. Normal language development is then likely to ensue.

The final observation visit

Acquarone (2004) describes a way of evaluating a mother's capacity to mother. In particular, she mentions the mother's ability to find relief, physically and/or verbally, for the baby's distress. She also cites the mother's ability to express her own emotional states of sadness, worry, anxiety, and happiness. In this final observation, one can see how far this mother and her two children have developed emotionally. We sense that the observer's compassionate comprehension of mother and her children, her silent interpretations, her modelling of a parent responding to a child's emotional experiences, have all led to a development of the mother and children's capacity to *concavely contain* emotions. Infant observation can provide the potential for mother and children to internalise the observer's containing functions. This is illustrated by an excerpt taken from the last weekly visit. After this visit, the observer reduces her visits to once a month as a way of gradually "weaning" herself from the family until Jon reaches the age of three.

Observation: Jess, six months, and Jon, twenty-nine months

> Mum apologises to the observer for how messy the house is. Both Jon, twenty-nine months, and Jess, six months, are sitting at the table. As mother goes into the kitchen, she asks Jon if he wants some raspberries and he responds clearly, "raspberries". Mother gives him the bowl. When mother asks Jon if he likes the raspberries, he responds, "yes".

The observer is aware that mother has been complaining about the mess in her house throughout the last year. It feels like she is spending more time being with her children and less time cleaning. Still we sense that "the mess" may be a reflection of all the different feeling states mother has to tolerate within herself as she opens herself up to painful emotional experiences in herself and in her two children. The observer has never seen Jon responding directly to mother's questions! She was amazed by his saying "raspberries", for it had never before been apparent that he was so verbally fluent.

> When Jon is finished with his raspberries, Mother hugs and kisses him. He smiles and squirms in her arms.

Mother is now more openly and more physically affectionate to Jon, but to some extent Jon is still protected by his omnipotent self, and it spoils the pleasure of their physical union. Mother seems to experience his ambivalence to her when he squirms during her physical intimacy with him.

> Jon then comes over to the observer and holds out two little cars, saying "cars". The observer talks to him about the two cars and when she finishes the conversation Jon sees her keys on the floor and picks them up saying "key car". The observer says, "Yes you are right". He holds out one of the keys and the observer explains that the key opens the hospital door. He picks out another one and shows the observer who says, "that key opens the car". He continues showing keys before picking up a large red metal key. He pushes the key into the wheel well of one toy car. He tries the key on several different cars. He then places the keys along the back of his neck, arching his back so they drop on to the floor. He repeatedly does this while laughing as the keys fall. Then he sees a play board with table legs, turns the table over and places one

> of the keys in each of the screw holes. The observer and mother talk to Jon about how the key doesn't turn the screws, so he will need a screwdriver.

This long conversation with the observer, which he is then able to extend to his mother shows how Jon wants to be the subject of mother's thoughtful reflection upon his experiences. He wants her to be intimate with his thoughts. The observer's presence provides an opportunity for a special play time in which both mother and the observer participate and reflect upon the significance of his play. He seems to intuit that the observer might understand some of the negativity provoked in him by mother's kisses and hugs. Much like in a dream, the car key play is used to dramatise Jon's experience of intimacy and separation. One can speculate on the various meanings of the play: 1) baby being joined to mummy–mouth and nipple; 2) perhaps he is talking about daddy getting inside mummy, baby getting inside mummy; 3) keys go with cars, so he is illustrating his cognitive development; 4) he has the "key", or power, to make things turn on and off. There is also a theme of "falling" represented by the keys being repeatedly dropped. Whatever the meaning of the key in the hole is, it is clear that Jon laughs when the keys are "being dropped". We sense that his ambivalence to mother is linked with feelings of being dropped: "dropped" in the isolated bedroom, crying alone at night, where his ambivalence and omnipotent defences increased; "dropped" by the presence of a new baby; and persecutorily "dropped" by his wish to have father and new baby drop away from mother, leaving Jon feeling that he will be "dropped" and punished for this wish.

> Mother is playing with Jess when Jon puts the keys down and flings himself sideways into the observer's lap, laughing and putting his arms around her neck briefly. The observer exclaims, "Oh, do I get a hug!" Jon then drops to all fours in front of her laughing. He gets up and runs back and forth between the hallway and living room making "uh, uh, uh" noises as he does this. Then he falls down next to the observer.

It feels as though Jon is splitting off his affection for mother and showing it all to the observer. Mother can be jealous, he has a new mother, a new girlfriend, just as she has a new baby! But then Jon becomes courageous enough to show his love and interest in having a space inside his mother's mind:

> Jon sees Jess on mother's lap and he tries to find space for himself sitting on the same leg. Mother says he isn't going to fit in and he can sit on her other leg. Jon takes the side of the board that Jess was playing with, turns it around and goes and sits on mother's leg. This means that both children can play with the buttons on "Jess' busy board". Mother says they have been learning the "abc song" together.
>
> Jess is playing with her favourite toy, a plastic Ninja turtle. She puts it in her mouth, bites it and gazes up at the observer and smiles at her when the observer says, "I want to see what you are doing." Jon finds a couple of coupons clipped together with a very large plastic clip

> and he brings them over to the observer, hugs her knees first, hears her say, "nice hug, Jon" and then he hands her the coupons and the observer talks about what they are for.

This is a very different boy from earlier observations! Jon no longer always evades the frustration of no one attending to him by turning away to inanimate objects and gluing himself to the television. Now he runs to the observer and hugs her. This is partially love for the observer's compassionate comprehension of his mind, and partially transference love, split-off from his relationship to his mother. He is able to keep hold of the frustration of feeling left out. Through play in the presence of the observer he is able to think of his conflictual emotional issues and create ways to find the good relationship with his loving mother, which he wants to have. He is a more hopeful boy. Now he has lessened his omnipotent protective mechanisms against psychic pain, for at last he feels he can be successful when he reaches out for an intimate relationship with a mothering person. Although his language is delayed, Jon wants to communicate through these prototype conversations, the basis of speech.

> Jon is engaged in symbolic play as he takes a box from a wooden cabinet and removes all the Star War videos from it. Then he tries to put his red car in the box. Mother says, "That is not going to fit", but it does.

Looking at this as symbolic play, we conjecture that Jon wants to be the only one inside mother's mental space, inside mother's body. All the rival babies, Jess, and daddy should all be removed. This phantasy becomes more apparent in the subsequent sequence:

> Jon then gets up and puts the box lid on his head and runs around the house excitedly. There is a sense that all the comprehending attentiveness which he has received from mother and the observer has made him elated. He runs around almost triumphantly with pleasure and then he drops the box in the entry hall by the door. He runs near the observer, points his finger in the direction of the door and says, "uh, uh". The observer questions, "Did you drop it by the door?"

There is a sense now that his play is about the shared experiences of being one with observer and mother and then losing them. Soon the observer will leave through the door. Jon is using play to elaborate upon being dropped behind the closed bedroom door without anybody coming to retrieve him, dropped by his mother and dad going to work, dropped by the observer going out of the door. Now, however, Jon feels "a mother figure" is more securely present both internally and externally to get to know the emotional experiences of his hidden infantile self. As a result of this internalisation of a reflective mother/observer, Jon has developed the internal mental capacity to symbolise, to attempt to work through his jealousy and his experiences of the absence of a fully attuned, fully present mother in his earliest infancy. But then jealous rage about sharing looms before him:

> Jon sees Jess playing with a small plastic lawnmower. He takes it from her and begins to strike it against the top of the busy board. Mother firmly says, "No, Jon, we don't want Jess or me

> or Jon to get hurt." She takes the lawnmower away from him. Jon collapses on the floor with his face pressed into the carpet. Mother reassures him that he can play with the lawnmower if he can be gentle. He retrieves the lawnmower and mother straddles Jess on top of him saying, "She wants to see you!" Jess tries to put his tee-shirt in her mouth, she rolls around so this isn't possible. Mother picks Jess up and says, "We are going to get you!" while Jon runs away squealing and giggling. All three, mother, Jess and Jon are playing the game of finding and losing mother, being in a rage with mother, mother turning into "the big monster" coming after Jon.

Mother now seems to be able to keep both children simultaneously in her mind as she joins their play. It seems an experience shared by the two children, but also by mother. It is the childhood nightmare of rage towards mother, mother turning into a nightmare monster through the rage, then the nightmare monster, the bad object, chasing and frightening the infantile self.

> Jon is still running back and forth when mother decides to nurse Jess. Jon interrupts this by bringing over a couple of cars and placing them on the couch next to his mother.

Jon *is* competing to be the baby with access to the two breasts, but he is doing this symbolically. At least he feels mummy should be nursing two babies simultaneously. There is relief present in the observer, for Jon has been successful in drilling his way into mother's mind, and this helps his mother to keep both children in mind. The theme of departures is in the air for the whole family because the observer's weekly visits are about to stop. As the observer is about to leave mother says, "Drive safely". We wonder whether this shows both her dependence on the observer for being reliably present for twenty-nine months, and also her rage about separation at the impending end of the visits. The ending of the infant observation visits may reawaken internalised fears of being "dropped" and abandoned by her own mother, and also of losing her, partly because of her infantile rage and need.

Conclusion

Many factors may have influenced the mother–baby relationship in these observations. These include mother's better identification with a girl baby, the other inherited characteristics of each baby, the birth order position of each child in the family, mother's own sibling relationships and her other internalised family relationships, mother's experience in parenting, and the capacity to bear emotions in the "supportive cradle" of the marital relationship and extended family. Alongside these variables, there can be a spiralling interaction of mother and her children's personalities that can influence a mother–baby interaction to "get better" or "to become more difficult".

The parents' capacities to mentally represent their childhood experiences correlate with infants' security of attachment. If the parents used primitive mechanisms of defence such as splitting, projecting, and massive denial in relation to their own emotional experiences, this would impede the parents from being sensitively understanding of their infant's "thinking, feeling, wishing, believing, wanting, desiring". If the parents are not able to provide this for the infant, he becomes insecurely attached and relies on his own primitive mechanisms of defence such as massive denial. This use of massive denial ultimately constrains the child's capacity to use his or her own potential to reflect on mental states and develop emotionally and cognitively. The parents' willingness to contemplate their own deep experience and reflect upon the child's emotional experience provides the bridge to attachment security, to a sense that there is "expectable and good-enough mothering" (Fonagy, 1993).

In the early observations, the mother was suffering from depression, for which she was taking anti-depressants. She had chosen a husband who thought thinking about dreams was ridiculous. She might have chosen a husband with defences similar to a kind of "autistic capsule" within her, in which her own longings, her own grief, remained enclosed. This meant mother frequently felt she was "living with her grief alone".

Over a period of reliable weekly visits for twenty-nine months, the observer's compassionate comprehension created an emotional space for the mother. Although the mother did not initially put into words some of her experiences, we felt she used what Fraiberg calls *re-enactment* in the observational hours, much like a young child playing out anxieties and working them through. For example, mother showed Jon to the observer saying, "I want you to see just how much he protests." We sense that mother needed the observer to see *re-enactments* of "a baby feeling frightened, enraged and angry with an uncaring, inattentive mother". The observer's compassionate comprehension functioned as a silent interpretation and acceptance, which relieved some of the mother's buried grief and rage. In this way, the mother was enabled to internalise a compassionately comprehending observer. As a result, mother used this emotional space to develop an increased reflective capacity regarding her own experience of mothering the children. She also became increasingly able to identify with her children's states of mind. In addition, the observer's presence allowed a transformation to occur: Jon was able to begin to courageously release himself from his autistic-like protections against grief, find the observer, reach out to her, and find her as a trustworthy, understanding, a secure object. When he had begun to form an internal picture of a securely present observer, he was able to initiate reaching out again, like in infancy, to his mother who was now not so insulated by a "thick skin" against her own pain. Her "buried grief" had resurrected itself at the time of her pregnancy with Jon. As Fraiberg (1982) said, mother had been frightened of her baby's "painful tears" mirroring her own. Despite this progress, Jon's emotional, physical, and cognitive developmental delays are a source of concern. Jon's "being with grief alone" occurred through a series of protective mechanisms which then interfered with his emotional and cognitive development and his physical health. Through the transformational process during the twenty-nine months of the observations, Jon's "being with grief alone" was transformed into sharing his pains and joys with the observer and with his mother.

This chapter has attempted to illustrate how the observer's weekly role of observing with compassionate comprehension and using an observation seminar to reflect on participant observations may have played a profound and significant therapeutic role in this family, especially for mother and her two children. This chapter also emphasises that, when trying to understand a child's mind, it is important to look carefully at the child's preverbal gestures while recalling Giorgio Morandi's statement "To achieve understanding, it is necessary not to see many things, but to look hard at what you do see" (Kimmelman, 2004).

CHAPTER SIX

Evolving patterns of parental containment of a young child communicating through not eating or speaking

Jeanne Magagna

The development of symbolic functioning, the development of language, and the capacity for play are all influenced by the way in which the child's caregivers, usually the parents, respond to the child's needs. Obviously the young child's way of interacting with the parents influences the arousal of tender feelings in them, and elicits their benign and attentive care-giving responses. My philosophy incorporates the notion that parental work should accompany *all individual therapeutic work* with a child. Parents are with a young child at least 17 hours daily and potentially can be very well placed to effect deeper and more lasting transformation in the child's personality. For this reason, it is important that they be helped to do so via family therapy or parental therapy, accompanying individual psychotherapy, and perhaps speech therapy for the child. This chapter describes family and parental psychotherapy when a child has difficulty with both speaking and eating. (Feeding/eating difficulties often accompany difficulties in speaking.) I shall examine three types of parental containment of a child's anxieties and show how psychotherapy can facilitate a transition to a type of parental containment that aids the development of the young child's psychological capacities to speak and to eat. This therapy represents the type of therapy that can accompany individual child psychotherapy in the presence of the mother, as described in Chapter Seven.

Stephen Briggs (1997) has described three different ways in which parents might relate to emotions of their young child. These include *convex containment, flat containment and concave containment.* This chapter will explore a way of working within family therapy to enable parental concave containment involving them in being more attentively observant and more appropriately and empathically responsive to their son's needs.

First, there will be a brief history followed by a description of three types of parental containment of the young child and how various forms of containment were present during different phases of therapy. This will be followed by illustrations of how parental concave containment of anxiety enabled non-speaking, non-eating Sam to lessen his defences against anxiety and build an emotional bridge for expressing a kaleidoscope of emotions to his parents.

Brief history

Sam was three years old when he was referred because there was a developmental language delay with autistic features, he had a very restricted nutritional intake and was underweight, being 80 per cent weight/height compared to the normal population his age. His parents were very angry about the medical confusion regarding his physical condition when he was *in utero*. An ultrasound scan suggested that he might be mentally handicapped and the parents were asked to consider an abortion. After much grieving, the parents made the decision to abort the fetus, but a week later, when they met the doctors, the doctors suggested that they had made a mistake regarding the severity of the damage and indicated that the parents should go ahead and have the baby. The parents were shocked by this advice, particularly since after much grieving they had decided on an abortion, but they followed the doctors' advice and the pregnancy continued. At birth Sam's heart stopped beating briefly. He became epileptic from the time of his weaning at six weeks. There were no siblings.

Both parents were depressed and angry about the doctors' advice to keep the fetus. Their family doctor had prescribed anti-depressants in separate consultations with each of them. The parents expressed blame towards the doctors, and ambivalence towards Sam who was delayed in language development, had autistic features, epilepsy, difficulty in eating, and failure to thrive.

Treatment

An assessment was made and a written assessment was sent to the parents and professionals involved. The assessment was one day long and involved a physical examination, including a weight/height percentile, an observation of the parent/child relationship including parent-child interactions occurring during a feeding experience, a complete developmental history from birth onwards, a family tree, family history, including psychological and physical health of all family members, the story of Sam from conception, through pregnancy, delivery and the child's relationship with the parents from conception to the present time. There was also an assessment of the couple's relationship with each other, to Sam and to the extended network. Included in this assessment was a risk assessment looking at whether or not Sam was being sufficiently looked after to be considered safe when living with his family and whether or not the family required additional support besides the weekly family therapy sessions alternating with couple therapy sessions (with accompanying play therapy sessions for Sam).

A treatment plan was then made stating that weekly family/couple psychotherapy sessions would be offered and six weekly progress reports and liaison with other professionals would be part of this. A letter was written to the parents and copied to the professionals describing the assessment and treatment plan. Sam's weekly hospital weight results in terms of weight/height percentiles and actual weight would be given to the parents and therapists since he needed to gain weight.

Three evolving phases of parental containment of anxiety

Phase one: convex containment

Obviously, we did not see the process of mother-child interaction leading up to three-year-old Sam's rejection of his mother's food. During the assessment, I was aware that the interaction which we saw between Sam and his parents was distorted by the very heightened anxiety in the parents due to Sam's not eating. Sam's failure to connect with them emotionally and to develop language skills were both deeply worrying and a source of their ambivalence, guilt, and depression. During the assessment phase, the intense feelings and heightened anxiety in the parents led to *convex containment* of Sam's anxiety. Characteristic of *convex containment* is excessive parental control, intrusion, and hostility bombarding the parents' interactions, as seen below:

> *Sam, three years old*
>
> Part of the assessment phase involved the parents in being asked to feed Sam. The more they approached him with food, the more he withdrew to the furthest corner of the room. As the fifteen-minute observation period lengthened, the parents felt so guilty that they had not been able to feed their son, so worried about being judged and being blamed, that they intruded upon their son with increasingly anxious, demanding requests that he eat. Sam's gaze avoidance, involving his not looking at the parent speaking to him, was painful to witness. At times, as he faced the corner, his body would become limp and he seemed to become *dissociated*, moving away from any perception of his bombardment by parental mental discomfort.
>
> As the parents unsuccessfully attempted to feed Sam, they spoke in a persecuted way to us, saying, "We have tried everything to get Sam to eat including coaxing, cajoling, bargaining, distracting, starving him for a day thinking he would get hungry, forcing food down his throat. Nothing works!"

Sam's response is similar to the "no-entry responses" described by Gianna Williams (1997b). Gaze avoidance, turning the head away from the parents, and closing the mouth are linked with the child's feeling that he is the receptacle of something bad emanating from the parents alongside the intruding food. Sam "cut his parents out" emotionally by not speaking and not eating.

When the weekly family therapy sessions began, I left toys for Sam in the centre of the room. A psychology trainee attentively observed his play and interacted with him at times, while I listened empathically to whatever the parents wished to spontaneously tell me about the difficulties that they and Sam were experiencing. I felt "bored into" by very painful stories of mother's postnatal depression, from which she had not fully recovered; by father's "difficult family life" that he wanted me to know was horribly challenging, but which he didn't want to talk about. Alongside this was the parents' increasingly potent fury with the hospital doctors who advised them to go ahead and have their handicapped son.

Under their fury about "the handicap" seemed to be an accompanying severe anxiety that Sam might die in the regular nightly epileptic episodes. Guilt about destructive feelings to their son led the couple to be defensively over-protective and over-solicitous. One of them slept in Sam's bed every night for fear he would die in one of the epileptic episodes. There was virtually no separateness between the parents and their child. They said, "We buy him everything he wants and do everything he wants us to do for him." Father spent most time at home playing with his son. Sam seemed the receptacle for all the parents' projected needy, vulnerable, damaged, depressed selves. Massive confusion between self and other was enhanced by intrusive feeding and clinging covering unconscious hatred to Sam. There was a split in the family relationships in that an abundance of consciously felt love was directed towards the damaged child while conscious conflict and anger were located in the couple's relationship. Father complained about mother's inadequacies as a mother and mother complained about father's attentiveness to Sam and neglect of her basic needs for physical help and emotional support and understanding.

The first stage of treatment was to allow the parents to "intrude into us" pouring into us all their anger, their hatred … to allow ourselves to become the container into which all sorts of repressed and unacceptable feelings from both the parents and Sam could be encouraged to flow. We accepted how awful the couple and Sam felt. We were part of a long line of specialists involved, and that meant we should keep in mind Betty Joseph's (1985) concept of the "total transference": we accepted their anger with the various professionals who each had looked at separate aspects of the child—the epileptic part, the not-eating part, the language developmental delay part, the depressed baby-part of the parents. A separate doctor for each separate symptom. No one had really fully understood either their child, Sam, or them!

In the early phase of treatment in which one sees intrusive parenting and a child trying to evade the projections of emotions and food, the therapist needs to become "the toilet-breasts" (Meltzer, 1967). As therapists, we are to replace their child, Sam, as the receptacles of unwanted projected parts of the parents. It would be simple if the parents simply complained verbally to directly to us, but many of the unwanted parts of the parents came out through criticism of professionals and projection into us of their despair, inadequacy, ineffectualness and even feelings of being possibly detrimental to Sam's progress.

Then the parents said to us:

> "Nothing has changed since we last met. Sam hasn't gained any weight. The advice to leave food available around for simply touching it, feeling its texture, looking at it, is useless. He won't even look at new foods!"

It is at this moment that we are particularly aware of our countertransference experiences. We can't simply pay attention to the details of Sam's restricted diet. In the countertransference, we are to feel the parent's experiences that are so hard to bear: We need to feel very inadequate, worthless, criticised for being "no good" and bear the guilt which ensues from feeling "a no-good parent". Little progress in therapy will ensue unless we can bear these weighty projections. Simultaneously, we are aware that the parents are still feeling very persecuted and guilty and scrutinising our every comment in order to find any implied criticisms of them. Progress in mitigation of the severity of the family's internal critic, the superego, occurs through our empathically understanding—without echoing the criticism of this internal critic. This is a difficult task, for it means that we have to become more deeply identified with the parents' psychic pain while at the same time fully identifying with Sam's emotional needs and the risk factors present in his family life.

During this first phase of the treatment, it seemed crucial to be emotionally present to receive and contain the parent's distress, their baby-selves. We felt that only when the adult-parental selves of the parents was not overwhelmed with unwanted feelings would the couple have sufficiently undistorted mental space for attentive attunement to Sam.

Phase two: the therapists' increasing awareness of "flat containment"

Flat containment (Briggs, 1997) exists when the parents hold themselves unavailable for the projections and communications of the child. The sequence may also involve father not receiving distress of mother, mother feeling unsupported and then offering the child a daily dose of *flat containment*. In *flat containment*, there is no space in the mother or father's minds to think about the child. Misunderstanding or lacking understanding of what the baby really wants or feels when in distress, the mother or father feeds the child to provide physical nourishment. In this situation, the child may take in the food, giving up control of the mouth rather than confronting the mother or father; however, the child may fail to put on weight. This is known as *failure to thrive*, where the body does not secrete the hormone necessary for growth or digest the food in a way that food can be assimilated as a source of nourishment to the body cells. The failure to grow physically, to translate food into muscle, is mirrored by an absence of a loving, protective internalised parent.

What one sometimes sees in the development of a child receiving an abundance of flat unattuned containment is a turning to achievement, mechanically drinking the milk, eating, holding onto one's own protective mechanisms like rotating of the wrists, fiddling with hair. Accompanying this is an underlying depression and lack of self-esteem. The mother and father may miss signals of distress because, instead of remaining attached to the parents, the child is attached to adhesive mechanisms involving control rather than concave containment *of* emotions. So, for example, repetitive play, rituals, non-stop rotating of wrists, or running, or even turning to rote learning as a way of soothing oneself can all be used in instances where there is a predominance of flat parental containment of the child. Flat containment also included avoiding the seriousness of Sam's lack of development of symbol formation evident in his repetitious, unimaginative play and in his delayed language development. Denying that Sam was becoming seriously underweight was part of the parents' flat containment. Lack of feeding of Sam occurred at times because the parents were trying to avoid a conflict with him which would stir up too many anxieties in both Sam and his parents. Lack of language development and Sam's serious low weight were denied and brought to the attention of the parents through the intervention of the neuropsychiatrist treating his epilepsy. To avoid evoking father's criticism of mother's mothering, at times the couple had resorted to unconscious denial of both Sam's severe developmental language delay and his feeding difficulties.

Phase one, in which we accepted the projections of the parents, is an essential phase of therapy, for it has often previously been an emotional necessity for the parents to split-off and project their infantile feelings into their child. They have done this because their infantile feelings were too overwhelming and they had no emotional equipment other than *splitting and projecting* to deal with them. Once some of the parents' traumatic feelings are accepted, thought about and understood by us, the couple could initiate the process of *internalising* perceptive, emotionally containing therapists. This internalisation of containing therapists frees some of their emotionally perceptive selves to look more closely at their interaction with their child and thus transform their *flat containment* into *concave containment.* According to Stephen Briggs's *Growth and Risk in Infancy* (1997), *parental concave containment* promotes the child's psychological development, including the development of symbol formation, as described by Alex Dubinsky in Chapter Four. The development of the child's wish to relate to the parents through talking accompanies these developments.

A child speaks to the parents when the child is developmentally ready and emotionally willing to do so. Asking the child to say something in a family situation filled with unconscious hostility can result in the child feeling "close-mouthed" out of anger at being controlled. Likewise, it is difficult for a child in family situation permeated with unconscious hostility to be willing to eat. I should explain that the family was referred to a team specialising in eating disorders and hence there was by necessity a focus on the symptom of Sam's not eating as well as a focus on the family difficulties which had not been addressed in the various other specialist clinics.

Here is an example from a family session of how we tried to help the parents move from *flat containment* of Sam's experiences to attentively observing, trying to step into Sam's shoes and imagine what he felt and try to become more in touch with their emotional responses to his behaviour:

> Sam rejected every attempt by his parents to feed him and also he rejected their insistent requests that he eat by himself. The parents and we, the therapists, observed that at present Sam seemed to feel that he had to take care of himself, he *had to be* independent of his parents when eating, even though he was just three. I silently wondered if his weaning at six weeks, accompanied by the beginning of his epilepsy, represented a basic trauma that he overcame through *omnipotent control* unconsciously involving a thought: "I will feed myself, I will never again be a helpless child, depending on others for food!"
>
> We discussed ways in which Sam could feel he had some choice, some control over the timing of his eating and the way in which he ate. (This isn't ideal as a permanent solution, but it represents our attempt to work *with* Sam's defence of *omnipotent control* rather than initially battling *against* it.) After some consideration of the noon meal during the family sessions, the parents decided to give Sam a little red plastic school box with salty cheese nibbles, chocolate pieces and tiny marmite sandwiches. Also in his lunch box was a Ribena drink in a thermos bottle with a hard small aperture through which he could drink his juice. Sam could now spontaneously feed himself! At 12 o'clock when the sessions began he would be given his little red container, it would be opened and he was told he could eat now. Every fortnight after about 10 minutes he would be reminded that after he ate he would go to the play specialist.

> Every fortnight at 12:15 he would go to see the play specialist for 45 minutes while I would meet fortnightly with the couple alone.
>
> Sam began to freely choose and eat some salty foods. Mother would make exactly the same salty foods and chocolate bar available every day. Mother observed that after a few weeks Sam would stop eating for a few days. It felt to me that Sam's repetitious pattern of eating and stopping eating recreated the traumatic weaning experience of the breast suddenly disappearing at six weeks. The parents would then panic because there was no other type of food that Sam would eat. They again tried out a lot of different foods until he discovered another food he liked such as houmous and then he would have that daily in his sandwich until he tired of it. Although Sam was placating the parents by eating, Mother and Father felt as though they were simply going through the motions of providing food. The atmosphere felt flat in the room and I experienced myself feeling that the couple were not really understanding what Sam felt or what Sam needed emotionally, they were just feeding him.

There seemed to be an underlying atmosphere of sadness, detachment and distress, with some tension which I felt might suggest repressed anger. Sam looked waif-like, too small, too short, sullen and pasty-white in complexion although he was eating a bit more. He did not have language, but there we felt some urgency to prevent hospitalisation by helping him to eat while helping his parents to closely observe his "communication without words" and think about underlying familial issues. Pondering on the atmosphere in the session I was reminded of Coleridge's poem *Ode to Dejection* (Coleridge, 1802, p. 575) in which he describes an "unimpassioned grief" that cannot be put into sighs or tears or words. This grief "without a pang" lives unexpressed, locked within the dark chambers of the self. Underneath the conversation about life at home with Sam and helping Sam to eat was a pervasive grief that had no outlet in words or tears. Father kept saying he wanted support, but he had no capacity or willingness to express his feelings of being vulnerable, frightened, angry, deprived, and needy in words that could be understood. Instead, he had built up massive debts buying things for himself, Sam and his wife. Mother's eyes drooped, her mood was sad and heavy, but she kept saying in a somewhat strained voice that she had to "live for the moment", she couldn't think of the past, couldn't think of big issues, couldn't think of the future, couldn't think of what she wanted from her husband. Stephen Briggs (1997) writes that flat containment exists when the parents hold themselves unavailable for the projections and communications of the child. The couple offered flat containment for Sam, but this was linked with their history of deprivation and trauma resulting in their lack of mentalizing capacities prompting only flat containment for their own inner experience, "the child within" and for each other.

After four months of weekly family/couple meetings, we felt a little optimistic that at least some progress in Sam's eating was being made and a therapeutic alliance with the parents was gradually being established; however, just at this time, our optimism was somewhat dashed when the psychology trainee, who observed and interacted with Sam in the sessions, announced her pregnancy and permanently ended her placement with us. Simultaneously I also had a regularly scheduled and previously discussed two-week Christmas break. The sudden departure of the psychologist and my absence felt like an abrupt weaning, like Sam's.

The parents returned after the two week separation saying that "they just had to stop worrying for a while and let Sam do what he wanted." There was just too much tension over food, the parents passively denied the need for Sam to eat more. Father complained that mother was with Sam all day and she should do something about the eating ... Mother said, "I give up. Although he is a good father when he is home, he expects too much of me, expects me to do all the housework and all the food shopping while he is away from the home."

The presence of loss was very powerful: The parents' early experiences of losing the first baby through a miscarriage and suddenly losing the pregnant trainee psychologist, accompanied at the same time by my two week break, had stirred up hostility to the therapists. During the separation, the parents' hostility felt towards the absent therapists was brought into the couple's relationship, and they began severely criticising one another. Moreover, although identification with the good containing therapists had fostered the parents' attentive care of Sam, now they were left with internalised attacked, bad therapists who let them down. The internalised therapists had turned bad partly through their going away but also through their goodness being spoiled by the parents' hostility regarding their absence. Identifying with these uncaring, absent therapists, the parents had "given up" on working as a couple together and had given up on helping Sam. He was losing weight!

Now, I began to raise the transference issues: I described to the parents how the trainee psychologist and I had let the family down. We hadn't provided enough sustenance for them to manage during the break from us. Instead of perpetuating their criticism of one another by focusing on their not adequately helping Sam (who was also experiencing our absence), I talked about their identifying with my not giving them enough, therefore, not being able to give Sam enough care and food. Somehow my understanding their sense of loss of support, their feeling that we had let them down, and their anger towards us changed the relationship between the parents and me. They felt I was stronger, more understanding of their deep rage, linked with being abused and deprived, that interfered with their functioning as a parental couple cradling Sam's emotional experiences.

We became closer and they talked with more feeling and detail about their extremely abusive and deprived childhood experiences, experiences which they had previously described in a somewhat distant, detached, brief way. The notion of "an absent mother" elicited the father, Peter's, story about his childhood that he had previously "not wanted to go into". I learned that Peter's two younger brothers had regularly slept in his room to avoid the systematic sexual abuse from their father. When Peter was about to leave home at age 16, he had to virtually force his mother to leave his own father in order that the younger boys would be protected. Peter, described his father as being a "brutal, military commander type of man" who lined the boys up, hit them and beat Peter. Peter's wife, Sarah, talked about how her family looked better on the surface, but her mother had stopped helping her out with Sam and this was a source of her great anger and sadness. It is important to note that parent-child relationships are strongly influenced by the relationship history of not only oneself, but also by the relationship history of the other parent (Dunn, Davies, O'Connor, & Sturgen, 2000). It became apparent that the parents lacked the necessary past and present external familial support required to meet the heavy demands of their difficult family life.

Thus, I became "a partner in their sorrow's mysteries" (Keats, 1820). Now, it was not only Sam, who in eating felt he took in the hostility and depression in the family atmosphere... now my soul could "taste the sadness" of the family (Keats, ibid). But I do not believe that this would have been possible if I had not worked with the process between the parents and me... Directly discussing my unavailability to them, my working on the transference relationship to me, the "unavailable mother", was the secret to deepening the intimacy within the therapeutic relationship. Once the parents' hostility to uncaring parental figures was unleashed in the transference, a deeper dialogue about their internalised and external parental figures had ensued between us. Now that the parents felt more open and verbal about their own emotional experience, there arose the possibility of reintegrating aspects of themselves and providing more concave containment of Sam's difficulties.

Phase three: concave containment

The *concave containment phase* is marked by more parent-child interactions which promote the child's development of symbolic functioning, the capacity to think and to speak about his experiences (Briggs, 1997). Anne Alvarez (2002, p. 242) suggests that the child's capacity to think and speak is promoted by good maternal functions which include the parents' "willingness to enliven, to seek out the child and when the child is depressed to reclaim him; their eagerness to return to the child after absence, and their ability to receive pleasure and delight from the child, to permit reparation, to forgive the child."

Therapeutic work is necessary to establish within the couple a capacity to mediate and modulate Sam's extreme communications, make sense of his experiences through this attention and give names to the emotional experiences that are otherwise unknown to him. This therapeutic relating to Sam is both mediating and integrating. Because the parents hold themselves available for their child, as it were, to "put into them" through what Bion (1959) calls normal projective identification, it follows that the parents become concave containers for their son.

The development of parents' capacity for concave containment is described beautifully by Daws (1989) book entitled *Through the Night*. Daws describes how the parents' childhood experiences are internalised and affect the way they look after their own children. For this reason, it is essential that the therapist listen carefully to the parents' accounts of their own experiences as children in order to help them understand some of the problems with their own child. Parents need to listen to themselves, to find in their relationship with their young child or in their own personal history, indications of solutions to their difficulties with their child. When this occurs the child internalises a couple bringing relief and sustenance and has both self-esteem and vitality in which to explore relationships and learn about the world surrounding him. Concave containment of Sam's anxieties, not only in relation to food but also in relation to all aspects of his life, enabled him to resume eating and develop physically and emotionally. The turning point in the treatment was when I could give names to the emotional experiences in "the hurt and hostile child" within the parents and give names to feelings in the transference of my representing "the unavailable mother". The key to my work is supporting the parents in listening to each other, thinking about each other's emotional experiences, helping them carefully observe their interactions and emotional experiences in being with Sam, discuss together solutions to their conflicts with Sam, not only in relation to his stopping eating for long periods and his restrictive eating, but in relation to all aspects of their family life (Dartington & Magagna, 1994). Here is such an observation:

> Sam avoided any direct intrusion from the parents while eating. He turned his back on his mother while eating and did not want food if his parents drew attention to it, looked at him or looked at his food. He still liked to eat, in his own time, through his own independent approach to food that was left available to him on a table, rather than offered to him by the parents. If frustrated by his parents, Sam pulled his own hair out. He held onto and showed affection mainly to a stuffed animal whom he treated like a loved baby. It was a Cocker Spaniel called "Danny" by the parents.

Through the nine months of work, Sam has begun spontaneously speaking some words to the parents and me. He does not yet utter complete sentences, but the gist of what he is saying is made clear through his increased use of facial expressions and accompanying gestures including greater eye contact with both his parents and objects to which he is referring. Sam seems more securely attached to his parents; however, I discover that because Sam cries when they leave him with someone to go out, they usually sneak away. I realise that I am having to help the parents wean themselves from "expedient solutions" to helping Sam work through the difficulties of separating from them. Part of helping the parents develop concave containment involved working through father's negative identification: he did not want to be the "cruel military commander enforcing rules" like his father. We embarked on a lot of discussion on the value of overt parental limits as necessary and helpful to Sam learning to regulate his feelings through thinking rather than being dominated by their intensity. When the parents began therapy Sam's cries and wishes dominated their behaviour for they thought obeying him was being loving to him, although he was only three!

Some specific factors helpful to the development of concave parental containment

Observing and attuning to the child's ways

During the first phase of therapy, we encouraged the parents to observe Sam's eating behaviour and note his difficulty in approaching food, unless he felt eating was completely under his control. We suggested following his rhythm, but trying to ensure that they would provide food high in calories so that he would have sufficient energy and gain weight. We also helped them think together about how to arrange the eating so that it followed Sam's preferences, while gradually adding variety along the same tastes of food that Sam liked.

Bearing distress, preparing for events, providing comfort, story-telling

We also focused on another issue which was preparing Sam for separations, particularly at night, but also when the couple went out together on different day-time occasions. We shared the notion that preparing Sam for a difficult experience of separation and accepting his distress was important. It was also more difficult for the parents who would rather sneak away or simply cuddle him all night. Sam's frustration of having the two parents together in bed while he was left on his own was extremely fraught, but the parent–child interactions were saturated with father's childhood anxiety that children alone were at risk of being abused. Part of Sam's anxiety about being alone was also that he was left with all sorts of undigested emotional traumas which seemed to surface in epileptic episodes at night. Initially, the parents' fear of his dying, linked with their unconscious hostility, pressurised them to sleep with him. They were given time alone, without Sam, to describe how angry and sad they were to have this child who disappointed them in so many ways. Gradually, separation between the parents and Sam became possible at night. We suggested that activities promoting Sam's capacity to mentalize, to think about his emotional experiences during the day, would lessen the intensity of his nightmarish experiences during the night. With my prompting father was particularly adept at creating little evening bedtime stories, describing Sam's different experiences of love, dislike, curiosity, anger and fear. The parents had never had stories told to them as children and I sensed that the process of creating and sharing these stories with Sam was somehow also healing for father as he identified with Sam's anxieties. As an unprotected child, father had lived in terror of his own father's abuse.

During the sessions, we observed Sam closely and tried to work on ways of giving a running commentary to Sam on what he was doing and perhaps feeling during a session. I then suggested that at home father and mother have a running one-way dialogue with Sam, tentatively describing how Sam was feeling, much as parents might do with the non-verbal communications of a baby. The parents hadn't had this experience as children, so, once again, they were on new ground, but somehow they felt stimulated by the challenge of developing more intimacy with Sam who did not speak to them. Before they didn't talk much to Sam, for they felt they would simply be asking Sam questions which would receive no answer. Now they realised they could use Sam's gestures, facial expressions, and activities as signs of what he was wanting to express to them and himself. The gate to a new form of intimate communication was now open to them!

In the session, as the parents and I shared attentively observing Sam with a running commentary, we became aware of Sam's fear of moving objects such as the curtains blowing, a mobile on the ceiling moving, or a telephone light blinking. Sam seemed an extremely sensitive child, who seemed traumatised by his hypervigilant awareness. Any movement or change signalled potential danger for him. I helped the parents create some "transitional security" for Sam by making story books with photos of Sam and his stuffed toy, "Danny". They were to tell stories about the puppy "Danny" and Sam in the pictures. This was a book designed to emanate the message: "We are thinking of you Sam, even when we are not present." Sam could have the photo-books made by the parents in bed with him at night. These concrete parental activities provided encouragement to the parents to become more observant and identified with the ways Sam experienced his days.

Finding ways of expressing rather than evading conflicts

I asked the parents to talk together to think of possible meanings of Sam's activity in the therapy room or in an activity at home they described. They were to find ways to work together through a difficulty with him. In doing this, I was fostering the notion that it was helpful for Sam to witness their talking together, rather than withdrawing, when they had differences. One issue they confronted was the question of how Sam could deal with negative experiences besides by pulling his curly dark hair out. The parents devised some methods and then I encouraged them to help Sam practice these methods and then use them when required. They helped him to play games which included toppling objects, tearing paper, shouting "hurt" or "cross", stamping his feet, banging on pots, shouting "away" to a playmate when he was being annoyed by him instead of pulling his hair out. Simultaneously I continuously looked with parents at what annoyed them and how they expressed conflicts with each other and significant others, including me.

Underlining and integrating parents' strengths within the therapeutic work

Research has shown how much parents' progress when not only their anxieties are understood, but also their genuine strengths are noticed, underlined and supported as essential parts of the therapeutic work with their child. Research has also indicated that parents feel letters after emotive therapy sessions are one of the most helpful aspects of their contacts with professionals. I wrote a letter to the parents after each fortnightly family therapy session which included Sam. My letters included detailed observations of Sam's interaction with everyone in the therapy room. In them, I specifically noted the parents' approaches to Sam which felt helpful to him and commented on his response to feeling deeply understood and helped by their efforts.

While in the sessions, Sam started spontaneously adding a verb and noun together, making half-way sentences describing his dog, "Danny's" experiences: "bumped head" and "sad, no Sam". The parents were thrilled, for it seemed that Sam had internalised their way of receiving and thinking about his feelings, and he was now doing the same verbally for his dog, "Danny"! In fact, we subsequently realised that Sam localised his own feelings in his dog "Danny" and was able to begin giving his feelings names if they were located in "Danny", for this created less of a sense of vulnerability than locating intense feelings in himself. All this occurred spontaneously without the speech therapy which we had contemplated if Sam did not begin speaking once a deeper, more loving, more attuned emotional bridge to him was built by the parents.

Promoting the notion that intimately understanding the child promotes loving feelings

As the parents described situations which had been difficult for Sam, I used little boy dolls or animals to re-enact the scene for him. I talked using the first person, as the doll, talking about how "the Sam doll" or some other doll might feel. For example, I talked in first person about the Sam doll having a very sore mouth, not liking mummy being away to visit her friend, not liking mummy being with others. Following this, Sam, for the first time in a family therapy session, went into his mum's arms and curled up like a little baby. During this moment, I talked about how he wanted to be mummy's little baby, how difficult it was to have mummy having friends outside the home and also going to work.

Concavely containing marital conflicts and the couple's individual needs

Working together as parents for Sam at times helped the couple to heal some of their marital conflicts. However, as the worry about Sam's problems diminished, I sensed that the couple accurately perceived that Sam was receiving more as a child from them than they had received from their own parents or from each other. Perhaps as a result, without my asking questions, gradually the couple trusted me sufficiently to discover ways of discussing marital conflicts and developing more intimacy. Painful aspects of their past and current personal depression had prompted the family doctor to give each of them anti-depressants. Meeting Sam's emotional needs was a demanding responsibility for them when they had received impoverished parenting themselves. The couple's neediness and resulting hostility to one another meant that neither of them allowed the other to go out separately or lie-in on the weekend.

There seemed to be a split within the family process, with love going to Sam as their lonely, vulnerable selves were projected into him, while the hostility got located in the interaction between the couple. This hostility to each other probably contained unworked through hostility to their depriving internal parental figures. It still felt safer to show love to Sam, to prevent suffering in Sam, to stay with Sam late into the night rather than work through developing more intimacy with one another. Sam was having a better life, gaining weight, developing language, now they wanted more for their lives! The work with the couple needed more time but they were now going to participate in therapy locally and travel a much shorter distance to find more support for themselves. Our specialist hospital service for children was limited in terms of the amount of time it could offer them.

Summary

Through supporting the parents in sharing their worries we have facilitated their offering Sam concave containment rather than flat containment. By concave containment, I am implying that the couple are beginning to face directly and bear Sam's distress and think about it. Sam, in response to their concave containment of his anxiety and richer attunement to his emotional needs, is growing physically and developing the capacity to put his feelings into words. In our nine months of therapy, Sam grew six centimetres and moved from a weight for height percentile of eighty per cent to a weight for height percentile of eighty-eight per cent. This is not yet a normal weight, however he is still growing and gaining weight, so he can no longer be considered failing to thrive. He also grew emotionally. He is hitting out or going to his parents to complain rather than pulling out his own hair when angry or unhappy about something. As a whole, the family experiences more pleasure in being together. There still remains an enormous amount of work to be done with the parents and Sam, but I feel that the beginnings of concave parental containment of Sam's anxieties provide a better base for improvement within the couple's relationship. The parents reviewed the work we did together with the Consultant Psychiatrist and said:

> What we found most helpful was the fact that the psychotherapists were not focusing on one specific problem, the eating problem, in our child. All the previous professionals had divided Sam up into parts and dealt with one symptom or another in him. We needed understanding, not simply instructions about what we should do, and we found that in the psychotherapy offered. What also seemed helpful was that the therapist was observing everything with us and thinking about the whole of our relationship with Sam and with each other. The result is that Sam is now able to tolerate mess, he is able to tolerate our pouring water over his hair and playing in the sand. Things he was never able to do before. At times he is willing to communicate more through sentences and he is more affectionate, approaching us to be with us and asking for things. He seems more confident and curious about things in a way which he never seemed to be before.

I shall now share part of the letter I wrote to the parents following our six-month follow-up meeting in which Sam spent half an hour in a play session:

> Sam was so affectionate to you, Mrs Brown, more so than I have ever seen him before. It was such a beautiful moment when, after his play session, Sam came into the room and rushed towards you and gleefully hugged you. When you walked away together your arm embraced Sam's back while he snuggled against you with his arm curled round your leg. You are close and Sam is now able to leave you because he carries a loving picture of you inside himself. He assumes that Maria, who was playing with him in the playroom, will look after him as well as you do.

I have attempted to describe ways in which the parents of a child with feeding/eating difficulties can move in nine months from convex containment, through flat containment of emotions and denial of a serious feeding and language problem, into becoming parents capable of concave containment of their own emotional experiences and those of their only son. Concave parental containment created an emotional climate in which the parents' son could be receptive to them, thereby not only eating, digesting their food, and growing in this benevolent climate, but also developing the capacity to symbolise his emotional experiences and express his feelings through symbolic play and short sentences. Feeding, thinking and speaking difficulties reflect problems in relatedness within the family. The difficulties involve issues of love, intimacy, separation, loss, hostility and guilt. Sam seems more confident now and curious about things in a way that he never was before. The currents between the couple create the air the child breathes. This emotional connection between the couple is so crucial. It is not simply the mother's state of mind, it really is the receptivity of each marital partner to each other that creates a concave container, the cradle for the child's growth.

CHAPTER SEVEN

The child who has not yet found words

Jeanne Magagna

A meeting of two
Eye to eye, face to face
And when you are near
I will take your eyes
And place them instead of mine,
And you will take my eyes out
And place them instead of yours,
Then I will look at you with your eyes
And you will look at me with mine.

J. L. Moreno (1946)

Moments after her birth, baby is resting in mother's embrace. Mother says, "Hello" and baby looks up and greets mother's eyes. Standing nearby, father also says, "Hello baby", and baby searches for and finds father's face. Baby's eyes are alight in the greetings. After a few moments, mother places the breast near baby and baby roots around until the nipple is found. Gradually, baby slowly begins to suck the nipple and rest her hand on mother's breast. Baby is held by mother's embrace, held by mother's nurturing breast, held by mother and father's thoughtful attention. The process of "holding the baby" involves an empathic attunement in which the mother and father must:

- *see* the mother and father with the baby's eyes
- *experience* the baby's bodily sensations and give them meaning
- *feel* what it is to be "the baby" newly aware of people and unfamiliar experiences

- *speak* directly to the baby with a mind, a baby with a unique personality
- *bear* the baby's dependence on them for every mode of emotional and physical survival

As I watch this scene I imagine how different baby Nina's experience must have been. Baby Nina had an innate desire to reach out to her parents, to get to know them and explore her new world outside the womb. She recognises her mother's voice, but her eighteen-year-old Brazilian mother is uncertain in her greeting of Nina, for she wasn't certain she wanted to be her mother. Nina was conceived from a one-night stand with Nina's father, whose whereabouts are unknown to her mother. Mother wanted to abort her baby and at birth she does not want to keep Nina, but the maternal grandmother persuades her to take Nina home and look after her. After six weeks, Nina's mother decides she wants to go to work to be with adults, and she leaves Nina home alone in the company of two German shepherd dogs, a few caged canaries, and a black cat. Nina is left to cry and required to wait until mother returns from her job as a cashier in the nearby village grocery store.

A young baby naturally reaches out for mother with her eyes, signals her, opens her mouth to receive mother's nipple feeding her, and upon hearing mother's voice, baby turns to look at mother once again. Eyes, nose, mouth, ears, and hands are all ready to greet mother's body and mother's mind. Baby has learned to know mother's voice from inside the womb. Waiting, waiting, waiting alone for five to six hours a day without any response from anyone but the two dogs leaves Nina's wish to greet mother to become muted. Having no mother to come in response to her cries, Nina gradually stops waiting for her, searching for her, and crying for her to respond. Nina's mouth stops showing upturned expressive lips, her facial expression seems to have lost its alive emotional responsiveness, appearing unresponsive and flat. Nina's innate desire to reach out to her mother diminishes as a result of mother's long absences.

Maternal deprivation and emotional neglect involving no response to either Nina's distress or her desires promotes Nina's loss of capacity for developing a thoughtful and meaningful relationship to both herself and others. Her capacity for symbolic function is impaired as she holds on adhesively with her ears to the sounds of the dog walking around, barking, and the canaries occasionally tweeting. At times, Nina uses her hands to finger her blanket, and at other times she sleeps alone, deprived of mother's presence. Gradually, over the weeks, Nina's innate bond to her mother weakens. Nina's mother is depressed, bearing the burden of raising a now unresponsive Nina on her own while working.

By the time Nina is two years old, she has had twenty hospitalisations for various physical illnesses, including epilepsy and asthma, and unwillingness to eat adequate amounts of food. She is underweight and developmentally delayed. She is put in a daycare nursery by mother. Doctors, nurses, and nursery workers fail to observe the mother–child relationship and note that *the emotional bridge* between Nina and her mother is broken. Nina's painful emotional experiences have been imprisoned in her body. When Nina's mother completely loses her own attachment to Nina, she abandons her in the social service office. Nina resides for some time in a residential nursery, and the social worker tells the potential adoptive parents, "Nina is a pleasant child who does not create difficulties and rarely cries." At age three and a half, Nina is adopted. She makes few sounds of protest, for she has closed her mind to the notion of a responsive mother. She has only a few words, for her terror of being left by her mother has meant a closure of the development of symbolic functioning and language development in general.

Nina's new adoptive parents are a Belgian couple in their late thirties. They have both been divorced and the father has a sixteen-year-old son from a previous marriage. The couple were furious with Brazilian social services when they realised they did not simply have a shy child, they had a severely developmentally delayed child who seemed basically negatively responsive to the majority of their overtures. Not only that, Nina expressed her suffering through not-sleeping, not-eating, and refusing, out of terror, to go near a toilet. Her asthma, eczema, and epileptic attacks continued to result in hospitalisations, where the neurologist recommended that she see a psychotherapist and speech therapist.

The aim of this chapter

I shall describe a particular way of working in modified psychoanalytic psychotherapy with a newly adopted child. I chose to work with both Nina and her adoptive mother. I did this because I felt Nina was so disappointing to her mother and father and thus emotionally at risk. The parents were very frustrated by her unrelatedness, her muteness, her physical symptoms requiring many hospitalisations and this frustration could impede the development of a truly loving attachment to her. Nina and her mother needed to develop a more intimate, loving, understanding relationship, and I felt the most efficient, effective way of promoting their relationship was to have mother and I work together to know Nina more deeply and respond more intimately to her *communication without words*. Unfortunately, father could not join us.

I shall demonstrate how psychoanalytic psychotherapy in the presence of her adoptive mother fostered Nina's desire to think with us about her emotional experiences. She gradually relinquished some of her somatic expressions of terror and pain and found ways of being understood through her play, gestures, facial expressions and a gradually increasing use of language.

Why isn't a child able to protest when she doesn't like what is happening?

One of the first questions Nina's adoptive parents asked is "Why doesn't Nina cry?" I imagined that Nina didn't cry for as an infant she did not have the experience of engaging with a responsive mother who responded to her distress in a predictable sequence of behaviour by picking her up, bearing her distress, comforting her, and trying to understand what was the matter. Mother was absent, and Nina's rage, terror, and despair led to an internalised bad, hostile mother. To express anger and distress, the child needs the experience of a reliable, trustworthy parent. If the mother is not reliably emotionally present, the child stops looking at the mother, holding onto the nipple and eating, and loses her hand-grip. Tronick and colleagues (1997) suggest it is that reliability and trustworthiness of the parent that allows affective repair of an internalised hostile, unresponsive mother after a disruption in a relationship. If direct expression of protest and distress is not possible, then the negative arousal will be in the body and somatic symptoms often occur (J. Symington, 2000). Nina's negative somatic experiences requiring frequent hospitalisation were connected with *flat containment* of her protest and distress (S. Briggs, 1997b).

How did I prepare Nina for beginning psychotherapy sessions?

A young child is completely dependent on the parents, and for this reason the child will be sizing up the nature of the relationship between the parents and therapist. I imagined mother feared that although Nina rejected her, she might get close to me in psychotherapy and not to her. I suggested to mother and father to tell Nina how her mother and she were going to come to see Jeanne, a lady in the hospital. They would come on Mondays, for many times, first thing in the morning at 10 a.m. on the day daddy goes back to work after the weekend. I also suggested that the parents say to Nina that we would try to understand what Nina was thinking and feeling, she would go home and not stay at night in hospital. She could play and draw, and we would try to understand what she was feeling and what she was thinking. She could let us know if something was the matter or if she wondered about something. In saying this, I am implying to Nina and her parents that there are ways of communicating without words.

I also told the parents that my contact with mother and father before, during, and after Nina's sessions would be mainly a "hello" and "goodbye", although I might ask mother a question or two while she was in the session. I added that other necessary communication between us should take place in scheduled meetings via our regularly scheduled phone conversations or with the colleague who would be meeting regularly with them. This method allowed Nina to feel the session was for her to discover her own relationship with me, her psychotherapist.

As I said before, with very young adopted children, I generally prefer the mother to be in the psychotherapy session with the child. I told mother I would like her to simply observe Nina and her interactions. We arranged that we would discuss what she observed at home and within the session in a regular, fixed weekly telephone appointment lasting a specific amount of time, say twenty minutes. I choose to do this rather than talking much with the mother within the psychotherapy session. I ask mother to collaborate with me so that we can both understand her child, Nina.

Why do I keep the mother in the room?

Mother felt she had been cheated of a normal child and I felt her disappointment was creating difficulties in forming an intimate bond with non-speaking Nina. The task of working with a child who is imprisoned by protective mechanisms is to help not only her, but also the mother and father who have become different, less adequate, less attuned parents after days, weeks, months of rejection by Nina. I do not want to take over the parents' roles. I want to support them to use and restore some of their capacities that are similar to those I am using as a therapist. After all, good therapy is simply using the essence of good, thoughtful intimate contact with primitive emotions present in the parent–child relationship.

It seemed important that I work as collaboratively as possible with mother as a participant observer in the session. She could feel almost a supervisor to my work, enriching my understanding of Nina by telling me more about what she felt Nina was experiencing in our relationship. Mother was virtually silent in the session, except on those occasions when Nina approached her directly or when I asked her questions in the sessions because I was really puzzled and needed her to help me understand Nina's mood or sounds. In the regular telephone sessions, mother told me what she was observing and thinking about Nina.

After a month or so, I invited the mother to make a little picture-book diary with drawings she made for Nina. The instruction was that each day she was to think about either a good moment or conflictual moment for Nina and make a drawing and read out a simple sentence below a drawing which she had made. Reading the story-book of Nina's life occasionally could help Nina could understand the gist of what mother was drawing. As she drew at home every evening with Nina, mother sat Nina near her, pondered over the day, and told her what she was writing and drawing for her. Gradually, by the end of one year of therapy, Nina felt she could indicate with one or two words something that was important about her day. Pondering over the day and story-writing became a daily ritual for Nina and her mother, and sometimes the father, and they gained both pleasure and knowledge from this way of being and thinking together. I also invited mother to make a daily journal for herself to use as a reminder of which observations of her interaction with Nina she felt would be useful to share with me.

In time, Nina also spontaneously contributed to what mother wrote, for when something was happening outside of our sessions that Nina wanted recorded, she would say "Jeanne", and mother would know that she should remember to tell me about the incident. When mother and Nina returned for the next weekly session, I invited mother to show Nina one or two of the weekly events in the "feelings picture-book" and describe aloud to her and me those moments which they had shared. I then commented directly to mother and Nina restating or amplifying some emotion present in their shared experience. Sometimes, later in the therapy, mother would suggest to Nina that she chose the page to show me. I would talk to Nina about this event, underlining the crucial emotional point that I was to comprehend.

Example 1: "Daddy coming home from work"
Example 2: "Picking flowers in granny's garden"

As newly adoptive parents, the mother and father were very appreciative of our collaborative work, feeling they too were an essential part of the therapeutic process designed to help Nina develop a capacity to think about her feelings and share her emotions with her parents. I should add that every four months, Nina's parents, the social worker involved, the nursery teacher, and speech therapist met together with the consultant child psychiatrist and me to review our multidisciplinary teamwork with Nina and her parents. While the "team" was together, we tried to think about what Nina's current predominant anxieties were and how each of us was fostering her capacity to work through her difficulties. We also each described to each other what one of us on 'the team', could do to understand and to help Nina with some of the obstacles to her normal development.

The first session

I shall now describe the initial session and then talk about the theory and technique of interpretation:

> Nina came into the room with her mother. I had placed a box of toys on the floor with some of the toys beside the box. I suggested that the mother just remain silent while she played. Nina became completely obsessed with trying to get into locked cupboards and then she found some string in her box. She became fascinated by the string. She rolled it out tangling it in my feet, then tangled herself in the string and had difficulty getting herself out and required help to get her feet out.
>
> She didn't touch the toys until mother gave her one of the dolls on the table. She held onto the doll for much of the session. She tried to wrap the doll with a string, but she was unsuccessful in doing this, so I helped her. She then ran around the room with the mother doll on a long piece of string that trailed behind her. There was string from one end of the room to the other. She then very forcefully threw the mother doll on the floor. I said, "Goodbye mum."
>
> The intonation of my voice was used to show how I experience the violence of throwing. I said, "Goodbye mum" in a loud, quick and somewhat harsh way which was attuned to the quality of her throwing of the mummy doll.
>
> Nina repetitiously picked up the doll and threw her down a copious number of times. I varied the pitch, loudness and quality of my voice to echo the emotion with which she was throwing the doll. "Go away, mum." "Come back mum." "Here you are mum." "Hi mum," I said, as she gently put the doll on her mother's lap.
>
> When she threw the doll down I also slightly varied the content of what I was saying according to the velocity with which she threw the doll. I said "Nina keeps thinking, 'Jeanne is coming to be with me' but then she thinks, Jeanne just goes away." I spoke to her in second person now, "You can't stop thinking Jeanne, like mummy, just goes away.' Nina is afraid that this new therapist, Jeanne, might just go away!"
>
> After a while Nina went to the sink. She put the plug in the hole and filled the sink with water. The presence of water in the room seemed an essential part of the play equipment for her. Nina emptied the sink and filled the sink repeatedly. I once again echoed the emotion present in her face, hands and body. I used my tone of voice, loud or soft, the pitch of my voice, high or low, the emotion in my voice, angry, sad, excited, frightened … to meet her, greet her emotional state, make a non-verbal comment about how I was attuned to her emotional experience. At times, I spoke in identification with Nina, in the first person: "I want to be in control of a never-ending Jeanne, never ending like the water." Sometimes, then, depending on the mood, I spoke as though I were the water: "Oh, oh, I am falling, I am falling, I am falling … help me!"

At other times, I felt it was important to speak in a conversation between Nina and the water, identifying with Nina, then the water, using different intonations:

Nina: "Hello water."
Water: "Hello Nina."
Nina: "Goodbye Water."
Water: "Help, help, I'm falling. Where am I going?"
Nina: "Hello water."
Water: "Hello Nina."

My comment to Nina: "Coming and going, coming and going, coming back again to be together."

> Nina subsequently joined the father doll to the mother doll. She then picked up two tiny stuffed animals: a friendly furry teddy and a tiger. She held them one in each hand and then brought them together onto her chest and hugged them. Then teddy and tiger fell down. Somehow Nina had dropped them almost inadvertently and then she quickly looked at me with a slight smile. I sensed she took some pleasure in secretly dropping them. When the end of the session came, Nina didn't want to go. She stood still, eyes looking down to the floor and cried in a painful, moaning way. Nina then ran around the room and got her feet all tangled up in the string. She seemed completely stuck in my room.

As Nina's psychotherapist I am trying to understand the feeling of Nina's bodily and physical movements. I speak in identification with Nina and acknowledge as precisely as possible the nature of feeling present in each gesture Nina makes. I also personify the objects with which she is playing, for example, I am "being the water" stating what it would feel like if the object were a person in relation to Nina. I am entering Nina's dream world in which phantasies underlie each of her hand gestures (Isaacs, 1952).

One technique which I use is to "talk for" Nina, trying to speak in the first person as if I were her. I use the rhythm and intensity of her hand gestures, her bodily expressions and facial expressions to inform my speaking. I make it clear that I am wondering, not definitely knowing, what she thinks. "Greeting her gestures" with my wonderings enables Nina to reach down to aspects of her inner life that have previously been unknown, nameless, frightening and chaotic. Some of her emotions will certainly contain aspects of emotions experienced in her preverbal infancy.

In my mind, I am naming the objects as the internalised mother, the internalised father, the internalised unborn siblings, and Nina herself. Nina has very few words. She basically exists as an almost mute child verbally, but non-verbally, through her actions and expressions, Nina is filled with conversation about her mental life!

How do I think about my psychotherapeutic encounter with Nina?

I have been influenced by the work of Dr Henri Rey (1994) who wrote *Universals of Psychoanalysis.* I am thinking about the feelings inside me and the feelings which might be inside Nina. These are *countertransference/transference* feelings from one to the other. Aspects of

Nina's *internal world* and aspects of my *internal* world interact with one another. A number of questions are important.

1. *Who is Nina in relation to her primary internalised objects—the mother, the father, her baby-self?* She is showing a sense of wanting to be enmeshed with the object... but then she is showing some abandonment, some pleasure, before moving to controlling the object with the water play. She has quickly transferred her maternal object onto me.

2. *In what state of mind is Nina?* Nina is often the controlling figure: abandoning, dropping, making the water flow continuously. Water feels like part of herself. Remember, Nina is terrified of going near a toilet, afraid to defaecate there as though she will lose part of herself in the toilet. Apertures are terrifying places into which bad feelings can come in and out of which parts of self can get lost. The toilet is a terrifying pit.

3. *What phantasies are connected to her specific actions?* *The string play*: She seems to want to make a connection with me, but then she gets enmeshed.

The cabinets: She wants to intrude into the object with the key, in control of the door shutting her away from mother, from the contents inside the mother, from what she wanted and is curious about seeing.

The doll dropping: Nina feels overwhelmed with abandonment feelings which she controls by identification with the aggressor, being the abandoning one while projecting into the other the feeling of abandonment.

The water play: She is saying "I have my own water" (symbolising the breast-mother) "and make it come and go as I please. I will have as much water as I want." This symbolises a never ending supply of the "breast-milk". She will make the "milk-water" return when she wants it to come back, as though she is "inside the breast" and controlling its flow, rather than separate from it. This is *primitive omnipotence.* Nina's bottom and its contents may somehow be equated with the breast that is controlled by her (Meltzer, 1967).

The protest at the end: Nina has loved the experience of being attentively attuned to by me physically through the tone of my voice in rhythm with her play and psychologically through my trying to understand "coming and going". By the end of the session, she has become rather enmeshed with me. Separation feels as though she is "torn off" me and she moans, something she supposedly "doesn't do" usually (Tustin, 1981).

4. *What themes are there in Nina's activities?* Nina seems to lack a sense of separateness. If she likes the object, she gets right inside. For example, in the water play she wants to possess and control the object. This is a way of "not-thinking", of evading the anxiety of abandonment which she depicted in the doll play. Also, in dropping teddy and tiger, Nina evacuates her own anxiety regarding abandonment by "being the abandoning figure" and projecting hurt, pain, and despair into the teddy and tiger.

There is a subtlety to Nina's emotions and it is important to link the feeling qualities of her eye movements, coupled with her mouth and her hand movements. For example, I can see that she is gentle when she hugs the furry animal and tiger. I feel her friendliness to the object. But then she is being thoughtless and dropping them out of sight and out of mind. Then I realise she is obtaining some secret pleasure when she drops the animals, for the very first time she looks at me and she smiles. At this point there is a cruel abandoning figure with whom she is identifying. As Nina experiences aggression, her eyes, mouth, and facial expressions seem to come alive slightly. This makes me remember that most of the time Nina's eyes seem lifelessly stuck to objects, she doesn't usually look at either mother or me.

5. *Which object is influenced by Nina's actions?*
Continually I am focusing on Nina's *internalised mother* representing nurturing, understanding, physical caregiving, and her *internalised father* representing rulemaking and providing the limits to the mother's maternal caregiving, understanding, and nurturing. Within this one session, I see a multitude of images of her infantile self. Nina is a girl who gets enmeshed with the object, wants to intrude into the object, feels abandoned cruelly by the object and then stays in a state of *primitive omnipotence,* which means it is very hard to explore and get to bear her sense of not knowing. Her motions reflect an omnipotent state of mind expressing, "I'm the boss. I am in control. I don't need a mummy. I can take care of myself with my water which I hold onto, which I control." Nina has to feel "powerful, in control" to survive psychically without good internalised maternal and paternal figures. You can understand how difficult it must have been for Nina to have to survive as an infant alone in a room without mother, with only the birds and the dogs present during the day.

Now it is difficult for Nina to depend on "the mother", her own mother, but also me, her therapist, standing for mother in the transference. Instead she uses non-stop movement "to hold herself together psychically", the adhesive identification described by Esther Bick (1968), and like "the daddy" she intrudes, takes control of the supplies of the mother, represented by the water. This is another method of protecting herself from feelings of being a lonely, helpless, vulnerable, abandoned baby. It is also a way of protecting herself from depending on unreliable figures like her biological mother and father.

6. *What is the consequence of Nina's turning away from the mother to material objects for comfort?*
When Nina's face is still, lifeless, her eyes are not open to receive or to say goodbye or to observe people. As a psychotherapist or parent the tendency is to feel disregarded, devalued and useless. Nina's adoptive mother feels continually rejected. So do I. It looks like Nina doesn't want a relationship with anyone much of the time. It is a dangerous situation unless I realise her use of *identification with the aggressor* and *intrusion* into the object, which involves massively projecting parts of herself into me. When she projects into me I should feel that I don't count, that she doesn't want me, that I am the abandoned baby.

I need to understand that these protective mechanisms have protected her from the terrifying experiences of infancy when she failed to have the intimacy or even maternal responsiveness during the day from her biological mother. Nina felt compelled to turn to material objects for comfort because unlike a mother, they can be controlled by her. Meanwhile, she has lost track of her infantile self which felt traumatised to such an extent that she gave up contact with this self, stopped crying long ago. Who has there been to ask for help? She has few words. To whom would she have wanted to talk? Her *"bridge to mother"* was broken by parental neglect and Nina's response to an unavailable mother.

By playing repetitiously with objects, Nina further blocked access to her infantile self that desperately needs love in an intimate trustworthy relationship. She requires intimacy with me, with the mother. She needs a mother and father, a mummy-therapist to whom she can attach herself, upon whom she can depend; however, no one hears her cry, not even her!

Initially, Nina responds to my presence in the session, but she very quickly imbues me with qualities of the internalised objects (the parents filled with the child's projections of love and hate). I was often "to be ignored". As her psychotherapist, I was required to have certain attitudes that could not be counterfeited. Nina knew if I was tired, depressed, happy, and was anxious when there was falsity present in my required attitudes of receptiveness and my capacity to modulate emotions through mentalization. In other words, she could tell when I was under stress, and she seemed rather overactive at those times. If I was momentarily distracted from her, Nina would move nearer to me or drop objects, as though her hand lost its grip as my mind had lost its grip on her. She could differentiate counterfeit from genuine interest as I tried to understand all her feelings—love, hate, hope, and despair. Nina projected feelings into me and I was expected to understand the emotions present in the room at that very moment in the here and now (Stern, 2004).

Gradually Nina came to know that I was reliably present at the correct time every Monday and a deeper dependent transference to me representing a mother evolved. The endings of sessions gradually look different from the beginning of sessions for *all* young children. For example, the child might want to stay in the session longer, leave the session early, stop being connected to the therapist, or run out to see the parent in the waiting room. All of these are defences against the therapist's "father's role" of saying that there is a limit to the "mummy-therapist" time for "the baby". For example, during one session, I say "it is time to go in five minutes". Nina takes out two toy cars and starts playing with them in the doll house.

Nina's response to ending the session and her response to returning to the next session are always a focus of my interpretations. The interpretation is designed to "gather the transference to the therapist" ... by this I mean I collect the feelings *in the here and now* in relation to Nina and me meeting, breaking contact and also in relation to her feeling understood or her not feeling understood by me. Both loving and hostile feelings emerge in the transferential relationship with the therapist.

I am looking at how she holds eye contact, holds the toys, dropped eye contact, dropped the toys, used the toys or didn't use the toys. There are innumerable phantasies which are linked with speech and movement. For example, throwing a pencil on the floor is accompanied by the possibility of an aggressive phantasy whereas gently putting two pencils together on the floor might be symbolising a friendly reunion between two people.

Nina had been severely emotionally neglected during her first two and a half years of life, so her responses to dependency are more marked than those of some children in more favourable circumstances. However, most children will generally show an oscillation between beginning to depend on the therapist's receptivity and understanding and using *primitive omnipotence* to "looking after oneself" and they will try to barricade the infantile self from having a trusting relationship with the therapist, until they are convinced the therapist is trustworthy.

What were the aims I had in psychotherapy with Nina?

For Nina, it was important:

- To have a feeling.
- To hold it consciously.
- To communicate the feeling through movements, facial expressions, play, words.
- To lessen the severity of the cruel superego so that she is able to integrate different aspects of her personality, such as aggression, which is split off and projected.
- To help her move from being a "placating, compliant child" to have the courage to "be herself" without the fear of a repeat of being hit or abandoned if she isn't good, or interesting (at the present time, she hits herself rather than get cross with her mother).
- To develop the capacity to think about her emotional experiences, pain, love, hate, hope, anger, sadness- all of them.
- And in time, hopefully, to develop a sense of loving concern for both herself and others.

To develop a sense of agency based on introjection of good internal parents with whom she identifies, thus she can be resilient rather than omnipotent.

What is healing in psychotherapy?

The *self* is healed in therapy by bringing the infantile conflicts and pleasures back together in their existence inside the relationship with the therapist. Estranged parts of right and left hand brain are integrated in this way. In other words, through the hippocampal processing in therapy the right half of the brain, the sensory motor cortex which encodes implicit experience of physical experiences, can be brought back together with the left half part of the brain, which has explicit declarative memory. Enactment through play and action in therapy can bring back the story of the self, overwhelmed by subjective states which were never given words or thoughts by the self, but were instead avoided by emotional numbing and avoidance through not thinking (i.e., dissociation and splitting off of this part).

The therapeutic process

Part one: gathering the transference

Gathering the transference would involve thinking about how Nina felt about my capacity to be present for her, to understand her and how she responded to separating and arriving from the sessions and how she responded to my understanding or not understanding her (Meltzer, 1967). In the first phase, some of the severest anxieties about separation and loss have begun to be modified through learning from experience present in the here and now of the infantile transference relationship to the therapist. This was assisted by Nina's experience of being contained by me through sufficiently correct and timely interpretations.

What is gathering the infantile transference?

The infant has experiences in relation to family members. These relationships are tinged with the infant's own projections of love and hate and form part of the current unconscious phantasy, which is re-enacted right here and now in the moment of analysis. Melanie Klein thought that play re-enacted the child's own worst fears and anxieties in relation to internal and external relationships to primary figures.

To understand primitive infantile anxieties present in the moment-to-moment interaction between child and therapist it is useful to undertake a year long course involving weekly observations of infants in their families (Magagna, 2002). It really does help one to understand the deepest root of transferential infantile experiences moment-to-moment in the relationship with the therapist, rather than just focusing on separation experiences between sessions. Let me give you an example of an infant observation to show you what I mean:

> *Example of eight-week-old infant Susan:*
>
> After changing Susan's nappy Mother began to put on her babygro on her legs. Susan began to scream and cry. Mother says she doesn't like to get dressed and takes her into her arms. Susan becomes still and quiet as mother holds her. Then mother lay Susan down and sprayed baby's stuffed up nose with some medicine. Susan shouted, fluttered her arms and legs, moved her head from side to side. Mother said, "I know you don't like this my little girl, but I have to do it, sorry" and took her into her arms again. Susan was still and silent once again as she rested against mother's body. Mother then put Susan back down into her bed to sleep. Baby Susan began to scream and flail her arms and legs. Mother took her to her arms again and put her onto the breast. Susan sucked a bit while making sucking noises and then pushed the breast away with her hands and began to scream.

What do we see in the infant's relationship with the mother?

The baby clearly has an experience of the mother as a safe, trustworthy object and she feels totally dependent on mother to feel safe. The spraying of the medicine feels like baby is being intruded upon by a "bad mother" and she protests at the *bad experience* and cannot settle until "the good mother" returns to comfort her. Separating from the mother is felt to be bad and terrifying, because the baby has not yet introjected a good internal mother who allows baby to separate from the external good mother. For this reason, she has to *adhere to the mother's body/mind*. It is not possible to suck interruptedly from the nipple of mother's breast because the breast is not simply *the good breast*. It is filled with *bad projections*. The nipple becomes spit out as a representative of the "intrusive bad breast" responsible for spraying of nose, putting baby down. Baby is able to be dependent on the mother but screams, feels helpless, angry, and terrorised when there remains only the bad persecutory world. Then the nipple becomes bad, persecutory, and she pushes it away.

There are two separate bad experiences. Both separation and nasty experiences with mother cause hostility in the baby. These experiences turn the breast in part to a good / bad breast. Likewise, *gathering of the infantile transference* will encompass fears and anxieties linked both to bad experiences in the session and separations when the transference is to a good object who is felt to be abandoning the child who has not yet *internalised a good object*.

Why do we gather the infantile transference as the predominant mode of work that accompanies looking at external relationships?

Klein says that if we just look at relationships with significant figures outside the therapy the risk is that the child will split off feelings in relation to the therapist. The therapist will be kept as either "the good or idealised therapist" or "the bad, denigrated therapist". Those splintered off parts of relationship to the primary figure need to be integrated into the whole relationship to help the child integrate infantile parts of the self (M. Klein, 1952). In the early assessment phase of the therapy, we are looking at the mobility of defences, the intensity of the drive towards integration, and the capacity to accept dependence.

Why do I use my countertransference when working as a psychotherapist?

The base of my work is observation, coupled with using the emotional resonance stirred up within myself during the encounters with Nina. The use of the countertransference is linked to the psychoanalytic approach of Wilfred Bion (1967) and the research into therapeutic effectiveness described by Alan Schore (2002a). Using the countertransference involves receiving verbalised and non-verbalised experiences—present in tone, rhythm, volume, and velocity of speech, the bodily states, pictorial images, gestures, actions, and play—and subsequently understanding the mood and meaning present in an encounter with Nina.

What do I mean by the terms "concave containment" and "mentalization"?

Both internal and external family figures form part of the therapeutic discussion. The process of containment (Bion, 1967) allow Nina to unite emotions with symbols, and subsequently words, to convey and contemplate upon a meaningful and truthful picture of her emotional life. This process is also now described more fully as *mentalization* (Bateman & Fonagy, 2004). The therapist's capacity for *mentalization* is similar to the primary task of the mother to mentalize using reverie to receive, experience, think about and subsequently meet the infantile needs of the baby: the baby's need to be nourished and protected, her coldness, warmth, pain, terror, and aloneness, her need to be safely held and her need for intimacy with the mother. It is through this process of collaborative *attunement* between mother and baby that the image of the body is constructed, during which the baby integrates perceptions and sensations of having her physical and emotional needs met (Stern, 1985). The baby also internalises her significant caregivers and forms different attachments to each of them (Fonagy et al., 1993).

The basic psychotherapeutic method with Nina involved being attuned to the emotional experience of being with her in the session and in the therapeutic milieu. It was necessary to make sense of Nina's experience, coupled with her thinking, and to interpret her projections of physical and emotional states. As a predominantly non-verbal child, Nina was specifically attuned to non-verbal aspects of our relationship, such as the tone of my voice and my mood

(Perry, 2000). The application of Bick's (1968) observational approach of empathic attentiveness to minute aspects of the nonverbal dialogue between child and others involved right-brain–right-brain therapeutic communication, which is considered by Alan Schore (2002a) to be the first point of therapeutic action. Schore considers that it is most important to have psychobiologically regulated affect transactions that maximise positive and minimise negative affect in order to co-create secure attachment bonds (Schore, 2002).

Shore (2002a) cites a body of literature which is relevant to working with emotionally deprived non-speaking children like Nina: Lewis (1992) points out that the therapist's use of her body is especially involved in the reception of right-brain–right-brain transferential projections of split-off part of the self, and this mechanism specifically mediates defensive projective identification. Friedman and Lavender (1997) conclude that the presence of the therapist's recognition of her countertransferential discomforting bodily signals are necessary somatic markers triggered by her perception of the protective identification. Muir (1995) adds to their thinking by stating that the both physical and psychological holding are important.

If I blocked the negatively valenced somatic markers—for example, by defensively shifting out of the right-brain intuitive state into a left-brain intellectual state—I cut off my empathic connection to my own, and therefore to Nina's, pain. I concur with Schore's (2002a) ideas that as a therapist I must by necessity act as an interactive affective regulator for the child in order for therapeutic transformation to occur. I, like Schore (2002a), notice that if I became too overwhelmed by Nina's state of mind she became disorganised and tentative in my presence as though she were worried by me. Sometimes this was shown by her making cups of pretend tea for me. Transformation within Nina's *internal world* took place through projective identification, creating a transitional space in which mental pain, hopelessness, despair and a flickering of hope could be explored first in me.

The consideration and later verbalisation of my countertransference responses to Nina's primitive experiences, including sensations and movement or stillness of her body, has been essential before Nina could put her experiences into a symbolic form for communication. Although I rarely asked her direct questions which required a verbal response, when I had too strong a wish for Nina to be open and receptive to me, she experienced me as intrusive and withdrew from me. Despite seeming to be "sealed off" with omnipotent defences suggesting she needed to be 'in control', in fact, she was in a kind of hypervigilant state in which she was acutely tuned into my innermost, unverbalised states of mind. She rested upon "the choppy sea" of my emotional turbulence or "the calm sea" of my more emotionally regulated, thoughtful states of mind. If I was distracted by a thought in my mind, she seemed to sense it and signalled to me by coming closer to me. She was secretly "dependently resting upon" my being emotionally present for her, but not too close and not too far away from her.

Part two: sorting of the geographical confusions

In this early second phase, every experience of separation at the end of the sessions, between the sessions and during holidays tended to dominate the transference. Of course throughout psychotherapy problems with separation continually threaten integration, promote regression and disintegration. In his chapter on "The sorting of the geographical confusions", Dr Meltzer (1967, pp. 13–22) highlights six major reasons for the tendency towards projective identification. These include:

1. Intolerance to separation linked with absolute dependence
2. Omnipotent control
3. Envy
4. Jealousy
5. Deficiency of trust
6. Excessive persecutory anxiety

Let us look at this second phase of Nina's psychotherapy and try to shed light on these six emotional issues.

> *Clinical example two:*
>
> Nina had missed school and therapy for two weeks due to a bad cold. When I went to greet her she hid under the table in the waiting room. I wondered aloud to myself, "Where is Nina? I can't find Nina. She is missing and I can't seem to find her." Then, I see Nina's head, peering very briefly out from under the top of the table. She is not gazing at me, her face is flat, devoid of any obvious feeling, as though paralysed. I speak as Nina, "Scared of Jeanne, Jeanne frightening. Don't see Jeanne I know." Mother pulls Nina out from under the table, she doesn't want to come to my room. She tugs on mother to walk slowly, pointing to each door along the corridor saying, "Not this one. Not this one." It is though there is "no place" for Nina. She has lost "the good Jeanne". I am filled with projections of hostility and she has to protect herself when she comes in by spraying water in to my eyes, as though my eyes are hostile to her. She then puts soap into a cup of water and starts drinking the soapy water. It must taste terrible! I say, "soapy water, Nina's soapy water, 'ikky soapy water'. Nothing feels good. Nothing feels right. Nina isn't responding, it is like she has closed me off ... eyes turned away, ears switched off, mouth filled with soapy water, hard back towards me to protect herself from me as she stands at the sink, I say, 'Nina, are you here? Can you hear me?' She feels deaf and not thinking, so she won't be able to make sense of my words, but after a moment or two they are registered and there arrives a loud shout, 'No!' She doesn't turn around and look at me, but very unexpectedly, for the very first time, she hits my arm hard.
>
> She subsequently goes over to the sink and washes her hands. She then tries to get into the blue wooden box under the sink. I speak again, this time as Nina, 'I don't want that bad Jeanne near me.' I will take care of myself with my own things."

1. **Intolerance to separation**

Nina's constant glancing at me suggested that she needed constant contact not only with my voice, but also with my eyes. In accordance with Esther Bick, I think that there is an absence of psychic skin to hold together the parts of Nina's self. In time, there should develop an internalisation of the containing capacities of the therapist. There will then be less need for Nina's *adhesive identification* with aspects of the therapist.

> *Example*: two and a half months into therapy, an unexpected separation from me led Nina to feel I was filled with her bad projections .... I was terrifying and terrible and her hearing was deaf, her eyes were averted, her mouth was immobile, drinking awful soapy water. It seemed very difficult to mitigate her sense of everything turning bad, "needing an emotional wash" with my understanding. With this experience, her newly gained confidence in sitting on the potty disappeared. The potty represented a terrifying hole and she was afraid of falling into it completely ... as she had done in the session when she stopped being with me for awhile and got lost in her autistic-like cocoon of not-thinking, not looking, "being deaf".

What is "adhesive identification"?
This concept was developed by Esther Bick (1968). She realised that before the infant had internalised a good mother who had received the baby's projections, the infant would *stick to the mother* using eyes and ears as *sucking tentacles* and would also *hold onto her own body* by tightening musculature, clenching fingers and stomach muscles or by using non-stop movement (Symington, 2002, p. 105–117). *Mimicry* of facial expression or behaviour is also another way of *sticking, adhering to the mother.*

2. **Omnipotent control**
When there is inadequate differentiation between good and bad parts of the object, psychosocially deprived children often use omnipotent control and Nina was no exception as shown in the first session.

> *Example*: Six months into therapy, Nina understands when it is time to go. She is beginning to know from a clock on the table and partly she may just have an intuitive sense of the length of the sessions. She starts playing with the clock, trying to make the clock ring. Unsuccessful in this task, she goes to the light switch and repetitiously switches the lights off and on. It is a sunny day and lights aren't needed. I suggest to her, "Nina is the boss-daddy. Nina-boss says I am in control of 'mummy-therapist Jeanne' coming and going. I am the boss of Jeanne talking to me, seeing me. *I* have the clock."

3. **The role of envy**
It is sometimes very difficult to differentiate protective mechanisms. They spoil that which the mother has to offer because the child is terrified of intimacy and spoils and attacks the good feeding breast because it is good. Envy is different from attacking persecutory bad objects. Envy is spoiling what is good and then feeling that one is devoid of anything good inside oneself. Only hostile relationshps are established with good objects when envy persists. Envy involves the attack on people with special advantages and qualities simply for the sake of their goodness. When envy is strong there may be a taking in of the object with such violence that the object is spoiled. Greed may result in accumulation of damaged objects, so there is greater demand for good objects to be taken in to alleviate the steadily worsening state inside. The problem after

envy occurs is that it is not clear what is good and what is bad. The child can't be sure she can trust the therapist, who may be reliable or unreliable.

> *Example*: Nina starts pounding on the boxes of the other children. Then she grabs a jug, fills it with water and pours it over me. I felt this was an envious attack on the other children whom I saw for therapy and on me.

4. **Two kinds of jealousy**

There is the kind of *delusional jealousy* that gives the sensation of feeling that "the other babies", the internal babies, are constantly being gratified inside the mother. The second kind of jealousy is a more *possessive jealousy*, which leads to regression. It is a kind of wish to sleep inside the mother forever. In *possessive jealousy*, there is a wish to remain infantile or die, and the result for the therapist and/or child is often to feel particularly withdrawn into a cocoon of sleepiness.

5. **Deficiency of trust**

This is a kind of secretiveness or trickiness and it is linked with projecting hostile feelings into the object and/or having had bad experiences as Nina did. As a result of a paranoid relationship to the object the child hides her destructiveness or has a perverse pleasure in sadistic excitement.

> *Example*: Nina dropped the teddy and tiger and slyly looked at me with a smile. I thought she had some excitement in this "abandoning" of these objects.

6. **Excessive persecutory anxiety**

A virtually unbearable terror of attacked and damaged dead objects or dread is present. In these situations, physical contact can feel like a portal of entry into the body of the therapist. Using the therapist's body, hand, glasses, pen, as though having it meant being inside the therapist and having the capacities of the therapist.

> *Example*: As Nina had experienced both relief and pleasure in the first session she seemed to get "tangled inside" the room representing the body of the therapist.

In summary, all these methods are used to avoid psychic pain through the massive use of projective identification which induce confusion between self and object, confusion between evacuative space of the bottom of body- expelling bad emotional experiences, and the good nurturing top space of the mother, her breasts, her mind, her voice, her eyes- all responding in a caring, nurturing, understanding way to the baby.

The therapist in this phase is not necessarily loved, but rather valued and needed as someone into whom one can massively project all hated, unbearable, painful unwanted parts of self. This interaction is what Dr Meltzer (1967, p. 23) calls the *toilet-breast relationship*. It was interesting to note that prior to having psychotherapy, Nina had had vomiting, diarrhoea, epilepsy, asthma, and eczema requiring twenty hospitalisations before she was four years of age. In the first year of psychotherapy, all these physical symptoms disappeared! (The epilepsy, which has always been helped with medication, also disappeared). I can only suspect that the adoptive parents' increased capacity to understand and bear Nina's states of mind and the interpretive, containing therapeutic interactions between Nina and I facilitated the process of establishing, first, an externalised, and, subsequently, an internalised, "toilet-breast". Nina's negative somatisation of pent-up emotional distress and hostile feelings was no longer a necessity.

The establishment of the toilet-breast is often accompanied by the therapist's experience that the child happily leaves the therapy having deposited all unwanted painful parts of the self *inside the therapist.* Dr Meltzer (1984) would often say, "In like a lion, out like a contented lamb". He was suggesting that a child may come "in like a lion" filled with pent-up fury, but he often goes "out like a lamb" if the session has provided him with the pleasure of an understanding encounter with the therapist. Meanwhile, good experiences are located in parents, other children, or a teacher. But there is a modulation of psychic pain through having the external psychotherapist functioning as the *toilet-breast* bearing the unbearable psychic pain.

With this phenomenon of *the toilet breast* being established in the transference relationship to the psychotherapist, the child is able to experiencing a splitting: there is the *bad, toilet breast* and there begins to be the *good, feeding breast* represented by the therapist's mind, eyes, and speech. Nina was keen to come to therapy rather than frantically bursting into a space in which there was no differentiation between good therapist/bad therapist or "loving self" and "hostile self".

One of the problems with Nina was that she was barely speaking. By age four, she had a very small number of words, which she rarely used: perhaps a hundred and fifty words at the maximum. When I first watched Nina, I thought, "She has life without the emotions to go with it". Her expression was immobile, flat, without sparkle in her eyes, without changing expressions on her face. But, let us just take a look at her mouth. Nina has not had a good experience using her mouth: she cried for hours, but there were no replies to her cries. She fed with a bottle propped up on a pillow, but there was no mother dedicated to her while she was feeding. Mother said she was bored with Nina. On second thought, what I saw was "a bored with life" Nina, perhaps a face mirroring her early experience of a mother who wanted to abort her, who was "bored with her". Nina had found the mouth to be a useless tool for achieving security, attunement, comfort, pleasure. It gave up evoking responses through smiling, laughing, or crying.

Once Nina projected her bad experiences into me, her therapist, and found the "good me" who followed her with my mind, with my eyes, with my words, and my heart, she found she could trust me to be with her. Interestingly, she began using more varied facial expressions accompanying her activities and she showed her wish to use her mouth to communicate with me. She spoke using a few words to share her thoughts with me. Simultaneously, she began chewing food, staying at the table and eating a whole meal. Within six months, she was considerably less behind in her capacity to use vocabulary: Nina began joining two words together and verbally asking for help. For example, she said "open box". She also opened her ears, rather than "being deaf". This meant that at home she was now able, for the first time, to stop restlessly wandering around and sit near mother or on her lap and listen to stories. In other words, Nina's heart, mind, ears, and mouth that had been shut in the face of trauma were gradually beginning to be open to experiences.

As time passed, because I gathered her aggressive feelings *into the transference*, she was able to integrate some of them within her personality. This involved her in withdrawing her hostile projections from the very children whom before she feared and avoided. As a result, rather than avoiding her classmates, Nina began to hug her classmates when greeting them. *Gathering infantile feelings*, particularly negative feelings. *into the transference* to the therapist permitted Nina to think better and behave better when in school, and at home, for she was not so overwhelmed with infantile emotions such as possessive jealousy (Meltzer, 1967).

Part three: differentiating good therapist from bad therapist

Without an emotionally containing mother and therapist Nina's hostile feelings were projected into internal objects creating nightmares filled with persecutory figures. When the accretions of hostility were too great, the nightmares broke down into fragmented sleep and non-thinking awake life resulted. Ultimately, at times, Nina seemed to enter a delusional world, like that of the mathematician, John Nash, in *A Beautiful Mind* (Nasar, 2008). Inhabiting the protective space of her delusional world led Nina to seem unaffected by what was going on externally.

The therapeutic work was *gathering all sorts of feelings in relation to the therapist*. This task involved carefully noting all sorts of excessive feelings such as her persecutory guilt, her fear, her longing and rage. In particular, I needed to talk about her reactions to my loss of attentiveness, my failure of understanding, and my leaving her.

I also needed to note Nina's desire and jealousy of "the other babies" and "the daddy":

> *Example*: Nina put herself with the mummy-doll or herself with the daddy-doll in the doll house... I say, "Just the baby and the mummy together, 'Just the baby and the daddy must be together. Nina doesn't like being the left out baby' when I leave her."
>
> Nina then moved walked quickly over went to the cars. She made them bump harshly into one another outside the dolls house. I say, "The mummy and daddy bumping hard together." She again bumps them together in a very harsh way. I say she is cross that mummy has gone to be with daddy and left her out. She is cross that daddy has gone to be with mummy and left her out. She crossly makes them bump together hard.
>
> After this play, Nina feels I have been "bumped" by her crossness and she doesn't want to leave. Mother takes her hand to lead her out of the room, but Nina stops and turns around twice and says, "Bye", while looking in my face to see how I feel about her now. She seems to be worried and unhappy. She turns to her mother and plaintively asks, "No Jeanne?" Perhaps what has happened is that when Nina, "bumps crossly" with her hands and in her heart she has damaged "the good Jeanne mummy therapist" inside ... and "the good Jeanne" no longer exists inside her. Then Nina may worry that "the good Jeanne" outside her, who is carefully attentive to her, will also disappear.

Gradually Nina becomes more clearly dependent on the reliability of the containing and nurturing functions of the psychotherapist. It feels as though she has begun to internalise "the containing therapist" and she begins to be more vividly represent her states of mind. I am more able to understand what feelings and anxiety-provoking experiences she wants to share and think about more with me.

> Nine months into therapy, Nina comes in the room, sprays water on the walls, makes a mess, then she gives me a drink and spits out some water. I suggest: "Can I accept a messing girl who is angry with me? Do you *just* have to be 'a good girl' giving me a drink, taking care of me?"
>
> Nina turns on the tap and fills the sink with water until it is going into the overflow hole. She then puts her whole mouth and face in the water. She does this several times. Then she reaches up trying to pull me into the sink. I feel she wants to put my face in the water. I put my head down, very close to hers and say, "Nina, I feel you are worried about drowning. Maybe something has made you very frightened of drowning ..." Nina stands immobile. There is a silence. Unusually mother speaks up: "Nina was at school. She got knocked over and fell into the pool. She nearly drowned! The teacher had to jump in the pool and rescue her."

Nina was narrating a story of her experience of drowning, almost suffocating. Before that though she was making a mess, giving me some water, spitting water out of her mouth. I then say, perhaps she wondered why she had been pushed over into the pool: was she being pushed into the pool because she was a bad girl? Nina's response was to search for a toy crocodile whose big mouth with teeth opens and closes. She holds it to my mouth and smacks her lips together. I think she wants me to kiss the crocodile's mouth. I say, "It is important that I love the biting baby Nina. It is also important that I love the good baby Nina." Nina's body feels more relaxed as she explores the different areas of the room with the crocodile. The epistemophilic instinct seems inhibited when aggression is inhibited (M. Klein, 1931). Somehow the trauma of being pushed, almost drowning, "pushed Nina" into creating a story of her experience of being "abandoned" .... Was she abandoned by her mother because she was "a bad girl"? Could she be loved as both a, "loving baby" and "biting baby", all of her?

A new development in her personality was present; Nina was *holding onto her own emotional experience* of being "a terrified child" and finding ways of sharing this experience with me through her dramatised story. Nina's mind was working! She could "remember" and "narrate" her story when she had an image of " a trusted, emotionally receptive and thoughtful mummy-therapist" present internally and externally.

Part four: working through hostility to the parental couple

The establishment of the good, feeding, understanding "mummy-therapist" brings forth new complications in the transference. For example, Nina has established a good "day-time mother with the baby" but she is in conflict with the "bad night-time mummy who sleeps with the daddy". She is opposed to "the parental-genital-couple".

Example: Nina takes out the doll house and puts the mother and father together in a bed. She places the baby doll briefly in her own bed, in her own bedroom. Then very quickly and repetitiously Nina keeps reversing roles and beds: for several times, Nina puts the baby doll in mother's place in bed and the mummy-doll in Nina's bed and vice-versa.

Nina's hostility to the "night-time mummy" and her jealousy of "the parental-genital-couple" threatens the establishment of good, loving internal parents. Resolving these Oedipal issues is facilitated by Nina's introjection of a sensitive, thoughtful "mummy-therapist". With some increased inner security she can gradually let the parents have their freedom to have a life apart from the baby, supporting one another and having their freedom to come and go.

Example: In the nineteenth month of therapy, when Nina is five and a half years old, she is allowing a loving, supportive relationship between the parents. In a later session, Nina makes "daddy" with cut out strips of paper cellotaped together. The father has a penis. I sense that she experiencing love rather than possessiveness to the couple; allowing her father to have a genital relationship with the mother, but I am uncertain of this development and further sessions would be needed to elucidate the notion of reparation of the father whom she has attacked for being "with mummy". What I do note, though, is that instead of saying, "Car gone" when she shows me the empty garage where her father's car would be when he isn't at work, she says, "Car missing". This suggests that she is allowing her father to come back in her mind, rather than making him "gone" which results in feeling persecuted whilst worrying that he isn't all right and won't be returning home.

Previously Nina suffered from a cold sweat, going white, not being able to sleep because of scary nightmarish monsters in her sleep. I think her hospitalisations involving medical tests and doctors' injections promoted fears of "attacks by the monster daddy"; however, I suspect that the presence of internalised nightmare monsters is due in part to her aggression to the absent biological mother and father, the present adoptive mother and father who were sleeping together without her and my absences between the sessions.

The establishment of a loving internal couple is important for this represents a good prototype for Nina's adult life. The type of internal couple with whom she identifies influences the nature of her choices and capacities in an adult intimate sexual relationship.

Part five: dependence on the therapist to hold and understand both loving and hostile parts of the self

When Nina feels less persecuted and more openly acknowledges the importance of the containing breast she is somehow freed both physically and cognitively at school. Fourteen months into therapy, Nina goes horse-riding and feels secure enough to trot on her horse rather than simply ride at a slow pace as before. She also begins to read simple words, tell the time, draw circles, cars, and people. She also follows my example and begins making commentaries on her play, saying: "mixing cake, water is cold". At this time, on one weekend mother puzzled over three new sets of words which Nina used: "in/out and gone/back and open/shut". Mother puzzled aloud about these words with Nina and discovered that Nina was referring to her going "in and out" of the therapy room, the therapy door being "open and shut", and my being "gone" and "coming back". A few weeks later, Nina comes home from school and says, "Happy .... friend". Nina's mother realises that Nina is now able to *play with* a friend rather than just *playing beside* classmates.

Nina's loved speech therapist left during the first year of her psychotherapy. When this occurred, Nina began biting, dropping most things in the room, saying, "Boomp". She was terrified that I too would leave her. It was a terrible time for both mother and Nina, for Nina was sad, angry, terrified anything bad could happen next. I talked about how it hurt her very much to lose her "Judy", her speech therapist. She was sad and hurt, like she'd had a big "boomp" in her heart. She said, "Yes". Her communication continued develop and flow spontaneously. She could say "cross", "happy", "sad", and through her play between fourteen months and twenty-four months of therapy Nina "found words". This was because she was able to work through communication of all her states of mind with mother and me, her psychotherapist, receiving ALL of her! She no longer held the identity of "the abandoned baby": she was now the loved and accepted child. Simultaneously, Nina's linguistic skills, although still developmentally behind, had greatly improved.

Conclusion

The experience of having internalised a containing "mummy-therapist" who can tolerate her painful and difficult feelings has enabled Nina to move to a level of emotional experience that takes away the needs for somatisation of her painful and difficult emotions. She had no hospitalisations for the first time in her life after the first nine months of therapy. She now kisses her mother goodnight and sleeps through the night for the first time. This is another sign of internalisation of a good containing object who bears her anxieties and allows her to dream during the night.

Although Nina is still one year developmentally behind her peers in terms of language, her comprehension is good. After twenty-one months in therapy she is beginning to focus on learning and reading some basic words. She also draws using basic skills of a three or four year old child. Perhaps what is most significant is that my gathering her terror, persecution, and hostility into the transferential relationship to me has permitted significant progress in her relationships with her parents and peers. She can show angry faces when kicking a ball towards me, but she can also show friendly smiles which extended to her peers. She was invited to lunch by several children, and she had some children over to her house to play. More importantly, Nina hugs her dolls, kisses her mother goodnight, and sleeps the night.

Nina was referred to us for feeding difficulties and she was able to gain weight, grow taller and stay at the table for a whole meal. Her trust in containing internal parents has enabled her to sit on the loo again, swim and trot on a horse. She has integrated her hostile feelings, and now she feels less persecuted and more physically integrated too. Her progress has been due to the therapy, but also to the improved relationship with her parents. I gave her mother a lot of homework to do each evening. The mother was to think about the day with Nina, draw story books of her life, play hide and seek, observe Nina and write a diary of her thoughts and observations about her. Here is one example of mother's writing:

> "I saw Nina was restless. I thought she might be cross, so I wondered aloud about what she might be feeling. She said, 'cross'. Then I wondered what it was about. "No school, no Jeanne." It was the weekend."

Noticing the changes in both herself and Nina, mother writes:

> "Thank you, Jeanne. The quality of our home life has been transformed during the past years. I have learnt an enormous amount by watching you and I can spot Nina's signals better even if I can't always resolve the problems. I am very grateful that you have allowed me in". Sometimes she is gentle, loving, rather than hyperactive (And mother clearly feels more she knows Nina better and feels more loving to her). She is happy to go to school. I responded, "In our telephone conversations you have given me suggestions and asked questions about the meaning of Nina's behaviour. Your knowledge of Nina is better than mine and I am grateful for the notes and observations you have made. It helped me to understand Nina and work with her. It also helped to have you wondering with me about what Nina was doing and why I was responding to her as I did." At the end of two years of therapy, Nina's father also wrote a note saying thank you and indicating he would like to write about what he learned about Nina during these years when the parents and Nina were involved in psychotherapy.

There are still numerous problems which Nina must work out both within herself and in her relationships with others. One thing that remains complicated for her is the acknowledgement that the mother needs the father, that father has a helpful function for the baby and that father is allowed to make babies with the mother. This involves giving up the notion: "Mummy is just for me." Nina will be able to do this as she develops within herself a definite inner presence of a containing and loving mother-therapist. *Introjection of a containing and loving mother-therapist* with whom she can identify encourages the capacity to be separate, to think for oneself, and to be fully oneself (Waddell, 1998). Maria Rhode (1999) suggests that enabling the child to become reunited with hidden parts of the self and find her authentic voice, permits the child to think and find language. Nina has indeed begun her journey towards *having a voice*.

PART III

YOUNG PEOPLE

CHAPTER EIGHT

Extended family explorations using dreams, drawings, and play when the referred child does not speak

Jeanne Magagna

Henri Rey in *Universals of Psychoanalysis* states that "what patients think they are coming to treatment for and that which emerges in the course of treatment could be very different" (Rey, 1994, p. 229). He goes on to say that people may be asking for "an improvement", while the real request is how to bring about reparation of some threatened and dying internalised family members. Without such reparation of some damaged mentalizing functions of the internalised parents, the individual referred child cannot function normally and happily. Psychic reparation of mentalizing functions may be required, not only in the individual child, but also within family relationships.

Most frequently, when parents perceive that their non-speaking child is having a difficulty or they are having a difficulty with their non-speaking child, they refer the child for individual psychotherapy and sometimes for speech therapy. They are bringing *something which needs repairing in the child.*

In this particular chapter, I am referring specifically to families where the severely regressed and withdrawn child is not talking, walking, or eating; however, the chapter is equally pertinent to families with children who are simply not talking for various reasons. Out of concern for the child, it is important to offer 2 or 3 individual psychotherapy assessments for a non-speaking child, who obviously may still be able to think, regardless of whether or not he is speaking and thus still deserves to have a thoughtful person thinking about the emotional situation in which the child finds himself. Out of respect for the nature of the difficulties which require repair, I believe it is also essential to create an adequate mental space for looking at family relationships within the entire family, including all siblings and anyone living with the family. Family explorations are useful to ascertain which aspect of the emotional relationships within the external and internal mental life of the family require repair. Family explorations are also useful to discover the family strengths which can be used to facilitate development of the family's capacity to think together about emotional experiences.

All of us know from our experiences in infant and young child observation that mental maneuvers develop as a method of dealing with anxiety. A mouth closed to speaking, closed to food and a child's legs that have stopped supporting the child are problematic symptoms indicating the child's failed efforts to deal with anxiety and overwhelming emotions. One of the primary aims of the individual assessment meetings with the child is to understand the nature of the child's *internalised* family relationships. I would like to stress that I feel doing this alone is inadequate! It is also essential to make a formulation of the child's *external* family relationships and anxieties which either support and or interfere with the child's normal psychological development. It is essential for the individual child psychotherapist to work alongside a colleague who will do the parental and/or family exploration and therapeutic work required to support the child's re-entry into his developmentally appropriate life in both his family and school.

The aim of the extended family exploration is to fully understand *that which the family brings for repair.* I also am a firm believer that, alongside individual psychotherapy for a child who is not talking, walking, or eating, it is essential to have ongoing regular therapeutic work with the parental couple, either alone or together, regardless of whether or not they are separated or divorced. I say this because children require their parents to not only nurture and protect them but also to hold their emotions, give meaning to them and help them to think about their emotional experiences day by day. The aims of individual child psychotherapy can best be met by parental work and some family work supporting the individual psychotherapy. With this in mind, I never offer individual psychotherapy to a child without stating that the way to repair the difficulties is for the parents and I to work together to help the child and themselves find ways of sorting out the difficulties which are occurring. I am firm that these are the conditions under which I work: a two-fold, effective approach rather than a one-armed, half-baked approach to problem solving alone with the child not talking, walking, or eating. I would say this regarding every child who is not-talking.

Now I shall explore some concepts in extended therapeutic family explorations designed to discover *that which the family unconsciously brings for repair.* Following these individual and family therapeutic assessments a formulation of *what requires repair* and *how it can be best undertaken* should be given to the family.

I suppose one can choose whether the extended exploration occur within one or two days or in several weeks of 1 ½ hour family therapeutic exploration sessions. I have worked in two institutions, *Great Ormond Street Hospital for Children* and *Family Futures Adoption and Fostering Consortium,* who offer extended therapeutic assessments lasting four to five hours in one day followed by another day or days in which the family feeds back their thoughts which arose. After the therapeutic extended family exploration there is a formulation of the family issues, a proposal for a therapeutic care plan indicating time, frequency, nature of therapy proposed and dates for regular reviews of therapeutic progress.

In an audit of family feedback, families have been very clear that the deep engagement with the professionals over an extended period time in two days has helped the parents to become more fully aware of some of the family's anxieties and ways of coping with them. They have felt more contained by the lengthier period of time during the whole day which allows an enlargement of the family *thinking space* without the interruption of a week between meetings which prompts the erection of defences linked with stopping the process of conversing with the therapists. In our work with parents, we have found that a letter following the assessment, rather than just a conversation, helps the parents to delineate what they need to work on during the course of therapy. Parents often told us that the *written letter* was one of the most helpful aspects of the assessment because they could refer to it again and again. It is helpful to address one letter specifically to the referred child who is not talking, walking or eating to read when the time is appropriate.

I shall now describe a basic structure for extended family explorations using twelve approaches, including *drawings, dreams, drama and play,* to engage with family members surrounding the non-talking, non-walking, non-eating child.

Aim of the family explorations

The aim of these meetings is:

1. To help family members *name and regulate their emotions*.
2. To help each family member to stand in the emotional *shoes of one another, and particularly in the shoes of the non-talking child.*
3. To create a containing space in the family to voice and to tolerate the hostility and other negative emotions which arise in intimate relationships.
4. To pay more attention to the *family patterns* of turning to each other for support or avoiding seeking help when in difficulty.
5. To think about how each person and the family itself processes emotional experiences.
6. To think about how intimacy is shown or impeded by various emotional issues.
7. To understand, using one's countertransference, how family conflict is evaded, projected into others or contained with family relationships.

(Magagna revision of ideas of Dallos, 2006)

Techniques that can be used in explorations with a non-speaking child's family

1. *Evenly suspended attention; giving attention to one's countertransference while each family member's contribution is observed*

Research into siblings of a very ill or problematic child, such as the non-talking, non-walking, non-eating child, suggests that the siblings will definitely require the parents or professionals to attend to how they perceive and are affected by their sibling's serious retreat from life. Otherwise, a sibling of the non-talking, walking, eating child may become the next symptom bearer. In fact, it does seem crucial to keep *an evenly suspended attention* during the family assessment to ascertain what psychotherapeutic treatment is required for different individuals in the family. Sometimes, the non-talking, walking, eating child presented for treatment *may not be the only child* in need of psychotherapy. For example, in the situation where the non-talking, walking, eating child has been bullied and hurt by a sibling, the bullying sibling(s) may also require some therapeutic intervention in relation to guilt about a sibling becoming so very ill. Siblings of the non-talking, walking, eating child are often traumatised by the parents' anxieties surrounding the child's difficulties, and for this reason it is essential to offer the siblings time to think about the emotional impact of the family crisis on them. The therapist's evenly suspended attention and use of the countertransference is required to intuit and to clarify in detail the repair work to be done for the inner child of each family member, and the repair work required within the family process of interaction itself. It is important to imagine that the child's not-talking, not-walking, not eating *could be* symptomatic of some overwhelming emotions needing containment within the entire family system.

2. *Description of the presenting problem and how it affects various family members*
Generally it is helpful to ask the parents what the non-talking, walking, eating child and the other siblings have been told about the extended family exploration. The speaking siblings can answer and then the parents can complete the information for them. It is useful to note if the parents have been able to adequately prepare the family members for encounters with the therapists or if they only told them at the last moment for fear of creating anxieties. Following this each member of the family can be asked the nature of his/her relationship with the non-talking, walking, eating child. It is useful to explore what the conflicts are between them, what the quality of closeness is between them and what the quality of their friendship is, if there is one. What impedes the creation or continuity of intimacy with the non-talking, walking, eating child? How does the child's not talking, walking or eating affect them?

> *Example*: A three-year-old non-talking, non-eating girl was referred to the clinic. She also masturbated. When the mother was asked about what she did about the masturbating, she said she shouted at the girl, stopped the masturbation, and felt very angry because her daughter would then resume her masturbating with more intensity. The father was asked how he responded when he saw this scene between the mother and daughter, father said he simply observed them both, but he felt upset with the shouting. When asked in what other ways the couple was affected by the child, mother said she and her daughter slept together, father slept elsewhere because their daughter cried if she was not sleeping in the parents' bed. Father was asked how he felt about this. He said he felt left out.

3. *Narration of the various stages of life of the identified patient and family members*
With older family members, each person is asked to draw a picture or show a photo of the non-talking, non-walking, not eating child from any age of the child's life. Then the family is asked to jointly tell the story of the non-speaking child's life from conception onwards with the therapists encouraging different people in the family to share details of what they remember about different developmental phases of the child's life from conception, to naming the child, to developmental milestones 0–5/5–11/11–16 years. Also, it is helpful to ask the parents and other family members to describe a little about what they experienced in relation to the non-speaking child during those developmental phases. Then the therapists can wonder how family life changed at different times during the child's life. If the non-speaking child is willing to signal in response, family members might ask the non-speaking child to signal through lifting

a finger or blinking twice if the family members are wrong about something. The family will know if there is any gesturing of eyes, hands, legs that they might use as a signal that they are on the right wavelength of the child as they tell the child's story.

It is also possible to look at sibling relationships through conscious messages to each sibling at different phases of one's life.

Example: The therapists can ask each child to make a family developmental relationship chart. Then *three developmental stages for the self* can be earmarked in relation to siblings each of whom can be represented by buttons:

- Describe how it was with Johnny (the non-speaking child) when you were one to five years.
- Describe how it was with Johnny when you were six to eleven years.
- Describe how it was with Johnny when you were eleven to eighteen years.
- What did you do together then, what didn't you like about each other, what did you like about each other?
- Write the major loving and hostile messages that you would give to Johnny at these three different times of your life.

The same questions can be asked about the siblings, apart from Johnny, in relation to each other. One can also ask the parents similar questions in relation to the non-speaking child.

Example: Ask each parent to describe their life at the age of the non-talking, walking eating child and describe their sibling relationships and relationships with their parents when they were the age of the non-talking child. Ask each parent: Which sibling position most closely represents your own sibling position in your own family of origin, for instance, were you the youngest child, the middle child, the oldest child? The main point of this question is "With which sibling roles taken by your own children are you most identified because those roles are most similar to your own roles within your family of origin?"

Maria, aged eleven, had one younger brother who was non-talking, non-walking, non-eating, Johnny, aged nine. The mother, Sarah, in creating messages for her own siblings in her own family of origin, identified with Maria. The mother, Sarah, also had a younger brother, and the mother felt she had been neglected when the younger brother was born. These are the words the mother spoke in imaginary conversations with her own younger brother:

0–5: You stole my mother and my playmates' attention away from me.
6–11: I knocked you down when you got on my bicycle or bike.
12–15: It wasn't fair that everything I did, you did better. I didn't want to talk to you much.
16–17: It was nice to talk about friends and school things with you.

Mother's dream: I recently had a dream I was in the plane with my younger brother and he fell out.

In this exercise, although consciously the mother, Sarah, has developed a more loving relationship with her younger brother, her dream expresses a residue of competitive and hostile feelings towards him (dreaming of the brother falling out of the plane) which might interfere with the way the mother, Sarah, protects her younger son, non-speaking Johnny, from his older sister Maria's nasty teasing of him. In other words, parental identification with the older, middle, or younger role of a particular child might create some obstacles in relating well to a certain child in the family. In this situation, mother had some unresolved competitive issues in relation to a younger brother, and these needed consideration in order that mother could become closer to her son, non-talking, non-walking, non-eating Johnny.

4. *Genealogy and family network: drawing the close family, extended family, supportive friends*
Encourage the children to make a joint family tree of all the family members and supportive friends surrounding the family. The friend network is especially important for single parents. How were the parents and other children impacted upon by the developmental changes of the non-talking, non-walking, non-eating Johnny? Ask the whole family about family deaths (including miscarriages), physical illness, psychiatric illnesses of family members in the extended family, including divorces. You can ask a family member, preferably a child who is old enough, to draw the family tree emphasising longer lines for distance in relationships, crosses for deaths, and the usual vertical line over a horizontal line to symbolise divorces or separations. Try to engage each family member in saying as much about other extended family members' personalities as possible.

The point in doing the genogram is to see family patterns of attachment in particular. Here is a series of questions to ask the family members, including parents and their children about the parents' family of origin (Dallos, 2006, pp. 166–167):

1. How would you describe the *emotional atmosphere* in the paternal/maternal grandparents' family? Cold, distant, warm? There might be disagreements requiring examples to facilitate discussions regarding this.
2. What happened when you were/are in distress?
3. How would you describe your relationship with your mother/father?
4. Who are you closest to in your family?
5. What happens when you are close? What happens when you are distant?
6. What is the difference between the paternal and the maternal grandparents' families? How do they show sadness or hurt, how do they show love? How do they show anger?
7. Ask each parent and the siblings: how are you *different* with your children to how your parents were with you? How are you *the same* with your children as your parents were with you?

5. *"Little chair" exercise in identifying with the non-talking, non-walking, not-eating child*
Sometimes, although extremely withdrawn and ill, the referred non-speaking child feels that meeting the psychotherapists is like being hauled into the court-room in front of the judge. The child feels his being very ill and not-talking, walking or eating makes his family view him as "being a problem" rather than "having a problem that needs repairing". Often, these therapeutic family therapy explorations free the non-talking, walking, eating child because the child feels the therapists are trying to get to know the whole family: their love, their hate, their hope, their strengths, their weaknesses and difficulties. Although the non-speaking child may remain sullen, he may feel grateful that the family's emotional climate is less blaming

and improving through the family explorations. The child's not-speaking may contain many distressing issues about which all the family feels compelled to be mute. At some point, the therapists need to note, "Even though your child is not speaking, there are emotional experiences which can be *given a name* in the family".

I will give you an example of how I work with the family of a non-speaking referred child. First of all, I always have a little chair in the room available to me to represent the vulnerable part of someone in the family. I place the little chair beside any family member and I might sit in it or ask a family member to place the little chair beside someone in the family.

Clinical example: non-talking, non-walking, non-eating Peter, 14 years old

Here is Peter, 14, in a family session with a younger and older brother and his parents. He is hunched over with his head in his hands, not speaking. Tears are rolling down his face. No one in the family answers my question: "I wonder what is the matter?" It is clear that Peter is in "not-speaking" mode. I position a little chair right beside Peter and I ask father to sit in it. I ask father to speak as Peter in first person. "Why might you be crying?" Busy businessman father changes from being rather cold and intellectual to saying in a softer voice, "I want to be understood. I want more time together with the family."

I then ask Emanuel, the sixteen-year-old brother, to "be Peter". "What are you worried about?" I ask Emanuel. Emanuel says in a younger-sounding voice, "I am worried about my parents not trusting me." Emanuel looks very sad as he is speaking. I ask Emanuel, being Peter, "Does your mother know why you are so sad?" Emanuel says, "All the others in the family are probably just as sad."

Mother starts crying and wiping away tears. I gently say to her, "Try to stay with the tears." Mother says to non-talking, walking, eating Peter: "Your illness is a reflection of sadness in the family." Father joins in and says to me, "The family has been sad since last summer." Father goes on to talk about himself, "No one is interested in what I am feeling. No one cares about what I am feeling."

As the session goes on, the family describes how the table at home is filled with mother's work and no one eats together. Academic studies, sports, music, and surfing on the web have filled everyone's life, and everyone in the family feels sad because each person feels no one cares about him or her. Alongside this is evidence that each of the parents are secretly thinking of divorcing the other. The family's unspoken shared sadness and loneliness has been projected into the identified non-talking, walking or eating child Peter, putting him into a hopeless, silent sadness.

Often a young person as ill as Peter starts out by getting a viral infection and stopping eating. Alongside this there is some angst, some trouble or depression and a feeling no one really understands what he is experiencing. If hospitalisation occurs and the child is separated from his parents, this is often traumatic in itself when the ill child does not have the psychological capacities to be separate from the parents. When the sense of despair is overwhelming the child collapses into dissociation, bodily limpness. Feeling helpless to make any change in either his external or internal emotional situation, the child gives up, not talking, not walking, not eating and in extremely adverse internal crises, maybe not even moving. Although the child may be given a diagnosis of *pervasive refusal syndrome*, I prefer not to use this term which may lead the child and others to feel that the child has had a choice to retreat, rather than feeling terrified and retreating from unbearable external or internal emotionally or physically turbulent situations (Magagna, Chapter Twelve). I say the child is *pervasively retreating from life*.

> The child gives up and retreats into not-thinking and not-talking in the context of family relationships. The child's non-speaking might be linked with denied feelings which can not be spoken about or have just been "sensed" by the young person who feels no inner freedom or capacity to think about the feelings and then put words to what is "being sensed" emotionally. As I reflect on the extreme behaviours of not talking, walking, or eating children who have given up hope, I become aware of intergenerational silences, family silences, and the child's dissociation, withdrawal from unbearable pain, and retreat from "family secrets".

I would like to stress that sometimes *it is simply* that the child has experienced a physical illness or a physical or social developmental crisis, bullying or change of schools and the child did not have the inner psychological capacities to bear these difficult situations and therefore retreated into not talking, walking or eating. But, it is important to keep in mind that there could possibly be abuse of some kind from inside or outside the family. When the family has no system of interaction which involves family members in being mindful of other family members feelings, trying to understand them and speaking about them, there is an overload of feelings which *drown the* referred non-speaking child.

One non-talking, non-walking non-eating young person lived in a family in which all members coped through manic denial of feelings. When she finally began to re-enter life and speak she said, "I felt like the toilet pipes were bursting. I felt I was going crazy. I was so confused, angry, unhappy I couldn't cope. I *had to* stop speaking, I *had to* stop eating. I *had to* turn away from others, my family, my friends." For this girl, she had "to close up"… for there was a sense of accumulating traumatic, destructive experiences for which she had no adequate inner psychic structure and no family mentalizing structure to facilitate bearing and understanding destructive emotional interactions in her shouting, quarrelling family.

The child who "gives up" and feels "dead-alive" may have experienced trauma from projections from the family or external people as well as feeling the internal trauma of being overwhelmed with feelings for which there is no adequate inner psychic apparatus to think about them and digest them. Such a child has sensations and feelings which cannot be symbolised, verbalised, described, or mastered.

There are major limitations to what can be achieved using ordinary verbal communication with such a child. The first therapeutic work involves receiving projections of the child's states of mind, holding the child's feeling in oneself, trying to puzzle over it and give it a name and then think about what the child is feeling.

6. *The use of spontaneous play by young children or structured drama in the session*

The unconscious mental life of the family, the anxieties and sentiments therein are often simultaneously given expression by young children's spontaneous play as the other family members are speaking in the family exploratory sessions. For this reason, I provide play materials in the centre of the room and comment on how the children's play or drawings may be used as a commentary on the nature of the interaction and the anxieties existing in the encounter between the family and the therapists during the exploratory sessions. In *Rescripting Family Experiences* (Hills, 2000), I provide many examples of the therapeutic interventions made in relation to children's *structured spontaneity* in the family session. Children's spontaneous play can *elucidate or can be used to evade or project* the family's feelings present *at that moment* in family's experience in the exploratory session.

I also ask children to dramatise what happens at home at a particular moment in time, say after school.

> *Example*: In the family exploratory session, asking family members to show a particular moment Daniel, ten, and Jack, six, began sitting on top of one another fighting and Shirley, eight, pretended to be in her bedroom stamping her feet because she was angry (Magagna, 2000, p. 100).

7. *Using dreams in the therapeutic family exploration*

Looking at dreams might feel weird to some families, yet there is nothing like a family member's dream to tell you more about the family's *here and now unconscious experience* in relation to your consultation. The dream represents a privileged opportunity to explore a spontaneous narrative of an individual's inner mental life. The dream can be seen as a moment when a family member's infantile part, connected with activated memory of the past, communicates and gains insight into a person's state of mind. Each individual's artistic capacity to use both poetry and art is shared through the dream's inner narrative depicted through coloured static scenes, dramatic moving-pictures and discourse or poetry. The exploration of dream-life is an essential feature of psychoanalysis and psychotherapy. Dr Donald Meltzer's books *The Psychoanalytic Process* (1967) and *Dream Life* (1983) are helpful in understanding family members' dreams. For some families, understanding arrived at in sleep may have a greater psychic validity than those derived from the process of questioning and intervention by the therapist and may be experienced as more "true" (Sanders, 1994, p. 369).

Sanders (1994) describes these five types of dreams in family explorations:

i. *Dreams that precipitate therapy*

The dream may present concrete and explicit distress or dissatisfaction that has been masked in daily life.

> *Example*: A man dreams of being shot by riflemen. His association was that he thought marriage was killing him.

The couple did not discuss contentious issues within their marriage, but the dream showed the need to do so. All the man's aggression about the marriage not working was projected into the riflemen who could also represent members of the family.

I would advocate that children tell their dreams in the family session and that parents tell their dreams in the couple's session *without the children present* in order to show different generational roles in relation to the emotional life of the family. Parents need to think about their children's emotional life; however, I personally don't feel that children should take responsibility for understanding their parents' dreams.

ii. *Dreams that provide hypotheses*

The symptoms of non-talking, walking and eating as well as other family issues can be given further understanding through a dream or repetitive dreams. Family members are asked to make dream diaries which assist them in sharing experiences with the therapists who can explore certain common themes in the family's dreams.

> *Example*: A child repeatedly dreams of falling down the stairs. A family exploration of parental depression leading to "not being able to bear" the the child's pain follows the child's description of this dream.

iii. *Dreams as memories*

Sometimes children are able to bring nightmares which contain not only their own aggression projected into wild animals or monsters, but also traumatic family experiences which can be hidden through a dream-telling, but not talked about explicitly in a physically and/or sexually, emotionally abusing family.

> *Example*: Sharon, aged fifteen, brought a nightmare of being a terrified child victim of aggression by people and a poisonous snake. Exploration of the child's fears and the poisonous monster's actions led to further family explorations of what happened in the family with a verbally abusive, mentally ill father.

Such nightmares can be looked at in terms of the horror and fear in the sleeping process of living through the nightmare. In an exploratory session designed for the three siblings without the parents, the speaking children in the presence of the mute child can think more freely about the quality of their external sibling/peer relationships and parental relationships.

> *Another example*: Sharon, fifteen, then brought into the family session a nightmare of being chased by a very frightening bear in the forest.

This dreamer, Sharon, is very angry with her father. In a sibling discussion without the parents, Sharon's older brother felt safe enough to describe how the father has been hitting Sharon hard as a form of punishment when, in a fury of anger, he is out of control. Watching the older sister being injured by the father has been very traumatic for the non-talking, walking, and eating youngest child, Gemma, aged nine. Until Sharon reported this second nightmare in the sibling group, no one had been able to talk about the father's hitting of his fifteen-year-old daughter. The siblings had only talked about father's abusive comments in the whole-family exploratory sessions.

iv. *Dreams as pictures of internalised family relationships*

> *Example*: The above fifteen-year-old, Sharon, reported another dream: "My head is on fire. My mother saw me and just walked away."

Here Sharon is explicitly terrified that if she expresses her rage she will be abandoned by her mother. Sharon's dream could be a clue to her nine-year-old sister Gemma's "not-talking and not-eating". As one not-talking, not-eating girl later explained to me, "not-speaking" is a way of closing her mouth to self-expression for fear her mother couldn't take it. She said, "I just listen mutely to my mother rant. She couldn't take it if I talked back at her, anyway, if I did, I would just get a crazily furious mother!" There is a sense that when the family does not have the emotionally containing psychic structure to modulate expression of emotions there is muteness or rage.

v. *Dreams suggesting transformation in the psychic structure*

After the family extended exploration sessions, it would be possible to look at one expression of the family's internal psychic change by looking at the transformation within one family member's dream structure. One example of development would be integration of the dreamer's feelings rather than seeing aggressive and loving feelings projected into other dream characters or family figures.

> *Example*: Comparing fifteen-year-old Sharon's dream of her head being on fire with her earlier nightmare of a poisonous fish chasing her allowed me to see that she was beginning to acknowledge her aggression rather than projecting her own aggression completely onto her angry hitting father represented by the frightening bear chasing her.

How to interpret dreams that are brought to the family explorations:

- What are your thoughts about this dream … knowing your child as you do?
- That dream showed fear … what else do you feel your sister is afraid of?
- What other things might be causing fear in other family members, in you?
- What is the theme in the dream? For example, a violent father, dictating and punishing and a flamingly angry girl with her head on fire.

If one is existing in such an external situation, it would be hard to talk about it … but talking about a drama in a dream space allows a certain safe *freedom of speech*. The non-referred children may give many clues to traumatising experiences which may be affecting the non-talking, non-walking, non eating child.

I shall now describe an example of how I would work with a dream in the family extended exploration.

> *Example*: In the therapeutic family assessment, I generally begin by saying "In some places, people are used to talking about the way they make sense of their emotional experiences at night through their dreaming about them. Everyone has three or four dreams a night, but sometimes one doesn't have access to them. When you awaken in the morning, if you ask yourself very quickly, 'What did I dream?', after some time a dream generally occurs. Who in the family remembers a dream? It would help me to understand your family more if you would be willing to share it." Then I invite the person to share the dream and, if children

want to draw a dream or draw a *pretend dream*, I suggest they do this. I create an atmosphere of curiosity in which the family members can search for a theme in the dream. Following this exploration of the dream's theme, I try to link the dream-theme to the family's experience of being in an exploratory family session with me. As mentioned before, I would not usually have parents bring their dreams to family group, but this dream was about the child brought for therapy.

Example: Sarah, the mother from the earlier example, who dreamt of her brother falling out of a plane, brought another dream. She said: "I dreamt I was in an old, broken down hotel in Greece. My child, Johnny, was playing around and he fell out the window. When I went to recover him, I found that his head had been severed from his body. I bent down to stick his head back on his body."

The whole family is then able to associate to the dream, and each member is encouraged to say something about what it might mean to try to put *a head on a child's body*. Before I give the family's associations to the dreams, it might be useful for you, the reader, to think yourself about the question, "What family processes might be reflected in this dream?"

The family's associations to this dream about Johnny who was not-talking, not-walking, not-eating included:

The oldest child, Roberto says, "Mummy is worried about Johnny, he seems so different. She feels he has lost his normal mind, and she is putting him back together."

Maria says, "We are worried about what Johnny will do next, he has been scratching himself too."

The father says, "We have been rather preoccupied with our own work and lives and maybe a bit detached from knowing what Johnny was feeling before he stopped talking, eating, and going to school."

I suggest that they have all come because they feel they need to keep more in touch with the feelings in the family. A dream is brought to show their need and wish to get closer to knowing and thinking about what each of them, represented by Johnny, is feeling. Losing touch with feelings in the family seems a dangerous thing.

I don't think it is always possible to make a group interpretation about an individual's dream. In general, I suggest to the family that the feelings expressed in the dream brought to the session could be a reflection of the family group process of experiencing and thinking about feelings. The family members were detaching themselves from emotional difficulties and they are now *trying to do repair work*—to connect their heads to their feelings ... to think about the feelings existing within the family.

8. *The acknowledgement of transference and countertransference experiences during the family session*

In *Psychotherapy with Families* (Box, Copley, Magagna, & Moustaki, 1981), and in Gianna William's (2005) chapter "The destructive super-ego, a shared object in the dynamics of a family", there are descriptions of the use of the transference and countertransference with the family members. Throughout the therapeutic family explorations, I would do the following:

- Note how the family are talking about each other and the problem. Is there a predominance of love and concern for the others in the family or is there an atmosphere of insecurity, persecution by problems and harsh super-ego like criticism of one another and/or the identified patient?
- Verbalise my experience of the family's transference to the therapeutic exploration process in which we are embarking.
- Note family atmosphere, mood, unverbalised emotional experiences that arrive through body posture, gesture, tone of voice, look of eyes and family feelings projected into me during the family explorations.

> *Example*: Two girls, Grace, aged eleven, not-talking, walking, or eating, Antonia, nine, and one boy, Michael, seven, are sitting with their parents. All the children are sitting unusually still. I ask, "Who follows rules in the family, and what are some of the family rules?" Michael, the youngest child, starts giggling and sets off the oldest child, Grace, so that she begins to giggle. The children don't answer my question about the family rules. I suggest that they seem worried while they are with me and their giggling seems a way of dealing with the worry, whatever it is. Finally, I uncover the worry: there is harsh hitting in the family. The father, who drinks too much, hits the children hard and fiercely shouts at his wife and threatens desertion. Terrified because she has no viable work or income, the mother remains tyrannised by her husband and unable to protect either herself or the children. She also does not have any effective discipline because she has projected all her aggression into the father, therefore there is chaos and sibling maltreatment of each other when the father is not present in the home.

This has happened in therapeutic assessments with three different families, and it makes me wonder if often there is some connection between giggling and secrets and/or giggling and terrifying aggression in the family.

> *Example*: Here is another strange incident: my old English sheepdog who almost never barked till I taught her how to, barked loudly and incessantly from the side garden when a family was being assessed by me. I finally said, "My dog rarely barks, you can hear her barking now, and she is worried. I don't know what she is worried about. Do you have any ideas?" There was a long pause in which no one in the family spoke. I am always troubled when there is complete family silence... . It feels as though people have been silenced and are afraid to speak. The father finally said, "I have hit everyone in the family and they are afraid of me. I love them too, but I make them afraid when I am in a rage."

9. *Drawing a picture of a moment in the family's life together or button sculpt of a moment of family life*

> Paper, a writing pad, and felt-tips are presented to each family member. Family members can also choose to use doll or toy animal families, buttons, or plasticene to make a family sculpt. Each family member is asked to depict a moment in the family's life. This *moment in the family's life* will be delineated differently by each family member, and each of them will be doing the task separately. It is important to remember that the drawing hand has not been forbidden to draw that about which the non-speaking family member has been forbidden to speak.
>
> When the family members draw the entirety of the family in relation to one another in the family home, they express the unverbalised nature of their relationships. Looking at the drawings together enable them to gain new insights into each other's experiences of being in their family. If people are reluctant to draw, you can ask them to make a *family sculpt* through positioning family members in relation to one another and asking them to put certain expressions on the face, arms, and hands to fit the picture held regarding the family constellation. The other option is for a family member to simply draw an image or mould a plasticine sculpture image that can be used to represent the family.

I also ask each family member to draw a picture of him/herself at any age he/she would like, in any situation with the family. Sometimes the personal drawing shows an age-fixation. Somehow the child's drawing shows features suggesting that the psychological development became fixed during a particular developmental period of the child's life when a child experienced an internal or external trauma which was not given sufficient mentalization by the parents to help the child continue his/her normal course of development. A drawing of the eyes on a human figure can also show unverbalised terror or hatred, sadness or joy. Also, the family therapist can become alerted to the risk of emotional, physical, or sexual abuse through a group of significant signs in the family drawings. For this reason, I suggest that children can draw freely during the assessment with some good pens and pencils and with a

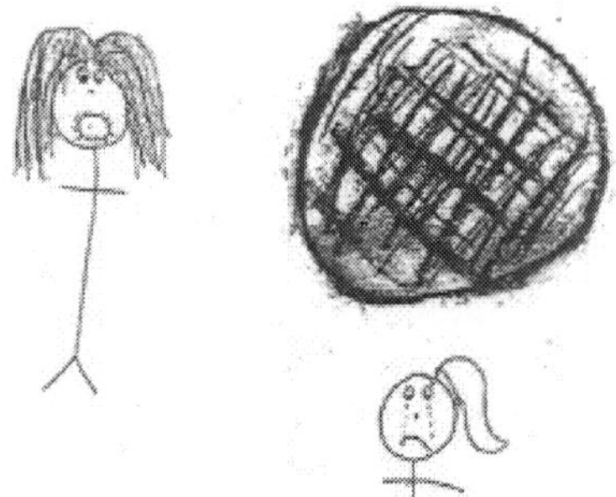

Figure 8.1 The sisters

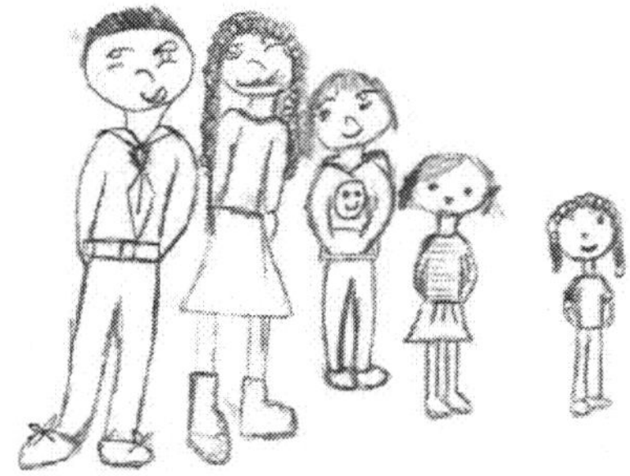

Figure 8.2 The family

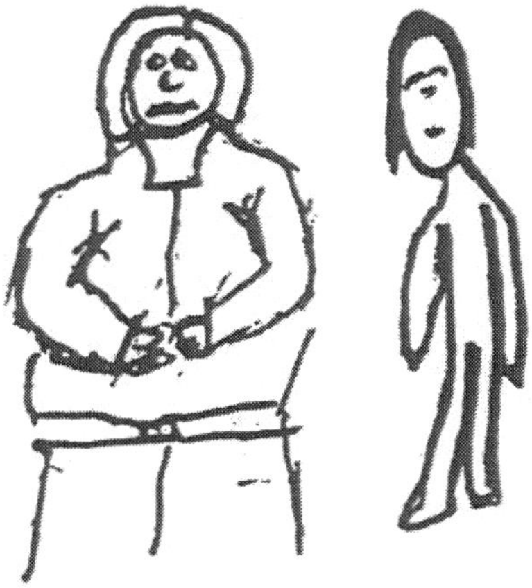

Figure 8.3 Inadequate self

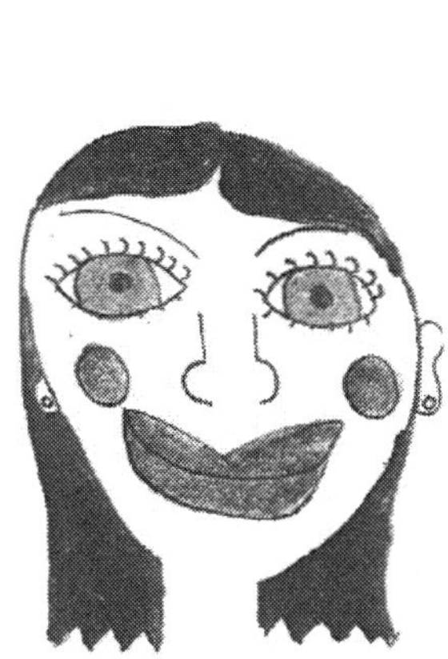

Figure 8.4 Traumatised self

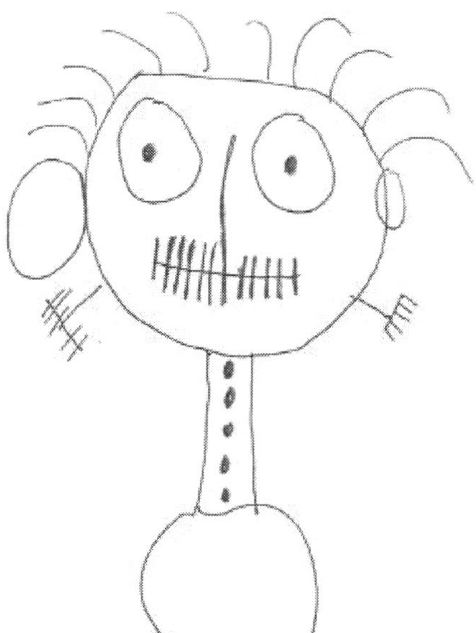

Figure 8.5 Scared self

writing surface provided or, if they are very young, a small table placed in the centre of the family circle.

The family will then probably need to think about making some depiction from the perspective of the child who is not talking, walking, or eating. Subsequently, each family member takes a turn describing his or her drawing or sculpt to the whole family group. The therapists assist by wondering about closeness, conflict, pleasure with each other. The *family home* functions as

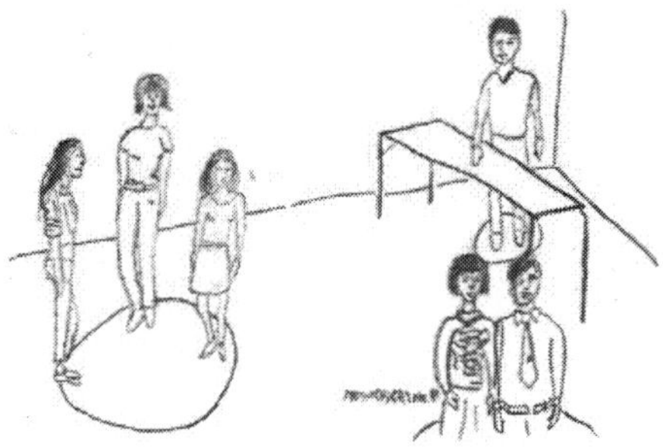

Figure 8.6 Isolated in family

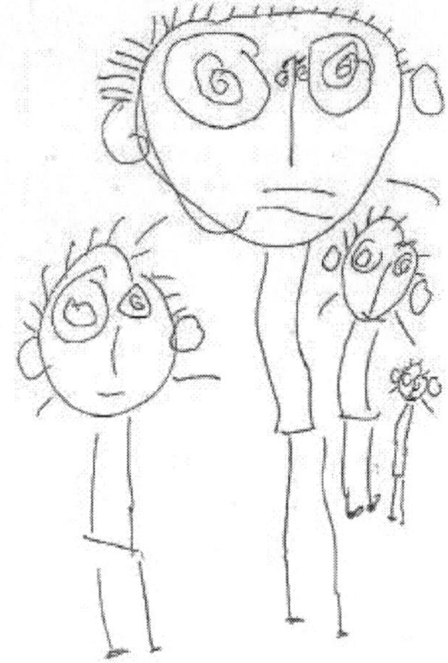

Figure 8.7 Worries in family

a containing space in which people congregate together or remain separate. In fact, these days, it is useful to describe the use of the mobile phone, facebook, texts, and how much these things keep the family members in touch with and/or apart from one another.

The therapists might introduce the task thus:

> "Before we talk any further, we would just like to get to know you as a family. We have brought all these supplies and we would like each of you to find a way of drawing a *moment in the life of your family*, or use buttons to place people in relation to one another, or use the plasticene, or the family dolls or animals. You may take five minutes or so to do the task. Then, can you share with the group what you have done. Afterwards, you will be asked to create some picture for anyone who has not contributed to this task. You can do this separately or jointly."
>
> The therapists could then explore. For example, using drawing (Figure 8.6), they could say, "How do you see Johnny's relationship with his sisters?"
>
> The therapists explore relationships depicted visually by each family member. In the exploration, it is important to ask each family member, "When you are distressed, what do you do?" (Note if the person doesn't trust any family member but turns only to people outside the family or only to the self.)
>
> - To whom do you turn if you have a difficulty?

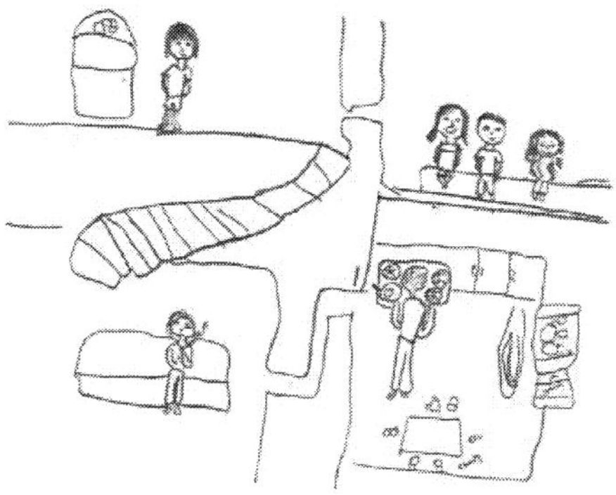

Figure 8.8 Not-together family

- If children are too young to answer questions, Jill Hodges's (2003) Story Stems can be used. The *Story Stem Approach* allows child to show attachment relationships using play scenarios set up by the therapists and set questions are asked.
- In what way does that person help you with your difficulties?
- In what other ways could family members be helpful to you when you are in difficulty?

Let us look at the ways of *helping the family* think further about the family drawings. I am implying that the task of the family extended exploratory sessions is to begin to develop a *family work group* (Bion, 1961) which engages in deeper thinking together about family relationships. The therapist's task is *not to interpret as much as to facilitate* the family members' capacity to observe and note the impact of a particular family artist's family drawing on other family members' perception of the family. The family artist can say some things about his/her own drawing ... but it is helpful to elicit thoughts from other family members, rather than simply asking the particular family artist to put words to his drawing which after all shows what he can't put totally into words! Raising some questions to facilitate the family members' observations can be helpful at times. Above is an example for you to consider (Figure 8.8.).

With the drawing above (Figure 8.8), I asked each family member why they had chosen that particular age, what their relationships with family and friends were at that age. I was struck by the fact that the drawing of the referred young boy and two sisters beside him were about five years younger than they currently were. I would ask people in the family to comment on the drawing and comment upon what they heard each person in the family saying about their own drawing. Once again, I am trying to help each family member identify with other family members' emotional experiences. As with the empty chair technique, I am asking each member of the family to stand in the other person's shoes and wonder, how does that person in the picture feel? I am also trying to facilitate empathy for the vulnerable part of each person and respect for each family member as an individual with strengths and weaknesses.

After spontaneous family responses, I ask the family to imagine what the not talking, walking, eating regressed child in the family might be feeling and thinking. I might then ask

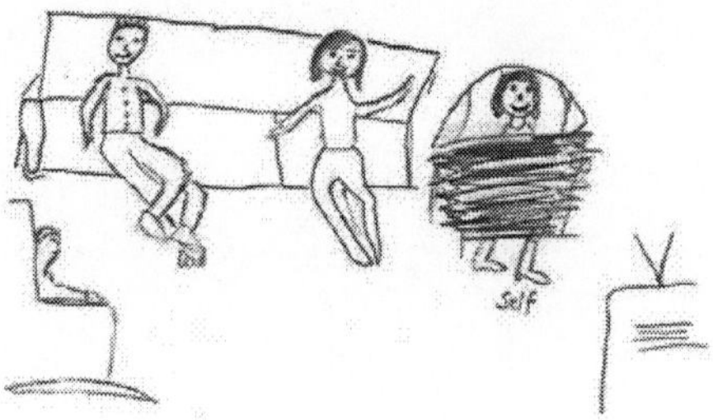

Figure 8.9 Scribble on self in family

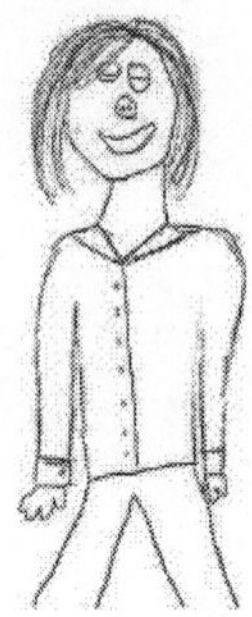

Figure 8.10 Unseeing self

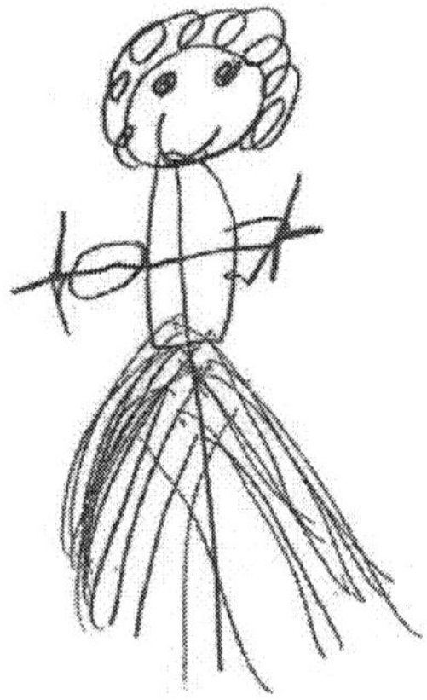

Figure 8.11 Conflicted body image

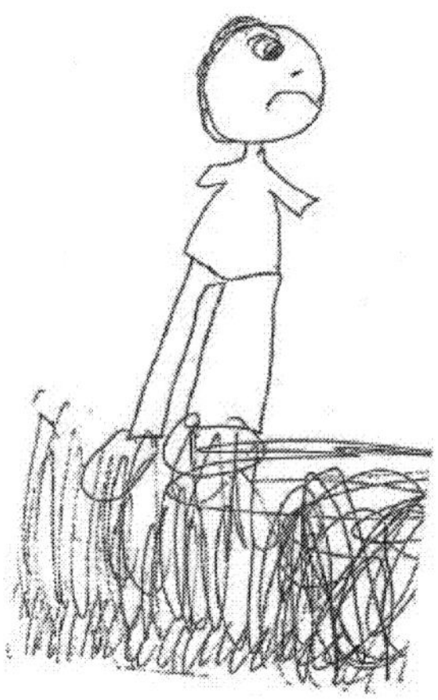

Figure 8.12 Aggression and fear

the not-speaking child, the boy in the centre of sisters (Figure 8.8), if the family understood, or was it something different from what they understood? The child may be able to nod or may remain completely unmobile (see Lask, Chapter One). Family members' human person drawings may be filled with body distortions based on projections of feelings which inform the nature of details in hands, feet, eyes, body size, and posture. Take a look at the drawings of the family and of the self on the next page (Figures 8.9 and 8.10).

Both dreams and drawings have been subject to research showing that they are good indicators of personal and interpersonal family functioning (Oster & Crone, 2004). Indicators of problematic areas in family functioning which require further exploration can be found in both dreams and drawings.

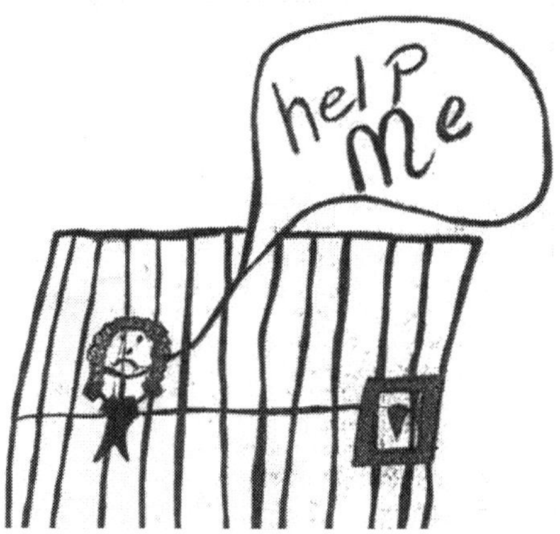

Figure 8.13 Alienation

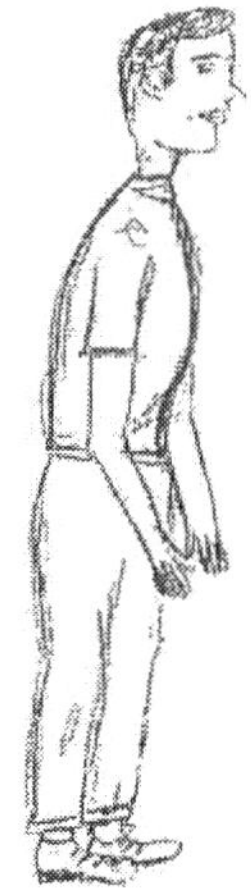

Figure 8.14 Older son showing identification with a loved, benevolent father

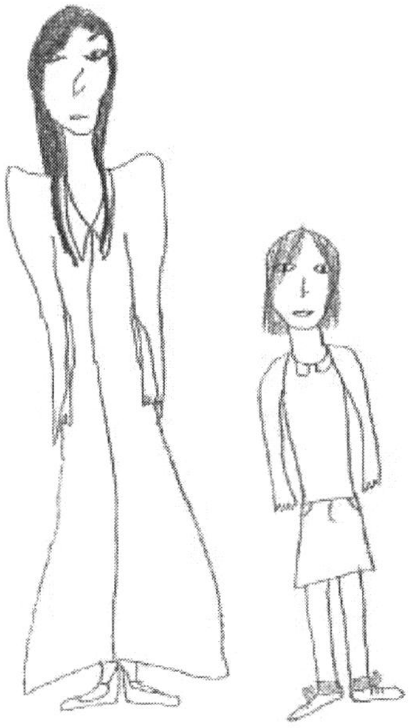

Figure 8.15 Sense of awkwardness in relation to a witchlike mother filled with girl's projections of hostility

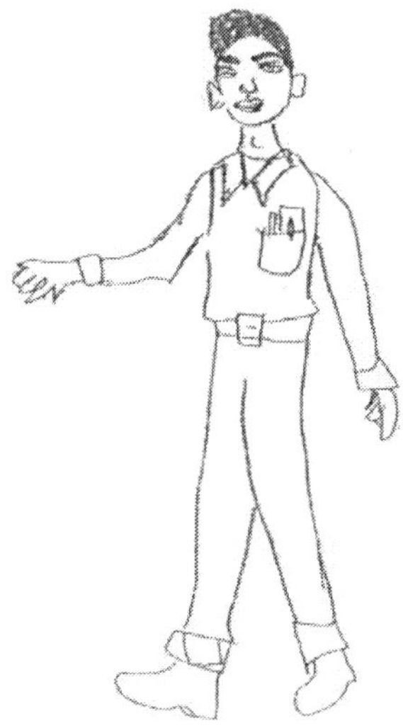

Figure 8.16 Older brother developing adequately

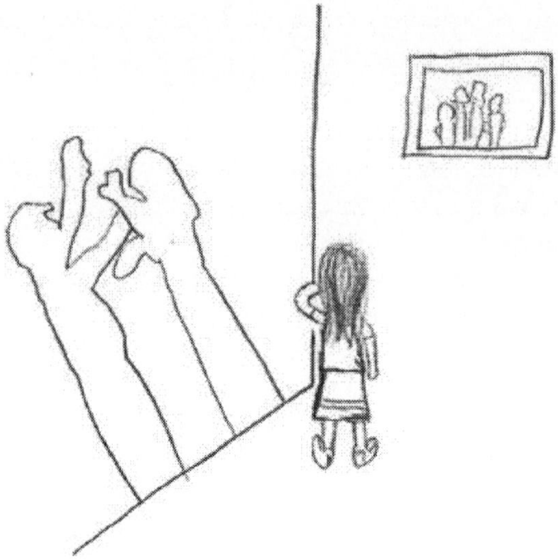

Figure 8.17 Parents physically aggressive to one another, neglecting child

Discussing dreams and drawings within the family can facilitate the opening up of effective communication and understanding between family members. The following indicators in dreams and drawings can be compared with later dreams and drawings in order to assess progress in psychotherapy (Kaplan et al., 1981):

a. the self-image of the dreamer or drawer if poor or inadequate or lacking in a positive outlook
b. the interpersonal relations of the dreamer or drawer if alienated, submissive, conflictual
c. the relation to role of the father, the paternal function, and to the father himself
d. the relation to the mother and to maternal authority
e. appropriate sexual expression, sexual development, and sexual identity
f. affect shown in the dream (too negative rather than reasonably optimistic); also note the capacity to show and modulate feelings, and the types of feelings such as anger, sadness, fear, happiness, and love

10. *Brainstorming by all family members*
I would ask each family member what else we need to think about in trying to gain a deeper understanding of the family.

11. *Making a formulation regarding family processes and referred child's individual internal world*
Before beginning to see a child for individual psychotherapy and the family for family work, a family formulation should be made to delineate those areas of family function which also *require repair* and firmly note *those family* strengths which can assist with the *work of repair.* The

McMaster Criteria of Family Functioning (Epstein, Bishop, & Levin, 1978, pp. 19–31) are useful in creating the formulation. These include:

a. The ability of family members to communicate in clear, concise and direct messages.
b. The appropriate allocation of family roles for effective problem solving. In particular, there should be a generational boundary in terms of assignment of appropriate roles for the children and the parents.
c. The family's capacity to respond with the appropriate emotional responses to individual family members needs for nurturance, protection and containment of anxiety.
d. The family members' capacity to be affectively involved and invested in each other's well-being as well as one's own personal well-being.
e. The kind of pattern adopted by the family to most effectively control behaviour and to establish clearly defined standards of behaviour and agreed-upon family rules.
f. I would like to add: the capacity of the parental couple to work together to meet each others' and the children's needs.

Conclusion

An offer of about four hours to six hours for various family group explorations allows a family way of thinking about emotional issues to evolve. In *Assessment in Child Psychotherapy* (Rustin & Quagliata, 2000), Beta Copley writes about "Family explorations". She describes how a family exploration is not only to relate directly to what is brought as a problem by the parents, but also to create a space in the family's mental life to gather together and think about shared and private personal experiences in family relationships. She describes how the reception and attention given by therapists to what is conveyed by the family draws on the model of containment. The therapist finds a space in her mind for the distress, conflict and family confusions and then returns them to the family, reconstituted into a more mentally and emotionally digestible form. (Copley, 2000, p. 126). Donald Meltzer and Martha Harris talked about positive family functions which include "generating love, promoting hope, containing depressive pain and thinking." (Meltzer & Harris, 1976, p. 425).

The intent of the extended therapeutic family exploration is to contain mental pain and understand the causes for hate, persecutory anxiety and despair. Hopefully there is also a diminution of projections of vulnerable or unwanted parts of the self into the non-talking, walking, eating child. The approach using children's drawings, family dreams and genograms, and dramatic techniques, like the small chair next to the identified non-speaking child, are designed for exploration and thinking about each family member's current preoccupations and strengths for promoting the well-being of the family.

> To be *truly myself*
> in my family
> What a gift that is.
>
> (Magagna, 2011)

CHAPTER NINE

Inpatient care of a child who does not walk, talk, or eat

Jo Guiney

> Michael lies motionless on the sofa, eyes barely open. He is discreetly watching other young people as they move around the room. He is crying a pained, repetitive, and rhythmic cry that has become an audible backdrop to daily life in the eating disorders unit he was recently admitted to. A nurse comes to gather the young people together as it is time for the evening meal. As the nurse approaches, Michael firmly closes his eyes and turns his head away from the room. His crying becomes louder, and he begins to scratch at his arm with the end of his naso-gastric tube. The nurse gently speaks to Michael, telling him it's time to go to tea. The crying becomes louder while the scratching becomes furious. The other young people look on with a mixture of expressions: concern, fear, curiosity, irritation, exasperation. Someone brings the hoist that is used to move Michael in and out of his wheelchair, and with its arrival, his body becomes stiff. The nurses struggle as they move Michael into an upright position. Some parents waiting just outside the room look silently on, their alarm barely concealed. As he is hoisted into the chair, Michael jolts violently. Tears run down his face as he shakes his head from side to side, silently signalling: "No! No! No! NO!"

When encountering a child who has withdrawn from the world, we naturally feel the urge to help, to do anything within our means to coax the child out of their entrapment, their shell. When attempts to do this are met with angry defiance, it can be quite a shock. The child's withdrawal from everyone and everything in life challenges us on many levels: it can frustrate, it can eat away at empathy, it can stir up wishes to retaliate with neglect or anger. Caring for a child whose capabilities are only utilised in order to fend off anything that might help him reconnect with the world can be baffling, disorientating, and deeply challenging. It can expose in sharp relief the usual nursing assumption about helping: that someone wants to be helped.

This chapter is based on my experiences of working as a therapeutic careworker and keyworker to children, like Michael, who were in various states of withdrawal from life.

All of the children resided in a child and adolescent inpatient unit specialising in the treatment of eating disorders. Refusal forms a fundamental component of the presentation of eating disorders, this much is clear. However, this chapter will be based on experiences of working with non-speaking children who profoundly retreat from life when feeling hopeless and helpless. This syndrome has been labeled as *pervasive refusal syndrome* (Lask et al.) but actually it is basically *a pervasive retreat from life* or *a pervasive regression*. The withdrawal from life spreads across multiple domains of eating, drinking, walking, talking, and self-care. The style of therapeutic work within this particular treatment milieu is explored in relation to a pervasively regressing child, Michael. In writing about my experiences with Michael, a particular approach to treatment will be outlined, which is based on *an acceptance of the child's current state of withdrawal from a terrifying world and the minimising of expectations placed on him over and above non-negotiables, that are clearly delineated, predictable, and consistent.* "Non-negotiables" refers to those aspects of care or participation in treatment that are held as an expectation of the child, in spite of the child's wish to completely withdraw from life. Such an approach might be utilised in approaching the care of silent children in widely differing states of retreat from life throughout their recovery. This is linked with the amount of terror and helplessness that the child experiences. As simple as it may at first sound, such an approach can go against the grain of the usual ways of caring for unwell children and cause a great deal of tension and anxiety in the multidisciplinary clinical team, and wider inpatient group. It is, however, an approach to a non-speaking, pervasively retreating child, Michael, that ensures physical safety while at the same time granting the space required to contemplate change.

I hope to capture two important aspects of working with a child who pervasively retreats. The first is to give a sense of the practical tasks involved in giving structure to the provision of sensitive care. The second is to provide an account of the subtle interactions that are the delicate fabric of such a structure.

With regard to the second aspect, it is of the utmost importance to make careful observations of the non-verbal interactions between staff and child. Only by maintaining curiosity about these interactions are the team able to reflect on possible meaning and gain insight into the child's experience. This understanding can then be used to gauge the child's needs and readiness for change, and the corresponding expectations that should be put in place by the nursing team.

To demonstrate the concepts involved in working therapeutically with a silent, pervasively retreating child, I shall provide scenarios of interaction between Michael and his therapeutic care workers and nurses. I will pay particular attention to the provision of care by a dedicated, patient, tolerant and persistent nursing team working collaboratively with a multidisciplinary team. A nursing team working in such a way provide a backbone of sorts to other therapeutic work, "holding" the child on a moment-to-moment basis.

Understanding pervasive retreat from life

At its most severe, pervasive retreat from the terrifying experience of living extends across the domains of nutrition, speech, movement, self-care, and social participation. Such presentations have been described in the psychiatric literature, and diagnostic criteria for a "new" *pervasive refusal syndrome* classification put forward (Thompson & Nunn, 1997). Lask and colleagues first used the term "pervasive refusal syndrome" in the psychiatric literature in 1991 when they described four cases of girls (aged nine to fourteen) who presented with "a potentially life-threatening condition manifested by profound and pervasive withdrawal from life. This includes a retreat from eating, drinking, walking, talking, or caring for themselves in any way over a period of several months" (Lask et al., 1991). Also noted in the subsequent literature (e.g., Graham & Foreman, 1995; Lask, 1996; McGowan & Green, 1998; Nunn & Thompson, 1996; Taylor et al., 2000) was the presence of a terror of treatment and dramatic social treatment and dramatic social withdrawal in these cases. Thompson and Nunn (1997) suggested specific diagnostic criteria for this syndrome, as detailed below.

Diagnostic criteria for pervasive refusal syndrome (Thompson & Nunn, 1997, p. 147)

1. Clear food refusal and weight loss
2. Social withdrawal and school refusal
3. Partial or complete refusal in two or more of the following domains: mobilisation, speaking, attention to self-care
4. Active and angry resistance to help or encouragement
5. No organic condition to account for the severity or degree of symptoms
6. No other psychiatric illness that could better account for the symptoms.

While causes for such a presentation remain unclear, they are likely to be complex and multiple. However, noted recurrently in associated literature are the themes of hopelessness and helplessness. For example, Nunn and Thompson (1996) have postulated that the child's *pervasive retreat from life* is a response to events perceived by the child to be uncontrollable (e.g., the death of a family member, abuse in any form, conflict between others, or family migration). Using Seligman's (1990) model of learned helplessness, whereby the learned expectation of having no control over events in the environment is met with a generalised passivity response, they speculate that interactions between the child and events in their environment can result in the child experiencing profound helplessness and consequently, a loss of personal hopefulness. If this is the case, the word "refusal" is misleading, for the child is terrified to stay in the world and feels impotent in facing internal and external experiences, which he encounters through being present in the world and thinking about his emotional experiences.. Such a model is useful in explaining the deterioration of these children in the face of active attempts to rehabilitate them. If the children are experiencing the therapeutic interventions as coercive, then their sense of helplessness is reinforced.

While questions of aetiology are of great importance to our understanding of these children, I will not dwell on them, for my present focus falls within the area of treatment issues and how they relate to the minutiae of day-to-day care. Lask (2004) has outlined six "mainstays" of treatment of treatment for children *pervasively retreating from life*:

1. Patience, time, and sympathy
2. Basic nursing care offered by skilled staff
3. The use of the therapeutic ward milieu
4. Physiotherapy

5. Individual therapy in which the child's feelings are expressed non-verbally, and later verbally, understood, accepted, and modulated through the containing functions of the therapist.
6. Parental counselling/family therapy in which the family is supported to bear the family members' feelings, to try to understand them, and modulate them in order that they can be thought about rather than covered with symptoms.

In this chapter, I will focus on the first three components of treatment as outlined by Lask (2004), and an approach to delivering this treatment which can be broadly summarised as:

1. Totally accepting the child's current state of withdrawal from life and providing for complete comfort and safety of the child
2. Minimising expectations placed on the child and bearing not-knowing
3. Creating clearly delineated, predictable and consistent non-negotiables.

Such an approach can be utilised throughout the care of a child who presents in widely differing states of withdrawal from life and gradually recovers a capacity to live according to norms appropriate for their age and maturity.

A therapeutic approach to working with a silent, pervasively retreating child

Phase one: "You say go forward, I'll go backwards"

> The young people are gathering in the sitting area getting ready for the Morning Meeting. Previously, Michael spent the meetings lying on a beanbag, but on this occasion he is sitting upright, supported by cushions, at the end of one of the sofas. A member of staff who has been on leave the previous week enters the room. Upon seeing Michael she exclaims "Michael how lovely to see you sitting on the sofa with the other young people!" Michael's head slumps to the side and within 10 minutes of the beginning of the meeting he has slid off the sofa and onto the floor.

It was a challenge to staff's sense of utility and professional pride when words of encouragement, usually effective with other young people, were met with Michael's marked regression of competence. Such is the recurrent experience of staff directly praising or showing pleasure in the development of a profoundly retreating, silent child. This seems to occur because the silent child is using *pervasive retreat* as a protection against becoming part of healthy life encounters. The slightest hint of praise or even a fleeting recognition of change can trigger its immediate disappearance. In this sense, the usual ways of working therapeutically with a child, using encouragement, incentives, and praise, are not simply rendered useless, but apparently toxic to progress. It follows that nurses involved in caring for such a child can feel truly at a loss and, like the parents, rejected, redundant, and hopeless.

The myriad responses to a silent, to a silent, pervasively retreating child naturally present challenges for any inpatient team responsible for his care. Responses can be as varied as they are intense, ranging from the wish to protect and cocoon the child, to feelings of intense frustration, to a desire to punish. Outside this range of feelings can be a dangerous *lack* of responsiveness to the child: the sense of giving up, feeling hopeless and futile, being unable to think. It is therefore essential to recognise and name one's countertransference responses (Heimann, 1950), and to try to think about them with team members in order to develop insights into the internalised relationships of the child. These responses might also facilitate some understanding of the parent's reactions to the child and those of the wider family. The silent and retreating child, by being in this condition, can be seen as providing a residence for projected vulnerabilities and unspoken feelings of family members. Since this is likely replicated in an inpatient setting, it is important to understand the projections of staff and other young people onto the child in order that they are not carrying such an emotional burden for the group.

Time and space therefore need to be given to those working with retreating children to carefully explore their perceptions of, and reactions to, the child. While this process must vitally involve the whole community, it is especially important for the nurses and carers who are at the front line of providing care. It is they who must bear the brunt of the near-continuous rejection of support that occurs in the care of a child retreating from eating, drinking, walking and talking. To take an everyday example, a nurse might be tasked with brushing a child's teeth. As straightforward as such an *action* may appear, it is in fact an *interaction,* and one that can be approached in many ways. The nature of approach and the interaction that ensues has an impact on both staff and child that should not be underestimated. Critically, it would seem that approaching such an interaction with a determination to "succeed" can trigger a more staunch retreat from life on the part of the child and, in turn, a sense of anxiety and having failed in the nurse. Giving space to reflect on these interactions, with attention to personal expectations and responses, can therefore serve to minimise the tremendous amount of anxiety such children can provoke in a nursing team.

Success is *not the child's compliance*; rather, it is initially *accepting a child's retreat from life* and simply *containing the anxiety* it provokes. Simple as this may sound, in practice it can be hugely difficult to resist the urge to "push" the child. Such an urge can have many motivations: the keyworker might feel desperate for the child and unable to seemingly allow her to languish in his condition; alternatively or together with this is a fear of appearing unskilled to other members of the team, and a wish to enable the child to "do" something. Such professional positions are to be expected in the climate of an inpatient setting where care plans are written, progress carefully charted and the regaining of health in all its senses is the explicit aim of therapeutic work.

However, expectations of success, of being able to "get the child to do something" can quickly corrode the sense of safety and emotional space so crucial in this particular therapeutic relationship. The setting of unachievable goals for the child retreating from a life which terrifies him can initiate a tug of war leaving both the therapeutic care worker and the child battle weary and hopeless. This being said, the idea is not to simply leave the child to his own devices, providing only physical care until he decides he is ready to change. While this stance would obviously remove any expectations that may have previously caused a regression, it could also carry the message that staff were giving up on the child. Such a message, while perhaps being in a sense congruent with how the child may be feeling, would only serve to cement the child's, the parents' and the multidisciplinary team's sense of helplessness. Rather, it is a patient, secure, trustworthy and understanding relationship that enables a silent, retreating child to begin to think and develop. It is such a relationship that allows a child to develop hope that life can be different from before and find the strength and ability to reconnect to life.

It quickly becomes clear that a delicate balancing of hope for health and recovery with low or even no expectation of progress is crucial. Such a balance requires continual adjustment of expectations according the to the child's shifting, developing and regressing capacities. Critically, the pace of change must be set by the child, and in most situations the child is not speaking and even if he were, would not initially talk about his feelings about changing. For this reason, those working closely with the child must utilise their responses and feelings in carrying out even the most minor tasks. It is through this attunement with the child's emotional state that a picture of the child's inner state can be painted little by little, guiding the levels of expectation, support and space required for both containment of the child's anxiety, wonderings, naming of feelings and curiosity within *both* the therapeutic care worker and the child.

Michael: early days

My first meeting with Michael was on his admission day. I had known for a couple of weeks that I would be his keyworker and, because it was important to work collaboratively with the parents, I had spoken to his mother on the telephone a couple of times in the weeks prior to admission. Michael's mother had given me an initial impression of Michael's emotional state during his current residence on a paediatric ward. The picture painted was sorry indeed: once bright and sociable, Michael had been steadily deteriorating over the preceding few months until he was not eating, drinking, walking, or talking. Currently, he was lying in bed day and night, either in an inert state or crying and scratching himself repetitively. Since his presentation was found to be disturbing to the other children on the ward, Michael had been moved into a private room where his state had remained unchanged for some weeks. His mother's outlook seemed one of battle-weary optimism. Her sense of desperation and impotence in helping her son were palpable, and yet she seemed to be approaching the impending transfer with hopeful anticipation.

Michael arrived at the inpatient ward in an ambulance accompanied by his parents and a nurse. I, along with some other members of staff who were to be involved in the admission, went out to greet them. Michael was taken out of the ambulance on a stretcher. Before I could see him, I could hear his loud, anguished cries. Looking worn and anxious, his parents were doing their best to soothe and reassure Michael as he was transferred, with a great deal of struggle, from a stretcher into a wheelchair to be taken inside. In the midst of this tumult, they somehow managed to greet me warmly. Michael's mother introduced me to Michael, saying that I was the "nice person" with whom she had spoken on the phone. At this point, Michael's cries became louder until they effectively drowned us all out. He looked about wildly, giving the impression of being in the grip of sheer terror about being separated from his family.

Michael's crying was so loud throughout the admission procedure that it split the gathered team and family into two parties: eventually his mother and the consultant psychiatrist met in a separate room, while I and a nurse remained with him and his father. Michael was intent upon sliding out of his wheelchair onto the floor, his cries filled with rage. His father would return him to his upright state and Michael would briefly cling to him before the process would begin over again. We helped his father keep him safely in the chair, something that caused Michael's cries to turn into piercing screams as though we were causing him some grievous pain. I was aware of feeling as though we should just step back, leave him to slip onto the floor, anything to lower his level of agitation and distress. I found myself exhausted by the noise and aware of its power of disruption, already evident in this breaking of the usual admission routine. At this point I wondered about how I might start to get to know Michael. For how long would he cry? Without the usual means of conversation, how might he get to know me, let alone trust me? I felt at quite a loss.

A subtle sense of contained chaos pervaded the first few days of Michael's admission: his mobility was far less than we had hopefully anticipated during the referral assessment, and his arrival successfully stirred up a flurry of anxiety in both the young people and the staff group. While the young people in the centre had been briefly informed about the forthcoming arrival of a new admission, something which always generated an atmosphere of curiosity and trepidation, some seemed quite overwhelmed by his presentation and repeatedly questioned staff about what was "wrong" with Michael. Some asked if he was "normal" and if he could hear and understand people. Seeing the naso-gastric tube in situ, others seemed alarmed or curious about his state, viewing it as akin to the "worst" form of an eating disorder. Answering such questions required a great deal of sensitivity with regard to his privacy and for this reason, to the young people he remained shrouded in mystery until some months in the future.

In the midst of the chaotic and anxious atmosphere, Michael's presentation stirred up, I began to notice that, in spite of his distress and his mostly keeping his eyes tightly shut, his glance did occasionally flicker across to me and then quickly away again. If our eyes met, he seemed to recoil into deeper distress, as though even this minute experience of social contact overwhelmed him. However, I detected a definite curiosity, a fleeting watchfulness that made me somehow hopeful that we could connect. It seemed that with unfamiliar people, the only level of interaction with which Michael felt safe was watching them, unobserved, from a distance.

Timetable—the importance of a flexible structure

By way of preparation, Michael's key nurse, the nurse consultant, and myself had worked on formulating a timetable of sorts for his arrival. This turned out to be a very useful endeavour indeed and a kind of "hook" to hold onto in the hectic first few days. Having some kind of written structure in place that could be referred to seemed to contain some of the anxiety around how best to approach caring for Michael. A clear, and detailed timetable was kept to hand in the nurses' office for quick reference purposes. "Timetable" is perhaps misleading in that at this stage it was more a plan of those activities in which we *would not* expect Michael to participate. It represented the bare bones of a structure that could be fleshed with our growing sense of his capabilities. This process in itself reflected the tone of much of the work to come: it was a seemingly paradoxical balancing act of tightly controlled structure and flexibility. For example, it was "non-negotiable" that Michael would be present in the morning meeting from the first day but would not be expected to attend school. The remaining time was left as "rest time" in which Michael was made comfortable on a beanbag in the communal sitting area. In this way, Michael had plenty of quiet time but was not isolated in his room all day and away from the group, who would come and go through the room throughout the day.

Each morning, Michael's allocated nursing team member would write up the timetable for the day while sitting with him, explaining aloud what would be happening. No changes to his own timetable would be made on a day to day basis but writing it up with him present was intended as a reminder of the structure of the general timetable and would also entail that he knew which staff to expect at which time of the day. This written timetable would then be left beside him and while he would not open his eyes to read it in the presence of staff in early weeks, he would glance at it when others were not sitting close to him.

At the end of the day, the same member of staff, who had spent most of the day with him, would sit with Michael and complete a Daily Review sheet. This consisted of a brief summary of the day along with something Michael had found particularly difficult (in the opinion of the staff member), and something that might have been experienced by him as less difficult or helpful. At the beginning of his admission, staff were careful not to point out any progress he was making but might write something about his having received a letter or a text from his Mum, or that he would be having a visit soon. Again, this process took place with the member of staff wondering aloud with Michael present, and it soon became evident that if we were off the mark with our ideas, his crying would increase or change to a more angry tone. With a little exploration in this way, it was an early way of communicating with him and showing him we were curious about his experience. This review sheet could then be used in the following day's meeting, a meeting based on the children and staff listening to one another's experiences. When it was his turn, Michael's allocated staff member would tell the community what they thought his previous day had been like for him, thus including him in the meeting, albeit once-removed, and this meant that the other children could also think about him.

Implementing Michael's timetable was far from straightforward. To begin with the amount of distress he showed at the smallest expectation of social involvement was almost unbearable for the group. The first Morning Meeting was as good as drowned out by his furious cries of protest. The staff held firm in spite of an overwhelming urge to remove him from the meeting, and persisted in trying to think about one another and Michael's state. By bearing and containing the anxiety his crying evoked and not feeling pushed into breaking the non-negotiable (that he would attend this meeting), Michael's anxiety diminished little by little. His crying continued in meetings for months to come, but its tone changed to become less disruptive before becoming patchy and intermittent, before stopping altogether.

Through such experiences, it became clear that in working with pervasively retreating children, the nursing team need to be supported to contain and reflect upon highly disturbing feelings that arose when one was being experienced as cruel, and to persist in spite of them. If this can be achieved, then gradually it would seem that the unshakeable consistency around non-negotiables (even in the face of rageful protests), coupled with space around these times when there are no expectations at all, enables the child to trust those caring for him while becoming desensitised to social interaction and being thought about little by little, day by day.

Like many young people with eating disorders, upon admission, Michael presented staff with a simultaneous fragility and hostility. However, unlike many of the children, Michael was without words. He was far from silent though for he protected himself with a formidable barrier of cries. In trying to communicate with Michael, the nursing team were often left with the feeling of being without words too and thinking could quickly become muddled. To illustrate this, I would like you to imagine yourself being tasked with taking Michael down to the dining room at a certain time. You are alone with Michael and he is sleeping. When awakened, he starts to wail loudly and scratch himself, saying *no* over and over while looking at you with a mixture of fear and pleading. If you stop moving him into his wheelchair, he falls back into a peaceful sleep. The temptation to leave him to rest in such a situation is close to irresistible, especially given how minor the task now seems in comparison to his distress. You might wonder how wheeling a child down to a dining room where he will sit in distress with the other children for ten minutes before wheeling him back again can possibly be justified in the face of such anguish.

Such thoughts were commonplace in my experience, and without the usual tools of sensitive conversation, gentle enquiries and reassurances, I and the other staff members moving Michael from place to place could be left feeling very disrespectful of his wishes. Without the usual means of negotiation with a young person refusing to do such things, physically moving a child into a wheelchair as he cries in protest, we could quite easily feel monstrous. It was in such situations that having clear, predictable expectations in place was invaluable. Not only in order that the transitions of the day would be handled in a consistent manner, but also in order that Michael would at least come to expect certain movements and their timing. Furthermore, one could put the interaction into a more long-term framework of treatment. It felt as though since Michael's protests were so powerful, and so muddling to one's thinking, that the thinking about how to manage certain interactions needed in part to be done *outside* of the interaction. In this way, one avoided the pull into either thoughtless action or inaction in response to his fury.

Allowing curiosity through giving emotional space

It became apparent very early on in his admission that Michael found direct attention, let alone assistance, deeply intrusive. While certain types of assistance were deemed essential and therefore non-negotiable (such as assisting with toileting and nutrition), any efforts over and above this with the intention of "pushing" Michael, no matter how gentle, were avoided. This entailed that Michael was not encouraged, verbally or physically, to do *anything*. Rather, the focus of interaction with Michael at the outset was the creation of a space in which his sense of safety and curiosity could grow without being too closely commented upon. While this might sound counter-intuitive, especially given that in these early days the agenda might have been to get to know Michael as quickly as possible, the team's sense was that this was a boy who was quite saturated by attempts to rouse him from his withdrawal. Comments on any of his capabilities or even his slightest movement were met with a marked regression of competence. However, while the approach was to back off a little as it were, it was not to simply leave him be. On the contrary, the team would hold out hope that Michael would, in time, become stronger and respond. But any sense of hurry was noted and avoided.

Within the first couple of weeks following his transfer, any direct attention in the form of sustained eye contact, looking and questioning seemed to cause Michael to recoil further from the world. It was as though he was experiencing it as an attack on the cocoon he had built around himself and so would double his defences. However, left with enough space, it seemed as though Michael would tentatively put his "feelers" out and allow himself to take in more of the world. Privacy in which to do this seemed essential, and privacy was what - as a fifteen-year-old boy being washed, dressed, and fed entirely by others - was alarmingly missing. An example:

A couple of days into his admission and Michael is lying on the beanbag during a free period. The other young people are in school and so the building is quiet. I enter the room to take over sitting with Michael, and as I approach I notice he has his eyes shut and is clutching his teddy bear to his face. He does not stir.

I sit down on a nearby sofa and quietly (but not in a whisper) ask the nurse how he has been. The nurse tells me that Michael is sleeping and has been for the past hour. As we talk, I notice Michael's eyes open a crack: he is observing us. After a short while, I look over to him and he quickly closes her eyes. I continue talking to the nurse, saying, "Michael does seem very, very tired. I wonder what it must be like for him, being in this new place and with so many different people to get to know. Must take a while to work everybody out." Michael continues to lie motionless as we wonder aloud together about his experience.

The nurse leaves, and I tell Michael that I'll be with him for the next hour before we go to lunch. I say it's been cold and rainy outside today and that the other young people had needed umbrellas and coats for the walk over to school. I comment that Sammy, his teddy bear, is looking quite snug and seems to want to stay close to Michael at the moment. I add that I'm not surprised, a lot of the young people here find it hard to be unwell and far from home, really quite scary. At this point, Michael stifles a sob, eyes still closed. He clutches Sammy even closer to him, a tear rolling down his cheek.

I am aware of an urge to physically comfort him, to put a blanket over him, to immediately soothe him somehow. I feel guilty that I seemed to have roused him from his quiet state into a painful one and feel responsible for the tear. I resist a powerful urge to do something to return him to his inert state. Instead, I tell him that I can see he is feeling very sad and that I'd like to sit next to him for a while. He does not respond. I sit on a cushion next to where he is lying. He continues to sob very quietly, his breathing ragged. I continue to wonder aloud how he might be feeling, going through a few events of the past few days. "It seemed so hard for you to say goodbye to your Mum and Dad, it must be strange being so far away from them. I wonder what it's like to arrive at a new hospital. Maybe it's hard not knowing who everyone is and how long you'll be here. Maybe you're wondering if you can trust anyone here to really understand what's been happening".

As I speak, Michael's cries become softer and I have the impression he is listening to what I am saying. I am quiet again and he cries for a while, holding Sammy close to his face. I tell him I'll get some tissues, and as I get up from the cushion, I notice that he watches me cross the room, shutting his eyes as I turn to return. I tell him that the tissues are next to him if he needs them, again resisting the urge to physically wipe his streaming nose as I had seen his mother do two days previously. He remains motionless but continues to cry for a while. His cry has taken on a mournful yet self-soothing and repetitive quality, and I am filled with a sense of exhausting sadness.

The young people start returning from school and clatter into the room in which we are located. A couple of them cautiously approach us and I ask them about their morning at school, again sensing Michael's furtive glances. When I turn back to him, I see he is clutching a tissue.

Being silently together

In the first few weeks of getting to know Michael, I found myself being careful not to speak too much as he felt so easily overwhelmed. Much of the time we spent together in these free hours would be spent with him lying motionless, gaining what seemed like much-needed respite from the world. However, it felt important to try and acknowledge how sad he was and to show him that I was curious about his mind. I did not want to appear simply as a passive therapeutic care worker supervising him, nor did I want to make continual attempts at conversation which had the expectation that Michael would respond, for I felt at this point this questioning would lead nowhere but to frustration and hopelessness for both of us.

I did not expect a verbal response or even a nod from Michael at this point and so I did not directly question him. I thought that in this first phase of getting to know one another he would experience a question as my trying to make him talk, and therefore, as intrusive. I wondered sometimes if he might also feel I was somehow stupid for thinking that he would respond. Instead, I hoped that he might begin to think with me as I wondered aloud, or as we sat together quietly, even if he would not or could not interact verbally. I found myself being careful not to make comments such as, "you are feeling…", no matter how obvious it might seem. This was for two reasons. Firstly, I imagined this could be really quite infuriating for Michael since I didn't know him very well yet. Secondly, I felt my talking at this point would conceivably be driven by the anxiety his non-responsiveness provoked in me. It seemed that there was an inclination in those of us caring for Michael to announce what he needed: "*You're tired aren't you? Time for bed*", or simply act on a perceived need, "*You must need the loo by now, let's go*". While this seemed perfectly understandable, at times necessary and probably in some senses reassuring for Michael, I also detected that in this early phase he felt irritated, and protested at others intrusively trying to read his mind. I often felt that announcing what he was feeling, whether accurate or not, stirred up resistances in him, creating a block in the interaction.

For this reason, I tried to allow myself to be with Michael while quietly observing and detecting subtle changes in how he was responding in each moment. We were often simply silently together, or together while I wondered aloud about how he might be feeling, or while recounting some event or other from the newspaper or magazine. In this way, without a pressure on either of us to *change* anything, we were able to become comfortable in this relaxed and very gentle interaction. It seemed that, having established that I wasn't going to spring a new challenge on him or praise him for doing anything differently, Michael's defences softened little by little. Gradually, I began to detect subtle changes in how he demonstrated his feelings about the people around him and his own emotional state. In the first few weeks of admission, this could be something as simple as a change in his posture and bodily tension, or change in the rhythm of his breathing and the tone and volume of his cries. In the absence of words, much was communicated in this way. If he seemed very tired and withdrawn (which I might pick up from his turning his head away as I faced him or even yawning when I came to say hello), I might just move about the room occasionally, looking at a few things along the way and passing comment. Michael would invariably watch me doing this, but only when I was not looking at him. In this early phase, it was very important for me not to remark on seeing Michael being curious about what I was doing. It felt as though we were involved in a dance of sorts, with Michael able to make a move of curiosity as long as he felt unwatched. In time, and as he seemed more at ease with me, I would occasionally hold my gaze on him for a few fleeting moments. I might also comment, not on the fact that he was looking at something, but rather I would describe the thing itself. For example, there were moments when, as though caught off guard by a noise or movement, he would turn very slightly to look at something. Rather than commenting on my noticing his responding to something I might say something like, "perhaps that was the shed door slamming, it's really very windy outside today". In this way, I hoped to balance giving him a sense that I was interested and attuned to his curiosity and interest without drawing too much attention to his doing something in the context of "getting better". I was aware that he was a bright student whose interests had far exceeded his development of inner maturity. We would therefore share time together without undue attention to "achievement". Rather, the focus was to enable him to feel comfortable enough that he might allow himself to open a little more to the outside world and tentatively try out engaging with it again in ways other than retreating from it.

As time progressed, my wondering was occasionally met with single words such as "home" or "mum" or "forever". We could then move on to where those words led, and with his increased responsiveness came a sense in me that Michael was a bit stronger and more amenable to me. In this climate of knowing each other a bit better, my questions seemed less of an intrusion. I was able to simply ask, "Are you missing your mum?", and my question might then be met with a small nod of the head or the holding of a mutual gaze. The first few times this happened I found myself fighting the urge to exclaim how wonderful it was to see him responding. Instead, I would make sure I acknowledged Michael's response while I left my hopeful excitement for sharing with his parents and the multidisciplinary team.

Bearing frustration: the role of countertransference

Our therapeutic approach of giving emotional space and not challenging Michael could strike visiting nurses as very odd. From time to time, I would explain to agency nurses that in working with Michael, we would not ask him to try harder or comment if he did anything differently, strange as that might seem. I and the other members of the nursing team would explain this in terms of his needing time to develop internally for his long-term improvement. We might explain that he had very particular difficulties in "moving forward" and showing us he was getting better. In spite of this, some of the nurses would quite naturally comment to Michael on his moving, sometimes warmly and sometimes as though catching him out. Typically, someone might exclaim that they just saw him move his legs and therefore he should try it again. Needless to say, after such occasions leg moving would not be observed for the rest of the day and Michael's general level of engagement would drop. The conclusion of some was therefore that Michael was "faking it" or "playing games with us".

I could see how, within the usual framework of care and rehabilitation, Michael could be perceived as harbouring malicious intent in deliberately being uncooperative. He could stir up frustrations in an interaction with lightening speed. I could not help but think how Michael and other mute young people such as him are at such great risk of being mistreated when they stir up such anger. My own feelings of irritation, impotence and impatience towards Michael on a daily basis and observations of such experiences in other staff served to illuminate this vulnerability vividly. Obvious as it may sound, I think it cannot be overemphasised that it is of great importance that those caring for mute, withdrawn, non-moving children, such as Michael, be given space to vent their frustrations *outside* of their interaction with them. Otherwise, since most of the nursing interaction with non-speaking, withdrawn children is in giving physical assistance, the frustrations could become manifest through a subtle roughness or hostile tone of voice. To promote optimal care for such children and to avoid hostile interactions, each staff member *must feel supported* in a staff support group, work discussion group, and individual supervision to share reactions to such a young person.

It is also important to allow a staff member to feel able to ask for a break if need be. In my experience, naming a "back-up" helper in the early days of Michael's admission, someone who was consistently available to take over, meant that I could continue to *think* and not *react*. It entailed that whoever was assigned to look after Michael on a particular day did not feel too overwhelmed or burdened and did not have to resort to becoming burned out, snappy, or to playing the martyr. Of course, this did happen, but in acknowledging feelings of rejection, anger, and despair which were deeply evoked, the possibility of negative responses towards Michael could be emotionally contained through thinking about them as a team.

A work discussion group with the consultant psychotherapist, Jeanne Magagna, involving our observations of the child and our countertransference responses, helped a great deal in this respect. It enabled the team to think not only of the negative attitudes towards Michael, but to acknowledge the anger and contempt that also seemed present in him at times. It seems that when faced with a child in such a profound state of illness and despair, the most obvious reaction is one of empathy and intent to help and nurture. Less expected is the reaction of aggression in the face of a child's retreat from life, which leaves a carer feeling rejected. Also, at times, there is a guilt-provoking, powerful sense of futility and hopelessness; of giving up on the child. Professional pride and convention often dictates that such reactions be strictly defended against (Menzies-Lyth, 1988). However, as has been said, bringing these reactions to light within the team was a powerful means of gaining insight, not only into Michael's internal world but also his relationship with his family.

Opening up a collaborative discourse with the parents

When a nursing team feel secure enough to acknowledge and reflect on their particular feelings in being with a pervasively retreating child, this atmosphere of emotional honesty can enable parents to feel comfortable in doing the same. I am not suggesting that I would recount, on greeting mother, that Michael had driven me to distraction by crying over the leaving speech of another young person earlier that day. I might simply give an observation of how Michael had managed to stir up irritation in me, which had made me wonder if anyone at home, or indeed Michael, had ever felt like that. Sharing feelings that had been evoked in me or other staff members seemed a good way to open up a dialogue about guilt-provoking feelings. Michael's mother in particular seemed to gain some kind of relief in hearing that she was not the only one who could experience Michael as infuriating and draining. While it might have felt more comfortable to present ourselves to the parents as all knowing and completely positive, managing "experts", this would have thwarted a great deal of insight which grew through conversations regarding our mutual reactions to Michael. His parents, being very sensitive and thoughtful, seemed able to use such conversations to creatively explore positive and negative ways in which they and their other sons responded to him.

In working with Michael, it seemed that the denial of conflictual feelings which provoke guilt would impede therapeutic progress with all participants involved in Michael's life: Michael, his family and the therapeutic team surrounding him. By denying such feelings, by settling into the more narrow but more comfortable position of thinking "poor Michael", we could all miss the point.

Phase two: moving forward, slipping back

Noting changes in countertransference responses as pointers towards psychic development

As time progressed, attention to the entire group's shifting countertransference responses was of great use in making sense of the developments within Michael. At the beginning of his admission it seemed that there was a strong current of avoidance in working with him. This was noted in seemingly small ways: staff avoiding sitting with him during meetings, finding reasons why they could not be expected to be his allocated worker for the day, disappearing when needed, feeling he was "talked about too much in meetings" and so on. For a time, it seemed like a small proportion of the nurses and therapeutic care workers were responsible for the lions' share of thinking about and caring for Michael and resentments inevitably ensued. The naming and subsequent exploration of this sense of avoidance, and the ill feeling it was creating, was vital in opening up a discussion about the anxiety Michael could instill in people. The worry of "getting it wrong" emerged, along with fears of damaging or upsetting him. Worries about losing patience and being unable to bear the painful intensity of his non-stop cries also featured and we thought about how Michael seemed to be simultaneously pushing us away and drawing us in. We imagined how worried and exhausted his parents must feel and noted how burdened his mother had seemed.

As Michael began to make progress and the team felt more at ease with his day to day care, the opposite phenomena emerged. Staff were eager to spend time with him and much of group supervision was taken up with issues of his progress. An excited atmosphere prevailed in which staff, much like proud parents, were keen to share whatever new step he had taken with them. While this was certainly an easier atmosphere in which to work, the side effect was the competition and jealousy it evoked in some of the other young people in the inpatient unit, and the way it evoked the staff's sense of possessiveness over who was responsible for helping Michael to develop. I myself was very much caught up in this, yet it would only take a rapid regression on Michael's part to remind me with a sting that I was investing too much of my own pride in his recovery. It seemed that personal investment in his recovery was a double-edged sword: on the one hand, it was in this phase that Michael created strong bonds with some staff members, who in turn felt a sense of responsibility for his recovery. Such bonds were vital in giving him security to make steps forward. However, Michael became very powerful in making it clear with whom he wanted to be and by whom he was most effectively helped by to recover, leading to the staff's renewed squeamishness in holding firm.

It is easy in this phase of a retreating child's recovery to lose sight of the role of boundaries. Despite boundaries having played such a vital role until this point, once a child begins to progress, it can be tempting to feel that upsetting the child should be avoided. In the atmosphere of relief when a child emerges from profound withdrawal from life, no one wants to be the "bad" one, the one apparently slowing progress or causing conflict. It is therefore of the utmost importance to balance an excitement about the child's progress with a realistic view that recovery cannot happen overnight. It may be that a few members of the team end up "holding the reins", and thus end up being viewed as the "baddies" - the over-cautious, the party-poopers - not just by the child, but by the other young people and the wider team. Such a split seems difficult to avoid at this stage while progress is so fragile and the team is adapting daily to the child's emerging personality. But, if at all possible, all members of the multidisciplinary team should be encouraged to contain their excitement and pride in response to the first changes made and, while remaining hopeful and conveying this, also expect progress to be slow if it is to be stable.

In this early phase of recovery, conflicts commonly lead to the child regressing and slipping back into a mode of non-thinking. The feelings evoked in staff when they are the ones involved in triggering such a regression can be very powerful indeed, the common wish to sustain progress after months of the child's inertia is fertile ground for a pernicious sense of failure. However, just as in the first phase, staff must be supported to contain such feelings and not be overpowered by them. If staff feel overwhelmed, then the child's sense of frightening omnipotence is reinstated and the child is at risk of embarking on a shallow course of recovery.

It is important to mention the role of the young people's group in this stage, since the group provides vital commentary and encouragement as a child emerges from the isolation of silence and retreat from life, which he experienced as traumatic. For even if their presentations differ, the other young people on the unit can feel a strong sense of solidarity with a withdrawn and mute child. In Michael's case, the group seemed able to voice their opinions on his progress far earlier than the staff could without causing him to regress. It seemed that as he felt safer and more settled within the group, his eagerness to be liked by the young people was re-kindled. Therefore, when a young person spoke of Michael in a group meeting, rather than drown out young people's comments by his cries as in the early weeks of his entry into the unit, Michael would become a little quieter and seem to tolerate their thinking about him. He was beginning to identify with his peers while making tentative steps away from the developmentally regressed interactions, in which he had been caught with the staff and his parents. Slowly, he was allowing himself to be in the young people's minds, increasingly as an equal rather than simply as a competitor through illness symptoms for the attention of the adults. In turn, some of the other young people could use Michael's struggles in this process to think about themselves and their own conflicts with adults, thus normalising this difficult phase of individuation for Michael.

While an important aspect of recovery, the role of the young people's group in the unit should be carefully thought about and reflected upon by the staff team in order that a child emerging out of his state of withdrawal does not become a container for the group's difficult feelings. For example, those young people who are struggling with frustration at not being allowed to move forward at the pace they would like (i.e., leave the unit and go home tomorrow) can end up projecting this anger onto the non-speaking child, talking on his behalf about how unfairly he is being treated and how frustrating the staff are being. While there may be an element of truth to their identification, it is important that a newly progressing child be protected from being used in this way, given how susceptible he may be to seeking peer approval in these early stages. Instead, the other children are best encouraged to own their frustrations and discuss them openly with staff in order that the adults can understand their feelings and bear their anxieties.

Phase three: the manic flight to health—holding the line

As mentioned in the previous section, once progress has started, the ensuing sense of excitement can, in its extreme, lead to abandoning being mindful of the child's need for slow, steady progress. The theme of wanting to avoid conflict with the child for fear of his regression is a thread that runs through into the third phase of recovery in which the child is more or less *physically* independent of staff. That is, he is engaging in age-appropriate self-care again, is physically mobile, and is no longer under the constant supervision of staff. Further, in this phase, the child has successfully established for himself a place in the group; links with peers have been made, conversations are taking place, and friendships are being formed.

The pace of these changes after months and months of withdrawal can appear to staff to be happening at a giddying speed. Indeed, there can be a feeling of a manic flight from illness during this phase, a presentation of competence which seems a brittle cover on a fragile, new, "healthy identity". Attempts to staunch the flow of progress at this stage can be met with not just frustration but also with contempt. Staff can be left feeling they are clipping the wings of the child; keeping him from making progress, but it is vital that they are keeping the child grounded. A child in this stage can struggle to think with staff about the advantages of taking things a little slower, but staff need to persist with him to do this in order to keep him working with them. A metaphor I would sometimes use to consider this issue is that of drying cement: while someone might want to build a house as quickly as possible, if each stage is not allowed to set properly, then the whole house is not secure. This kind of thinking seemed to help a child in the final stages of admission to think about more long-term goals while acknowledging his desperation to leave behind the long, arduous illness from which he was recovering. Staff were prevented from becoming caught in fruitless battles if they could help the child to understand, through metaphor, the reasons for the adults' caution and concern.

In Michael's case, it felt almost as difficult to communicate and feel connected with him in this phase as it had in the beginning. Partly, this felt like an appropriate teenage rejection of me, along with an embarrassment on his part about the state of the old "ill" self. However, another part seemed to be driven by a wish to totally disconnect from thinking about his traumatising illness that, while understandable, did arouse some concern in me. Gently exploring his memories of when he had been at his most withdrawn formed much of our key work together prior to his going home. Initially, his memory was very poor and patchy. However, we persisted, and as uncomfortable as thinking through what had happened was for Michael, his putting the experience into words or drawings felt like a vital phase of processing and gaining insight. As his memory improved, we explored his impressions of being unwell and how it related to his healthy self. Despite squeamishness about looking backwards while he was progressing so well, it seemed important to keep a sense of continuity and not stop thinking just because Michael was "better".

Out of these conversations came Michael's ideas about why he had been so afraid to get better for such a long time: fears of not being cared for if well (which were partly realistic); fears of being overwhelmed; fears of not being special; fears that people would be angry with him for being OK after all the worries about him. We thought about how his illness had given him a sense of safety which had been difficult to leave behind, how being better meant taking risks which he still feared. It would have been all too easy to skip over this phase of work, given the pressure I felt to speed things along, to "make things nice" for Michael, just as I had felt when he was not speaking and immobile. Tolerance of distress and its containment is vital at all stages of work with non-speaking children, as in all therapeutic work of course, but it felt important to bear the notion of being mindful of Michael particularly at this stage. After months of working implicitly towards Michael's regaining of health, the switch to then putting the brakes on his progress when he is speedily moving along towards recovery can feel almost sadistic. Likewise, "slowing down progress" can be perceived as not having recognised the child's work thus far, or as being punishing for him having been so ill. Such perceptions are usefully explored with the child and the young peoples' group in order that ideas about what it means to be "better", or at least "better enough", can be considered. This is a more useful focus than looking at differences in perception as to whether or not the staff are being punitive by suggesting slow, steady progress.

Such caution, though unpopular, is crucial if the progress made is to be sustainable. The pressure to send such children home once they are "better" neglects to take into account the inner psychic developments that need to be consolidated alongside their physical progress. A flight away from the illness, while something to be celebrated, can also be a repeat reaction of dissociating from difficulties, albeit in a different, more acceptable guise. It is vital, therefore, that the child's family are involved in thinking about the pace of recovery and in considering the familial adjustments that will need to be made when the child is back home and well again. Long months of anguish and fearing that one has "lost" a child can lead to a natural impatience to finally have the child home again. However, thinking with parents about the advantages of a child remaining an inpatient for a little longer, in order that he might develop more adequate internal capacities to have a better chance of sustaining his recovery was, in my experience, well received, even if a little reluctantly. It also means that the parents are strengthened in holding firm with the child should there come a likely phase of pleading to be taken home.

At this stage, once the issue of keeping a child engaged in treatment has been addressed, work can be done with the aim of sufficiently preparing the child for the return to family and school. One approach is to try to help the child to think about possibilities of what might occur at school and at home in order to pre-empt potential stressors that he feels he may encounter. It was sometimes the case that children who had emerged from silence and retreat from troublesome life would claim they felt absolutely ready to jump back into their old life and had no hesitations about doing so. However, with a little exploration, it would often emerge that such a stance was motivated by a fear that acknowledging difficulties would extend the admission. Reinforcing that being able to think about difficulties and bear the feelings they bring is a sign of getting better seemed to help free up the child to think about that for which he did not feel sufficiently prepared. Alternatively, running through scenarios with the child, such as explaining ınd teachers at school what had been wrong with him, would often expose a "blank", .. ɔeing unprepared and a fear of being overwhelmed.

Another scenario that seemed useful to explore was the issue of how the child would feel about not being "special" in the way he had been previously, that is, being ill, worried about, constantly focused upon in the family. Without an illness, once the excitement of recovery has died away and "normal" life resumed, how would the child get his needs met by his parents? How would he communicate when things weren't going well? Thinking such things through felt like such vital work, not just with the child, but with his parents and siblings too. It may be at this point that guilty feelings emerge in the child, a recognition that his siblings may have suffered. It may even be that siblings now feel it is safe to vent their own frustrations about having felt so worried yet simultaneously overlooked in the family. If this is the case, having some time to adjust to and bear these feelings before the child returns home can help the family work through the inevitable fall-out following such a protracted and painful illness. It can also help the child readjust to being exposed to the painful and hostile feelings of others, which have been held quietly in a protected position for so long.

Conclusion

Working closely with children who have withdrawn themselves from the world highlights and challenges personal and institutional assumptions about helping. The extent to which we invest our own pride in another's recovery, what we define as health, how we react to being experienced as cruel - these are but some unexpected issues which can arise out of caring for a child who counters help with silence, fear and fury. Staying with, and staying attentive to, the complexity of feelings that working with such children evokes can grant precious insight into the myriad aspects of a child's personality and situation. Bearing uncertainty and confusion whilst simultaneously holding onto and protecting a sense of hope and utility can feel at times like a tightrope act. But it is this attitude that, if engendered in a nursing team, can provide both the containment and space for a child who is not talking, walking, or eating, to slowly let down his defences and start contemplating health again.

I was fortunate enough to work in such a team, and it was only with their patience, insight, and humour that I could tolerate and then think about feelings of being overwhelmed, unskilled, and at a loss. I was also fortunate enough to work with many parents who, in spite of feeling redundant or even responsible in the face of their child's state, persisted in thinking with us and shedding new light at times when we all felt in the dark.

I would like to acknowledge my gratitude to those children on whose experiences this chapter has been based. The road to their recovery was long, rocky, and in parts completely out of sight. I have learned much by hearing their experiences of their journey through such a severe illness to recovery and accompanying them on it for some small steps along the way. It is these shared insights that have been most illuminating and for which I am most grateful.

CHAPTER TEN

Collaborating, containing, and inspiring confidence: physiotherapy with a child who does not talk, walk, or eat

Jeanne Magagna and Melanie Bladen

This chapter describes a collaborative effort between a physiotherapist, Melanie Bladen, and a child psychotherapist, Jeanne Magagna. We have been working together in Great Ormond Street Hospital for Children, a paediatric hospital for 300 children. Children are sent to this hospital when their local hospital has not been able to offer them the specialised medical attention required for their particular illness. The children with whom we have jointly worked have been suffering with a combination of physical and psychological problems, which require an inpatient psychiatric admission. We shall illustrate our thinking through our work with a fourteen-year-old long, dark-haired, emaciated girl, Rosa, suffering from what Lask (2003) called *pervasive refusal.* We prefer to call it *a pervasive retreat from life.* She initially was completely *unable* to talk, walk, eat, open her eyes, or move her body. Rosa, her four-year-old brother, and her Italian parents had been living in Italy until recently when their father's work transferred him to England. Family therapy, individual psychotherapy, and physiotherapy comprised part of Rosa's care plan. In our roles as a physiotherapist and psychotherapist respectively, we helped Rosa accept and use a multitude of psychotherapeutic physiotherapy interventions.

Six concepts boldly insert themselves in every facet of the psychotherapeutic physiotherapy interventions. These elements of good physiotherapy practice made it possible for this fourteen-year-old non-speaking girl, Rosa, and many other children with whom we worked, to make sufficient progress during the course of one year to return home and resume a normal life with their families and friends at school. In the year following admission to hospital, a child who was previously severely regressed should be offered psychotherapy on an outpatient basis.

The six concepts informing the collaborative effort between physiotherapist and child are:

1. Collaboration
2. Curiosity
3. Containment
4. Confidence
5. Creative imagination
6. Surprise

You can remember them if you think of "The Six Cs'".

The "Cs'" are designed to seize hold of the healthy aspects of the personalities of both the physiotherapist and the child.
The "Cs'" facilitate therapeutically meeting the aims of the physiotherapy encounters.
The "Cs'" create a beneficial experience for both the child and the physiotherapist.

The "Cs'" will be explored in more detail below:

Collaboration

The family, physiotherapist, child, and multidisciplinary team have a continuous reciprocal interaction and influence on one another. For example, the feelings of the multidisciplinary team and the parents towards the physiotherapist influences how the young person receives and responds to the physiotherapist. These factors also influence how the physiotherapist relates to the young person. How the physiotherapist helps the young person influences how the multidisciplinary team and the family relate to the young person and the physiotherapist. In the case of young children, the parents can frequently resent the physiotherapist for getting close to their child's body when the child is an inpatient, for during this period the parents are deprived of many parenting functions, which they usually assume for their child.

Rosa became very engaged in the physiotherapy with Melanie and excitedly anticipated the physiotherapy sessions; however she *split off* any good feelings, which she might also have for the nurses, and placed them all with Melanie. Rosa complained to her physiotherapist that the nurses were depriving her of everything she wanted (not to eat, not to have to go to school, not to be able to stay sleeping all day in her room). For this reason, Rosa wouldn't show the nurses the progress she had made moving her limbs in physiotherapy. The rejected ones, the nurses and the school-teachers, became angry with the physiotherapist because they wanted her to offer physiotherapy during her non-working hours, which were times which would suit the teachers' main teaching programme.

Collaboration implies working out a mutually agreed timetable with the families and child, as well as with members of the multidisciplinary team who also work with the family. In *The Child, the Illness and Others*, Maud Mannoni (1973) suggests that the family members may project a multiplicity of feelings including their own neediness, sadness, rage, and feelings of impotence in relationships onto the child suffering from a physical immobility. Over time, as the physiotherapist collaboratively works with the child, a close emotional rapport is formed. This feeling of being excluded from a helpful relationship sometimes leads the parents to feel their own neediness, and they become aware of how they need more supportive understanding themselves. They also require some regular reviews with the physiotherapist so they can feel connected to her and her work with their child.

In fact, every six weeks there is an Inpatient Unit Review Meeting attended by the parents and the multidisciplinary team, including the physiotherapist. The Review Meeting enables the multidisciplinary team to share their views with the parents. The parents are able to express their sentiments to the physiotherapist and other members of the team. For example, Rosa's parents were at first horrified that the physiotherapist was creating some expectations for their very ill and very withdrawn fourteen-year-old daughter Rosa. Later, they were able to share with the physiotherapist how grateful they were to her for engaging Rosa in physiotherapy exercises, which she both appreciated and used to recover the use of her limbs.

Curiosity

Rogers and Hammerstein (1951) wrote an old familiar love song about "getting to know you, getting to know all about you". These words echo our thoughts that the best working alliances occur when the physiotherapist and the child find a way of getting to know one another.

"We don't know each other yet... why are you touching me in that way?" said one speaking child to the physiotherapist. A *pervasively regressed* young person will not verbally say this, but rather gradually just freeze or withdraw from the physiotherapist if, before touching the child, the physiotherapist has not spent sufficient time making herself known to the fearful and perhaps curious child. As a physiotherapist you will touch the young person's body in a particular way, you will also talk to the young person with a particular tone of voice, in a particular selection of emotionally distant or close phrases. The way you are depends somewhat on whether or not you have taken the time necessary to get to know the young person; her story, her past, her present and her attitude to her future. Of course, all this is very difficult when the young person is not speaking to anyone!

Being curious about the young person involves getting to know the young person's story from conception onwards. Some of the young person's story will have been obtained by the other members of the multidisciplinary team. But generally, being curious involves finding the missing pieces of the puzzle until you have an emotionally complete developmental narrative of the young person and have intuitively grasped, through the young person's non-verbal communication, how she *feels in your presence from moment to moment.*

Aspects to be curious about

1. In what ways is the child disabled?
2. Is the child's intellectual functioning impaired?
3. Does the child have developmental gaps or family difficulties that might promote a wish to remain regressed in hospital? Is this shown through not facilitating physiotherapy assistance for the limbs to move?
4. Is any part of the body capable of being moved through the child's conscious volition at this point?

5. What are the emotions within, and surrounding, the body and the unused limbs?
6. How does the child feel about being in bed and not using the limbs? Some children do not want to get back on their feet!
7. What does the child feel he or she could, or would, like to do differently with the different parts of his or her body?
8. In what way would the child prefer to take care of his or her body's progress and care today? Having a few possibilities to choose from leaves the child feeling less imprisoned and controlled.

But more importantly, *what is the emotion behind the unused limbs?* Why did the young person continually break an arm or a leg before she stopped speaking? For example:

- Is it because the young person is feeling emotionally dropped from the family's mind, or depressed, and can only feel looked after when a physical illness prompts more family concern?
- Rosa broke her limbs four times before her *pervasive retreat from life,* which left her completely incapacitated. No one understood that underneath her seemly upbeat and confident manner she was miserable and needy.
- Each time fourteen-year-old Rosa needed to move and later to go to the loo, it was her father who was involved in her physical care. His involvement with her body perpetuated an already present Oedipal issue in which she wanted the father for herself and competed with her mother for his company. It was developmentally inappropriate for the father to be having so much physical contact with her even though Rosa required physical care.
- Rosa arrived using only the top half of her body. She felt she had no control over the limp bottom half of her body. When she trusted us, we learned she had been sexually abused at a party of drunken young people. She had to withdraw from her current peer group who were behaving in a too developmentally advanced sexual way for her to manage in her social peer group. Unconscious withdrawal through conversion disorder enabled her to have time to meet more of her emotional needs at home and in hospital. For this reason, physiotherapy, which helped her to get better, was initially a threat to her *need to be ill.*

Young people who are high achievers scholastically or through sports, drama, dancing or music, may reach a point where the competition is creating too much expectation, fear of failure and anxiety. Being curious about the child's current life situation enables the physiotherapist to avoid the assumption that the child wants to get better. It is important to be curious about how motivated the child is to help his body that isn't able to function adequately; the body that needs help to at least improve circulation. Being curious about how motivated the child is to work with you in physiotherapy immediately promotes the idea that you are not doing things *to* the child, rather than being together *with the child* to help her body function.

When the child experiences herself as paralysed in a conversion disorder, a *pervasive retreat from life,* or has a permanently incapacitated body, it already feels to the child that something horrible has been done to her. Unless trust in the physiotherapist has developed, having "help with the body" can be experienced as an unwanted intrusion, as something nasty, painful, and demanding. These attitudes of the child will undermine any attempt to help the body move.

The child has a completely different experience if the physiotherapist demonstrates interest and curiosity about the child as a person, not just as a malfunctioning body. If the physiotherapist can demonstrate genuine interest in the child by getting to know the child, the child may cooperate with the physiotherapist to do "something for the body".

Melanie, the physiotherapist, said, "With another child I lost so much time. I went in too quickly. The other child, Andrew, didn't like my coming. I needed him to develop more trust in me. We needed to get to know each other more so that I would be experienced by him as being present *with him*. He just felt I was someone '*getting at him*', intruding upon him. I had to start all over and use the insight I had forgotten about... You need to develop a child's trust first... and then do the work with him."

It is important to remember the child may not wish to get better. Something else, such as changes in his/her life in school, in the family, or within his/her self may need to be occurring before he/she will feel that recovering physically is either what is wanted or even what is important for his/her emotional wellbeing.

So, it is important to be curious, not to make false assumptions that everyone wants physiotherapist to help! The young person may want the physiotherapist to comprehend the whole self, and to understand exactly what it is that needs to be helped.

Speaking of *curiosity,* a vulnerable, physically disabled child is certainly going to be very curious about you. The child will get to know you by observing your face the first moment that you enter the room. The child will evaluate the the look on your face the minute you lay eyes on him. How do you greet her and her physical problem?

In his book *The Diving Bell and the Butterfly,* Jean-Dominique Bauby (2004) movingly describes some of the emotional experiences of a person whose body cannot move. He says, "... his mind intact, imprisoned inside his own body. He was unable to speak or move. Blinking his left eyelid was his only means of communication" (p. 12). Bauby helps us identify with such paralysis as he says, "Becoming aware of my physical condition was... as blinding as an atomic explosion and keener than a guillotine blade" (p. 17).

Bauby (2004) continues with a description of his relief in having a physiotherapist regularly visiting him, saying, "Her warm fingers travel all over my face, including the numb zone... I can only half-smile... but this experience (with the physiotherapist) can trigger the most varied emotions" (p. 24).

Although he is accepted by the physiotherapist for who he is and his physical condition, Bauby feels the cruelty of disgust and rejection saying, "As I direct my one eye towards them, the young man, the grandmother and the homeless man turn away... " (p. 41).

They cannot bear how the paralysed Bauby looks. Bauby casts a cynical glance as he goes on to say, "... and then there are the less conscientious minority, who make their getaway pretending not to notice my distress signals" (p. 48).

This experience could be unbearable to someone unable to move, but Bauby describes that there is a way to survive emotionally when he states, "I keep my mind sharp, to avoid slumping into resigned indifference, I maintain a level of resentment and anger, neither too much nor too little, just as a pressure-cooker has a safety-valve to keep it from exploding" (p. 63).

The question the child asks as he/she looks into your face is: "Can you be curious about all that I feel, not just smile and be jolly and pretend I feel okay being like this?" Each moment of interaction you have with the child will be a time when the child will be curious about your physical and emotional response to her sensations of fear, pleasure, pride, pain, anger, encapsulated in the physical movement in which you are engaged. It is in this way that the child gets to know the depth of your compassion and sensitivity to his plight, but also gets to know your attitude to acceptance of life, courage and hope. The child will also be curious about whether or not you are bored with him and about how you experience any lack of progress: will you be critical, will you be too passive, will you be gently supportive or appropriately accepting of lack of progress depending on the child's current emotional state?

Some of child's curiosity may be too possessive of you and intrusive into your personal life. You need to be aware that you can meet the needs of the child without feeling you must satisfy all his curiosity. Curiosity about facts of your life can also reflect the child's experience that you are not sufficiently emotionally responsive to his feelings. He may try to satisfy his anxious curiosity about what you are like through asking personally intrusive questions, for which you may feel it is not appropriate to answer or answer in any detail.

Mainly the child wants to hold onto you and be curious about you if the physiotherapy is going well. You can accept this fact and comment upon this wish to be connected to you without agreeing to an unhelpful invasion into your privacy.

Containment

Hospital staff have all learned a cheery message, "Good morning, how are you today?" "It'll be okay." "Oh, don't worry, it will change for the better." This forms part of a protective repertoire against the overwhelming burden of sadness, despair, rage, discomfort and loneliness of the child in hospital. Isabel Menzies-Lyth (1959) illuminates the hospital staff's use of this protective armour in her paper entitled "The functioning of social systems as a defence against anxiety".

Menzies-Lyth describes how anxieties arise in the personal relationship between the professional and the child. The professional erects defences against the anxiety of being intimate with the child's painful feelings and fears. Working in a defensive rigid social structure in the hospital and within oneself leads to job dissatisfaction, low morale, and staff burnout. No one can be truly satisfied unless there is an opportunity within the institution and within himself/herself to bring the emotions to consciousness, and feel they are accepted, thought about, and understood. Containment of anxieties within the institution is essential to prevent the erection of social defences in relation to the child's and parents' feelings.

Daniel Stern, in *The Interpersonal World of the Infant* (1985), describes selective *attunement* between the child and the caregiver as being one of the most potent ways that a caregiver can shape the development of a child's life. He says that attunement permits the caregiver to convey to the child what is shareable and which experiences are "beyond the pale of mutual consideration and acceptance" (p. 208). Stern indicates that "for a child to be a subjective partner only in enthusiasm will place the more depressive-like states of enthusiasm outside the pale of shareable personal experience. And, on the other hand, to be a partner only in enthusiasm will place the positively exciting states of enthusiasm outside of shareable personal experience" (p. 209).

Physiotherapists exert some degree of selective bias in their attunement behaviours, and in doing so they create a pattern for the child's shareable interpersonal world in physiotherapy sessions. This applies to all internal states; enthusiasm and exthusiasm are only examples. I have used them, because enthusiasm is overused in situations when attunement to the child's present emotional state would be better.

Attunement involves being curious about the state of mind of the child each moment you are present and modulating your tone of voice, the speed of your actions, the soft or lightness of your touch, and the expression on your face to greet the emotional position of the child at that particular moment.

Attunement also involves being aware that the child is curious and wants to know about the what and why and how of your aim in being with her on that particular day. In being attuned to this need of the child, you find yourself describing the task the two of you are working upon, and of course you owe these explanations to every child whether or not the child is mentally disabled or a baby, for mentally disabled children are still emotionally curious and a baby understands words at three months. Being attuned to the child involves also showing you are curious about the child's response to your shared activity.

Being available to receive the present emotional state of the child, giving time to hold and experience the emotions of the child present in both the body and the psyche, giving thought to the emotions evoked in you by the child, giving meaning to child's emotional relationship with you; this is *containment* of the child.

Containment of the child's emotional relationship to you and his/her body promotes the growth of the child's curiosity, vitality, and growth of loving feelings and dedication to work on the mutual aims of the physiotherapy experience.

There are three different periods in physiotherapy which should be considered: they are the beginning, middle, and end of each physiotherapy session, as well as the beginning, middle, and end of each stretch of physiotherapy sessions before and after you have taken a holiday.

Here are some illustrations taken from the work in physiotherapy undertaken by Melanie and Rosa.

Beginning of therapy

Physiotherapy provides an intimate encounter with both the body and the inner self. Enabling an experience of the physical depths within the therapeutic encounter can facilitate a sinking into the most painful and repressed levels of the infantile psyche. The split between body and mind, with its capacity to think, find meaning, feel pleasure, and accept pain, can be healed through helping the child recognise the underlying feelings, images, and thoughts which spring from a particular bodily experience (Bloom, 2006).

At the beginning of physiotherapy, even if they are hidden, the child's primitive fears of being with a stranger are mobilised. The child is experiencing loss of a part of the well-functioning body. This gathers phantasies about loss: *loss* of the perfect body, *loss* of the being the perfect child in the eyes of the family. The family and child, regardless of what they are told, may expect the physiotherapist to restore the body's function more than is possible. The physiotherapist needs to prepare the family and child at the beginning for the limits of what is possible. Even if the body may recover, the recovery time will not be instantaneous. For this reason the physiotherapist has to bear the child and family's sense that there are limits to what the physiotherapist can do in terms of speed of work with the child. Accepting feelings around loss, such as sadness, despair, and hopelessness, are present in the first encounter with both the child and the family. These feelings might be linked to feelings of separation and loss, which originated in early infancy.

Melanie, the physiotherapist, said: "At the initial assessment there was an element of apprehension regarding what Rosa would think of me, and what I would make of her. Since Rosa was trapped in her bed, I made conscious attempts not to take even more control away from her. I spent time talking about who I was and why I was present, attempting to establish a framework for my presence. As I tried to engage her, because Rosa had no verbal communication and her eyes were tightly shut, I was fearful that I might cause her to suffer, so I had to deliberate over everything I said or did with her. I was able to discuss my feelings about this initial contact with Jeanne, who reassured me to go with my instinct. Although difficult to engage with a person who offers little feedback, I realised not to expect, but instead just to feel and be emotionally present. A small finger movement or facial change I described and attempted to interpret, rightly or wrongly. From day one, I endeavoured to have a structure to the sessions, so that Rosa was able to anticipate my appointment. In addition, I described everything that I was doing or I was about to do, with the hope that in some way Rosa could and would collaborate with me."

Middle of therapy

The child wishes that the physiotherapist will hold her as long as needed, but never too long! During the middle phase, the physiotherapist becomes *a cushion* holding the discomfort of the body and the anguish, futility, humiliation, and resistance of the body. Being very appreciative of the containing functions of the therapist, the child can become very "hooked onto the physiotherapist", and it is important to acknowledge the growing attachment.

Melanie describes the experience of physiotherapy with Rosa, saying: "As treatment sessions progressed, Rosa began to take more control over the sessions, often initiating activities. At times we sat and chatted about where she had come from and how she had progressed. These sessions were often her way of slowing her physical recovery down. In addition, I also had to allow Rosa the time to consolidate her physical progress, allowing herself the time and emotional *space to be at one* with her physical progress. As well as clearly anticipating setbacks, repetition and practice appeared to be the keys to progress. This I found hard at times as the pressure externally for Rosa to achieve was often placed on me and at times I felt a failure. When new steps were taken Rosa often would complain of new pains or old ones would resurrect themselves. These were acknowledged, but we didn't focus upon them."

Ending of therapy session, holiday break, and complete end of the physiotherapy contact

Melanie describes the difficulties of endings, saying:

> "It was apparent that Rosa and I had established a therapeutic alliance and the prospect of my holiday loomed. It was important that Rosa's continued progress was not dependent on me, so a third person, her keyworker, was gradually introduced as I gradually reduced my leading role in providing the physiotherapy sessions. I found this difficult as this need that Rosa had for me to help her was also what fed our relationship. I realised, however, that my need to be needed was not going to be good for her continued health. Rosa's recovery needed gradually to be self-driven and not dependent on me.
>
> At the end of therapy sessions Rosa would often complain that she hated the nursing staff, that they were cruel to her. She dualised physiotherapy and the ward as 'heaven and hell'. This was distressing as Rosa was often upset at the prospect of going back to the ward. This feeling of 'good cop-bad cop' felt good as I was the person she liked and needed, but I had to take a step back and realise that this relationship needed to be part of an alliance between all of us, not simply an idealised dependence on me. We talked about what the problems were and I suggested that she broach them with her keyworker. Physiotherapy needed to be kept separate from the problems on the ward.
>
> Over the forthcoming months, Rosa was encouraged to take an increasing responsibility for her progress, setting herself goals that were realistic and measurable. In addition, her goals were increasingly directed to activities that she participated in outside of the physiotherapy session. For example, sitting up in her chair for increased periods, transferring from bed to toilet, and going swimming with the other children on the unit.
>
> Rosa eventually was weaned from physiotherapy in hospital as she increasingly spent more time at home. No follow-up physiotherapy was arranged for Rosa at home. Instead, Rosa thought about this and chose to continue helping her body through engaging in swimming activities, which she loved.
>
> Throughout my time with Rosa, I experienced a roller-coaster of emotions. I expected myself always to greet each session with 'my glass half-full', but despite a good session, I often came out feeling exhausted and with 'my glass empty'. I even at times felt slightly hysterical. I spent time with colleagues discussing my sessions and the transference feelings, which felt like 'a bleeding dry' of my emotions. The importance of talking with colleagues and the multidisciplinary team, reflecting and being listened to, cannot be underestimated. I felt that I was getting in touch with feelings of loss linked with the ending of physiotherapy."

Confidence

First, it is confidence in your self as a person, with good self-esteem, and with experience in using your physiotherapy skills that is essential. This confidence in yourself is essential because at times negative feelings of the child, the parents, and the multidisciplinary team will gather around you. You also need a group of colleagues with whom you can discuss your work to help you to be confident of the path you are travelling with the child.

"You are moving too fast with my child, it is too difficult!"; "You are working too slowly, you need to do more with my child even though he is reluctant"; "You aren't doing a good enough job with the child, there is not enough progress". These are all potential comments that will land on your shoulders. The physiotherapy space is a space in which the multidisciplinary team can locate failure, rather than facing the impotence of not yet being able to comprehend and sufficiently heal the psychological problems between both the family and the non-speaking child, and within the child's inner experience of the disabled part of her body.

But also, to work well, you need the child and the family and the multidisciplinary team to develop confidence in you. The child's confidence in you is promoted when, alongside containment and other factors previously mentioned, you provide the following:

1. A reliable setting.
2. Sufficient notice of the rhythm of working days and your holidays.
3. A regular time for which you arrive promptly and end promptly.
4. A good state of mind to greet the child's attentive spirit.

Here is an example of where confidence in the physiotherapist is essential:

> Rosa is very appreciative of Mel, her physiotherapist. The nurses start criticising Mel, for unconsciously and perhaps not so consciously, they are feeling jealous of the good relationship Rosa has with her physiotherapist. In contrast to her good relationship with Mel, Rosa is showing a very difficult uncooperative stance towards the nurses. Mel is confident enough to be curious about what the issues are. She has listened attentively to Rosa. She confidently says to the nurses, "I wonder if it might be helpful to think of ways of talking with Rosa and perhaps even accommodating Rosa. I think there might be ways that you could put things so that she would not feel too controlled, but rather have more say in the time she is allowed to rest and time she needs to be active on the ward". Melanie is able to identify that at least some of Rosa's criticism of her is linked with some of the nurses' envy towards how attentively and cooperatively she has been able to work with Rosa's resistance to getting better. Melanie is a physiotherapist who has developed because she has been able to spend time getting to know Rosa and found courage to work alongside the multidisciplinary team and say what needed to be said to them.

Creative imagination

> You can learn more about a person in an hour of play than a year of conversation.
>
> Plato (429–347 BC)

Bauby (2004), mute, half-deaf, every part of his body paralysed, describes how his "cocoon becomes less oppressive... when his mind takes flight like a butterfly" (p. 13). It is crucial that the physiotherapist helps physiotherapy to move out of its confining prison of the disability and into the realms of imaginative play that can truly acknowledge a child's individual physical and emotional developmental stages.

Movement both in the mind and in the body is motivated by curiosity and unconscious phantasy. Play in physiotherapy is an opportunity for the child to integrate experiences from both her internal and external worlds. Although the body may be immobile in some ways, the child can still feel some freedom of movement through the use of her imagination. Children experience the spontaneous aspects of play and the use of the imagination as fun. So the practice of various skills and roles in physiotherapy can be a pleasure rather than a tedious activity.

Acknowledging where the individual child is both physically and psychologically at the present moment is crucial in planning the physiotherapy sessions. For example, Rosa, in her early completely immobile state, was not at the stage of physical or emotional development to do much of anything, never mind sitting up or walking.

Time needs to be spent building a trusting relationship. Time needs to be spent on establishing routine. Just as a mother has little or no expectations of her newborn child, Mel talked to Rosa and guided her through her sessions, moving Rosa's body with no expectation of Rosa's active participation. As time progressed, the verbal dialogue expanded into what Rosa might be thinking or feeling, especially in response to hydro sessions in the hospital pool.

Imaginative play became more important as a vehicle of guiding the sessions. Mel suggested that Rosa try to imagine what it was like on a desert island, and which items of equipment she might be able to use to move away from the island to the land of people. This imaginative play gradually progressed as Mel, the physiotherapist, acted out the scenario of moving away from the island with a gradual increase in Rosa's participation in the journey; a journey that symbolised moving back into life outside the hospital bed. The sessions were structured, but always with the freedom of choice regarding which pretend activity to dramatise, how to do it, and when to do it.

To enhance interest in the physiotherapy sessions, a problem-solving approach was added. This problem-solving approach often involved figuring out how exactly the same game could be played differently. This meant allowing for some familiar sameness in the activity while adding a little that was new. For example, on dry land a basic obstacle course chosen by Rosa. She negotiated this initially on her hands and knees. The obstacle course was combined into an imaginative story structured by Rosa. She placed hula-hoops on the floor to symbolise water pools. Coloured rings became magic rings that needed to be collected and foam wedges became mountains.

This game was at times played with her physiotherapist, Mel, with a competitive element. For example, they raced against a certain amount of time available on the clock. Sometimes, music was added or pictures were created to generate a livelier, more imaginative ambience. At times, a problem was posed, such as, "How can you get across the 'mountain' when you are unable to use your hands because they holding the 'magic rings'?"

Other creative problems were posed to enable Rosa to think of ways of moving different parts of her body, which she had barely been using. After residing for months in a wheelchair or bed, Rosa now had the psychological and physical strength to decide which part of her repertoire of body movements she would initiate once again.

Additional creative ideas have expanded upon children's individual interests, for example, imagining that one is an animal exploring the land. Dens have been created in the physiotherapy department under the child's architectual instructions. Subsequently, the child moves alongside a physiotherapist who narrates a story. For example, the physiotherapist and child imagined they were animals going through a tropical rainforest searching for hidden creatures. In addition, the use of food, water, and different textures are used during the physiotherapy sessions.

Creating problems, with the physiotherapist's assistance, to be solved through her innovative physical movements allowed Rosa to put her body at the service of her imagination. Rosa greatly enjoyed using her imagination, much more than she enjoyed exercising her body, and this fuelled her enthusiasm to pursue the physical activities.

Surprise

When all is said and done, helping the body exist in a different physical state can be painful and can create fear, because the child is fighting against the wish of "Just leave me alone. Let me be." There is also a natural wish of "Just accept and love me *as I am*." Also, the child is very worried about relinquishing being looked after "like a baby" who has the continuous presence of a thoughtful adult.

Adding an element of surprise to a physiotherapy session can be an unexpected gift, like a Christmas or Hannukah present or birthday gift. Creating surprise in the session suggests that the physiotherapist has really thought of the child before the session and brought the gift of an imaginative, engaging session rather than just another boring task to be done together.

Psychoanalyst Dr Meltzer (personal communication) often said:

> You may have to say the same things again and again... because the child requires the same understanding yet again. However, if you have said something once and the child has heard you, then she will not listen. She will experience you as boring unless you find a way of saying the same thing just a little bit differently, with something new added.

Adding something creative and new is what adds an element of unexpected pleasure within the physiotherapy encounter.

Conclusion

What can you do when you feel overburdened, defensive, and reach an impasse in working with a child, or you are with a child for an extended number of years, because the child's disability will last for life?

Julia Cameron's book *An Artist's Way* (1995) suggests that you find a way of creating more space for your own emotional life. It is this that you can change more than you can change anything in the child's attitude to your physiotherapy. Cameron suggests that each day you write four pages by hand, not on the computer, to let out the emotions, dreams, and thoughts you have upon awakening.

You might also want to do another exercise which is to write honestly to yourself about how you feel about being with this particular young person. Often, it is your repressed anger, hostility, and frustration that drag you down and inhibit the flow of warmth and closeness to a child (Winnicott, 1949). So be honest with yourself about how you feel!

We don't see how anybody can work as a physiotherapist without having some regular supportive supervision groups or a supportive team. If you don't have one, set one up with a facilitator, or join a "work discussion seminar" similar to those offered by the Observation Course at the Tavistock Clinic in London (Rustin & Bradley, 2008). This might be another way of thinking about your relationship with the children with whom you work, and also a way of examining your relationship with yourself in the role of a physiotherapist.

These questions are useful to ponder throughout different stages in your professional life, for the answers to the questions may differ at different times in your life. The questions are:

1. Why have I chosen the field of physiotherapy?
2. What in my personal life has influenced my choice of career?
3. What about my work gives me personal gratification?
4. What am I trying to repair, not only in the child, but also in myself?
5. What factors impede my sense of fulfilment in the role as a physiotherapist?
6. What impeding factors can I locate in myself rather than in others?
7. How can I get help or create a situation that can modify these impediments to my work as a physiotherapist?

Answering these questions can be a way of enhancing the quality of your rapport both with yourself, and with the children and families you see. Remember, you might not be able to change a very disabled child's physical capability dramatically, but you can change your attitude to your work!

Our purpose in presenting this work has been to inspire you to think more deeply about the personal encounter you have as a physiotherapist engaged in an intimate relationship with the child and the family. We have shared a few concepts important to your task: collaboration, curiosity, containment, confidence, creative imagination, and surprise. Hopefully, this will inspire you to appreciate how much you have to offer to the non-speaking child and the family.

CHAPTER ELEVEN

The silent child in school: teaching a child who does not talk, walk, or eat

Sarah Dixon

Introduction

As a teacher I am expected to provide learning experiences and to evaluate whether or not I have achieved my aim of helping students to use their mind to learn and to be curious. A teacher is an acknowledged guide in the process of learning.

There is a code of conduct in place to ensure that the students have the responsibility for meeting the expectation which the school, representing society, places on them in order that they can become responsible citizens in the society. When confronted with a non-speaking, non-walking, child, this point of view with regard to education is severely challenged. Initially, because the non-speaking, severely withdrawn child does not want to be present in school, he is not interested in what is being taught and is non-responsive to any questions (even via a nod), or not willing to engage in any school tasks. The teacher feels that the non-speaking, severely withdrawn child is not allowing the teacher to function as a teacher. If as a teacher you are faced with a student who does not comply with the code of behaviour, you would refer the student to the Head of Year to be sanctioned. None of this is relevant when working with a non-speaking, severely withdrawn child apart from expecting the child to be in the classroom. In the school in which I work, I have been presented with a number of severely withdrawn students who could not follow the code of conduct as they were not speaking and would not or could not participate in any school tasks even by looking at what was being presented. At the severe end of the spectrum of not-speaking, withdrawing, not eating, not walking would be those children who have been given the psychiatric diagnosis of *pervasive refusal syndrome* (Lask, 2004). I use this term in this chapter hesitantly, for *refusal* implies that the self has an active choice in rejecting others' overtures, yet the way of behaving is much more like that of a terrified, traumatised child who feels helpless in the face of either or both an internal emotional experience or external trauma. We prefer to say that the child is *pervasively retreating from life*.

A non-speaking, severely withdrawn child has taken refuge in primitive protections by initially closing his eyes to people, closing his ears to the teacher, and turning away when approached. He has closed many doors to relationships and communicating via speaking or looking at the teacher. A teacher will rely on some means of communication to understand and work with the individual. A teacher could find herself in a place where she is not able to fulfil her duties. If the student doesn't give some feedback it is difficult for the teacher to assess whether or not learning is taking place. This can leave the teacher feeling helpless and challenged in her work.

When I found myself in this situation, with my first severely withdrawn, non-speaking student, Tony, I was advised to consider that communication is always taking place although it is silent. I needed to look closely at the position of Tony's child's eyes, hands and body and note the moment of changes which might occur through gestures such as turning the head or moving in the chair. I was also told that I needed to rely on my intuitions, my feelings from moment to moment when I was with the non-speaking child. This would be the communication upon which I would rely while teaching.

I have found it helpful to reflect upon how it might feel for the child to be in the classroom and think about how I feel from moment to moment with this child. It was very easy as a teacher in such a situation with a non-speaking child protectively cocooned by his back and initially looking away from me, to feel nothing was happening, because initially nothing apparent was being learned.

To assist me in this process of teaching and understanding the non-speaking child in retreat, I decided to write a diary in order to reflect more carefully day by day on any subtle changes between the child, myself, the teacher and the other students. This wasn't a simple diary like one might write about one's experience. As I embarked on the task of diary writing, I realised I wanted to bridge the gap between Tony and me. After all, even though he wasn't speaking to me, this wouldn't prevent me from speaking with him through writing my thoughts to him in the diary, that was, until he was sufficiently robust for me to speak more directly to him. Just because he was rejecting me, I didn't have to stop thinking and communicating with him! Through this diary, I was able to share my feelings with Tony. I would not necessarily share this diary directly with a non-speaking child, but the diary functioned as a bridge to help me to develop a shared understanding and connection with the child.

In the following section, I am sharing pages of my diary notes to non-speaking, severely withdrawn Tony, and I am accompanying my notes with a commentary regarding how our multidisciplinary team evolved in its own thinking with regard to helping Tony and other non-speaking, severely withdrawn children whose unique personalities were hidden under similar symptoms of retreat from relationships with the external world. As a teacher I was confronted with the emotional experience of feeling rejected by Tony's long retreat into not looking, speaking, writing, listening or thinking.

Tony is a fourteen-year-old Irish boy whose divorced parents are the second generation of their Irish family to live in Brighton. Tony has three younger sisters including a set of eight-year-old twins.

Week 1

Tony, you are going to take a new step in your journey to recovery in hospital by attending school. It has been a long time since you have done this. Perhaps one of your memories of school is that it is a very large space with different rooms and a lot of people being very noisy. It is a place where you are expected to learn, take notes, answer questions, and move from one classroom to the other. But most of all, it is an environment in which you are expected to speak with your teachers and peers.

At the moment, I expect you do not want any of those things: you want to be left alone. You feel frightened and anxious as it is a new place with new people. Maybe you feel angry that no one is listening to your silence, your inability to take part. You do not feel ready to be in school.

As your teacher, my role is to be the person who will try to make you feel safe and comfortable. I need to nurture and care for you, to show you that even though you feel so unwell, you can be in school. I can look after you and try to understand how difficult this new step is for you.

We decide that to make you feel safe, we will introduce you only to one teacher, me. I will be with you at all times. I will talk to you; describe this new environment to you. I am going to tell you about who is in your class, what lesson is taking place and what the other students are doing. I am going to describe what is going to happen next so that you know what to expect. I will reassure you: you are not expected to do anything, resting and relaxing in this environment is safe. I will find you a comfortable chair and cushions for you to sit on. You can go to sleep if all becomes overwhelming. This will be your seat and classroom for the next few weeks. I will not expect you to talk to me or your peer group or to use any resources to occupy your time. At this time being in the classroom is all you can manage.

You were brought to school by one of the nursing staff. You were crying, hiding your face with your hand. I could not see your eyes, but could only hear your sobs. Your neck looked tense but at the same time too weak to carry your head. Your head was bent forward, so you needed to use your hand to help support it to keep it straight. You looked so unhappy and frightened; it seemed you did not want to be here. You would not let go of the arm of the nurse who brought you to the school. I introduced myself to you, explained who I was and what I would be doing. I also told you about the other people in the room. You cried, showing me all that was hurting inside your body. You rubbed your hand in circles on your tummy, shaking your head at the same time. As I acknowledged how difficult this might be for you, you embraced yourself, holding your tummy, whilst retreating into a curled up position. You did

> not look around. Did you want me to see that your stomach hurt, that you did not want to be here, that you wanted to be left alone?
>
> I gave you some space and walked to the other side of the room. After a while, I came back and started talking about the pictures on the wall, wondering what you liked, what your favourite colour was. You did not look at me. I suggested you have a rest by pulling the blanket over you and arranging the cushions on the table so that you could rest your head on them. You refused the cushions by pushing them to the floor. Your gesture was very abrupt and it looked angry; maybe you thought I was not listening to you. Are you trying to tell me that you do not want to be here, you are ill; you want to be in bed? Because you were crying, I placed a tissue box in front of you, but you did not take any tissues, and tears streamed down your face. At the end of the lesson, I offered to help you out of the room by placing my arm underneath yours and gently pushing you off your seat. You did not move and I felt the tension in your body growing. Your arm became rigid while you curled up more on the chair; you wanted a nurse to take you. You don't know me and don't trust me and making changes is anxiety-provoking.

When initially working as a teacher with a non-speaking, severely withdrawn child, it is important to take away all expectations. At the beginning of entry into the school, as a teacher, I am not supposed to be teaching and expecting achievement. Knowing this helps to lessen the guilt I might feel. The beginning of school for a non-speaking, severely withdrawn child should be the start of building a trusting and reliable relationship, for the child might lack any internal trustworthy experience.

In the teacher's role of nurturing the child, we need to acknowledge what he is doing in such a vulnerable state of mind. Acknowledging anxiety about every little change that occurs in the classroom is important. This includes preparing the child for any transition by always warning the child of any change in the day, describing what will happen next, and reminding the child that there are no expectations in relation to the change.

Week 2

> Tony, this week I decide to meet your parents. I want to get to know you a little more, so I ask them what you were like in school. Did you like attending school? What was your favourite subject? What were your hobbies? I ask your parents to bring in some of your work, so that when it feels right, we can look at it together.
>
> I used this information to talk to your peers during the lesson so that they can get to know you. I tell them about your school and what year you are in. The students tell you what their home schools are like and what they enjoy. This gives an opportunity for you to meet the students in your class. We talk about your timetable and the different lessons that take place in the school. I reassure you: you are not expected to take part. You are not crying now.
>
> Towards the end of the week the other teachers in the school come and introduce themselves to you. They tell you their names and what they teach. I am still at your side. You don't cry in school anymore. When I ask you a question, you now respond by lifting your shoulders

> and letting them fall, while holding your head with your hand. It is still a very discreet gesture on your behalf. It looks to me like you are shrugging.

At this point there is no clear "no" or "yes", just what looks like a shrug, the beginning of a response, but it is unclear what it means. At times Tony is not using his mind to think. At other times Tony fears that his mind will be intruded upon by the teacher who is aware of anything he experiences in this environment. He seemed not to want to make a link that would help him develop in school or within himself.

Looking at Tony's life before he was so obviously ill helps to make connections with his previously healthy functioning self and thus reminds Tony that he has some potential. This link with the student whom he was can be achieved through discussions with both his parents and his peer group.

Because non-speaking Tony has given a little response to me, rather than acting as though I do not exist at all, which sometimes happens with other non-speaking, severely withdrawn students. I feel I can take the opportunity to try to take another little step with him by expecting a tiny step forward, while at the same time keeping very low expectations. It is difficult to know if what I am doing as a teacher with Tony is right or wrong, because there is so little response from him which indicates either a positive or negative experience. Sometimes I feel his body is present but his mind has left the classroom and moved into a blank state. He rarely shows a gesture which says things are okay, but when he dislikes something I do see him withdraw with a closure of his eyes or with a turn of his head. There is no prescription for how I, as a teacher, should proceed, but there are two things which help:

1. Observing Tony, putting myself in his shoes, seeing how I feel at that moment, and using my intuition.
2. Thinking with the multidisciplinary team, finding ways of being involved with members of team working with Tony. Developing a sense that they and I are supporting each other through our observing Tony, thinking about our countertransference experiences, and trying to make sense of them together.

As any progress or change occurs in the child there arise different and sometimes conflicting emotional experiences in working the different multidisciplinary team members.

For example, competition can set in and one professional may try to assign or take credit for the child's progress depending on to whom Tony is responding positively or negatively. If Tony responds positively to me and not to my colleague, then I sometimes must face the other teacher's rivalry. Part of working within a multidisciplinary team means that team issues surrounding the progress will occur. There are controversially different points of view in the multidisciplinary team regarding how much to encourage Tony to move forward. It is important for us to acknowledge both Tony's fear and his hostility. It is not helpful for us to simply see him as a delicate and loving child.

Colluding with and exploring Tony's hostility

Week 3

The nurses are still bringing you over to school and helping you sit down. We decide that we will introduce you to the rest of the school. I show you your timetable again and explain that this week we will move you from classroom to classroom so that you can follow your peer group. The nurses will help you sit in the appropriate room and collect you from it. I will be in the same room as you, sitting next to you. After each lesson, I indicate in which room you will be sitting next, so that you know what to expect. I will also tell you that I will be waiting for you so that you know I will be in the lesson with you. The teachers greet you at the start of each lesson; however, no material is placed in front of you. Sitting in the room is all you can manage. I cover your body with a blanket and put some cushions on the table. I suggest that you can put your head down and have a rest if you feel unwell, for you often complain of feeling tired and unwell.

During some free time in school, I decide to show you some of the work you completed in your home school before you became unwell. I make you aware that I am getting this work for you and I go to your drawers to pick up your books. You are sitting in your chair, holding your head up with your hand while your elbow rests on the desktop. I cannot see your face. Once I open the school-book, you start hunching your back a little more. You bring your second hand up and hide your face completely. I decide to ignore the fact that you seem to want me to leave you alone and not do something new. I look at the book and describe to you what I see. I notice that you turn your head a little away from me in the opposite direction.

I suggest that looking at your old school-book might feel difficult as it is a reminder of your life before you became unwell. (I am also aware that at the moment your mind might not be functioning as it was in the past for your mind is filled with worrying experiences.) I try to imagine what you like, leafing through the books, and I wonder aloud with you. With your head turned away from me, you stay completely still through this. This makes me doubt whether I am moving too fast with you, however I decide to persist, taking into account that you are not crying.

I spend my time with you wondering what you are like. You manage to shrug at times. I wonder out-loud inviting you to reflect silently alongside me as I consider your past experiences in school. Later, at no time do I acknowledge all the work you are doing to be present in our experience together. If I notice you are managing something differently because you are not crying and you are responding to me with a glance or facial expression, I don't give you feedback about this. I will acknowledge that you might be finding things difficult but I will not praise you. For some reason I don't understand, praise makes you go backwards to an earlier phase of your illness.

I continue to engage in conversations with the other students around the table while trying to include you. I share with the students some stories of your life in school in the past and describe how I feel you are experiencing the classroom experience with them. The students ask you questions and you manage to respond this week by very discreetly shrugging or shaking your head. The students try to imagine what you might be feeling in relation to whatever

> thoughts they may have about you. They also wonder aloud about how you might feel in the classroom at that particular moment when they are with you.

Praise is usually one of the main ways a teacher encourages the students' progress in the class. But Tony has different ideas about praise. He is not only turning away, shrugging or shaking his head to say no. He is signaling that he is not going to accept any suggestion of progress in school. Tony does not want to work alongside me or anyone else in the school. At this stage Tony simply does not want to have anything to do with his school from the past or his present life in our school. If I suggest that he is interested in what I, the teacher, am saying, interested in working with me, Tony worries that too much will be expected of him. If by some chance a teacher or student forgets and praises his interest in school life or any progress whatsoever in school, Tony retreats to an earlier phase of development! A non-speaking, severely withdrawn child such as Tony, has a defensive side that attacks any sign of life going forward.

Week 4

> I set up regular meetings with your parents to keep them up to date with your progress in school. I describe which lessons you attend and explain to them that our only expectation is for you to be in the room with us. I also explain that I don't praise you, as I don't want you to think that I believe everything has become easier for you. Your parents and I decide to keep in regular contact so that I can let them know your progress and let them receive any praise I might have for you. Letting them know even the most minute movements which suggest you are managing gives them some relief and hope that you will return to your life outside hospital. I ask your parents to describe in more detail what your likes and dislikes in school were. They are encouraged to tell me which subjects you felt enthusiastic about, which after-school clubs you joined, if there were particular teachers you liked and why? What didn't you like about your teacher? What was it like with your peers in the classrooms? I use this information to keep wondering with you about what kind of person you once were.
>
> I also keep talking to you about how difficult everything seems at the moment and how much you feel you cannot or do not want to be part of school.

As only non-verbal communication is taking place between the child and the teacher, and often only non-verbal gesturing is occurring between the child and the parents, it feels important for the teacher to work closely with the parents both to support the parents but also to gain assistance in understanding Tony. Once Tony's parents are aware that he was attending the inpatient unit school, they developed a new set of expectations. At times, because Tony was so very regressed within his pervasive retreat from life, the approach teachers had with him could come across as cruel. They would wonder at times why in the world we thought he should go to school! We had different expectations in school than those the nurses placed on Tony within living quarters of the inpatient unit. Also, for the weekly reviews and the six weekly meeting with the referring team, there was a certain style which was used in the teachers' written reports on Tony's school experience. In particular, there was no praise or expectation written in the report; however, this did not mean that no progress was taking place. The parents and professionals needed detailed discussions to understand the concept of "no praise" and why it was used for Tony in the school environment. The parents realised that usually both they and teachers would praise Tony and yet they also saw that praise set Tony back. By withdrawing praise and comments on progress, we realised that we were all collaborating in doing something that goes against the educational philosophy that praise supports a child's progress.

The inpatient unit school teachers also had the task of collaborating with both the parents and the home school teachers *to pace* Tony's progress. Our primary message was that Tony needed time to heal his emotional self. The work that was taking place in the school involved addressing some basic emotional developments which needed to occur before any learning could take place. It was important that Tony developed trust in us and confidence that we would not require too much of him next time round if he did participate in any school activity at any particular moment. Tony had a history of achieving very good marks, but perhaps he was not equally emotionally equipped to deal with the pressures involved in making social and academic progress in school.

Week 5 to Week 8

> It feels more difficult for you to settle in school. You seem more upset and spend a lot more of your time crying. You are hiding your face with your hands and it has become more difficult to engage you in conversations. At times you look like you are trying to curl up inside the chair, retreating into your own space and not wanting to let anyone in. You are no longer responding to questions from the other students. You stay immobile with none of the previous usual movements of your head or shoulders when they try to talk to you. Through your posture I can see that you are trying to retract yourself as much as possible. It feels like you are closing yourself down.
>
> We continue to make sure you are sitting in the correct room so that you are part of the relevant lessons. We continue not to expect you to use any of the resources. I continue to sit next to you, try to identify with you and speak on your behalf to the group. I'm trying to role model a little of who you might have been in the past. This can be difficult when I have never met you before you became non-speaking, not-walking, not eating and so very ill, pervasively retreating from life.
>
> The teachers have provided something safe and comforting through the cushions and blanket, which can be used like a turtle shell, to make you feel secure. When you become upset, I place some tissues on your lap. You take and use them. However your crying does not cease or calm down. I try to understand why things seem more difficult at the moment.
>
> We start talking about the school holidays approaching and the change of structure. I wonder whether or not this change is scaring you. You have become used to the school routine; maybe starting a new summer routine outside school feels unbearable at the moment? Too many changes!

Sometimes things become worse for a while. Why? There is no answer to this question. All that is known is that slow, steady progress feels like too much. I wonder whether Tony fears that he might leave the inpatient unit before he feels emotionally ready to do so. Maybe there is something which is simply "not-good enough" in his life outside the unit. I know he had felt hurt by his peers, but I don't know much about his family relationships, except that he is very close to his divorced mother. Is it simply that the change of routine is very troubling? Is it hard to be involved with peers because of unresolved peer issues? At this stage I just have to live with not-knowing and hold onto the hope that steps backward will be followed by steps forward. Tony is not talking, walking or eating yet! I need to trust that this way of feeling by seeing, through the window of Tony's eyes and using my intuition in relation to what I feel with him, is a way of helping his move forward. I need to realise that sometimes I may feel helpless, and I need to bear the fact that feeling uncertain and curious about him is appropriate at this time. I am encouraged by the multidisciplinary team to find some trust in this method of work. Tony's recent regression could be the result of too much social and academic progress too quickly. His regression does not necessarily mean that I and the other teachers are doing the wrong thing. Patience, persistence, and carrying hope on behalf of Tony might be the work that is necessary at this stage.

Week 10

> It was half-term and it has been a week since you were last in school. We decide to support you with making a change in school. I reassure you that we will only be making one change at a time. It was decided that we would help you sit appropriately on a chair by enabling you to straighten your back. This posture will give you a more secure base and perhaps more confidence when sitting in the classroom, but if nothing else, it will also help you look around so that you can take an interest in your environment.
>
> It is decided that I will be the person who will support you with your posture. The other teachers will continue greeting you, but will place no expectations upon you. As I am sitting next to you, I will remind you to sit straight. I will do this non-verbally, as I do not want you to feel that I am pressuring you by evoking the other students' attention. I will use gentle rubbing on your back. I want to give you the privacy to do the work you need to do.
>
> The teachers also decided to introduce one-to-one time with you. Every day, I will be spending time with you to complete a task on your behalf. I choose a picture to colour in, trying to pick an image that depicts things you like, so that we will have an opportunity to talk while I am colouring in for you. I choose a picture representing "T" the first letter of your name. The letter is made up of different animals. This enables me to connect with you, but also it gives a focus to the work we are doing. I suggest that we will decorate the picture so that you could use it at a later time as a poster for your room, or maybe offer it to your parents. I describe the shapes and the different shades of colours. I might say: "This is a horse. A horse can be many different colours, black, brown, white or grey. I wonder what your favourite colour would be for a horse?" Or, as I am looking at the other colours we have chosen, I wonder aloud to you, "I am thinking, which colour would look best for our picture". This gives me an opportunity to wonder who you are behind your illness.

I contact your home school every six weeks to update your teachers about the progress you are making. I use this occasion to ask your school to send a picture I could colour in with you, to keep a connection with your school-life outside the unit.

You feel more settled in school and you have started walking with assistance. I decide to take you outside in the garden to walk you from the inpatient unit school to the entrance of the inpatient unit. I place my arm underneath yours and pull you up gently. You respond to my support and grab on tightly to my arm. We walk together at your pace. It feels to me that you are starting to trust me, and you understand that I will not try to push you to do things you don't feel ready to do.

It is always difficult to know when the right time will be to introduce something new in the non-speaking child's timetable. Working with a multidisciplinary team means there is close observation of Tony in all the different activities and settings throughout the day. This close observation and discussion of our observations in weekly reviews and small core team meetings, as well as in the multidisciplinary work discussion group with a psychotherapist, helps all of us to become aware of Tony's emotional, physical, and intellectual development. At all times, the multidisciplinary team members were encouraging me to trust my instincts. If I felt that I had taken a wrong decision to encourage Tony too much, then it felt appropriate to openly discuss this with Tony. The teachers had regular school meetings to discuss the peer-group relationships, but I also found it very helpful to rely on the support of the multidisciplinary team. This was particularly important when Tony was having to manage the transition between the summer holiday timetable and the school timetable. It is at this time that the team might think it the appropriate moment to introduce something new, but actually there are enough changes at this point, and more significant changes could be encouraged when not so much external change is occurring. Tony's managing transitions was felt to be a sign that his emotional robustness was developing. More inner emotional stability and trust in staff permits a greater tolerance of external changes. We were also becoming more confident in refining the ways in which we could help Tony to work.

Week 11

In the previous week, you managed to accept the change we made, by setting the expectation upon you to sit up straight during the lesson. When I rubbed my hand onto your back, you would respond by lifting your chest. You relied less on the hand upon which your head rested. It did not seem that you complained about this new expectation because you persisted with correcting your position and placing your body in an upright position. After a few minutes, you managed to communicate that this task was too demanding for you by falling back into a hunched position. As in the previous week, you had allowed me to walk you to the door of the inpatient unit; from this, I understood that you were now allowing me to encourage your progress a little more. It seems to me that, as you trust me more, you will feel able to let me know when to stop encouraging you to move forward. I feel we are developing a shared understanding, a way of communicating with each other.

Due to these changes involving your walking with assistance and sitting upright for some time in the school chair, I sense that it might be the right time for a new step. From now on,

> I will take part in *all* the lessons on your behalf. I will no longer spend private individual time with you every day; however I will meet you on a weekly basis to reflect on how school-life is for you. I will wonder aloud to myself about whether or not there are educational tasks that you might feel able to do on your own, and question myself about which educational tasks which will be too demanding for you at this point.
>
> During the lessons, I will be given a notebook by the teachers, *as if* I am substituting for you. In this notebook, I will take class notes for you and complete your homework. The teachers will talk to you, looking at you directly, when asking a question, but I will respond on your behalf. We will become a twinned pair in the lessons, and I will do for you the things you cannot manage. The teachers will set an academic task to be done in the classroom, and I will do it on your behalf, speaking to you as I do it. They will address us as a team, and I will become your voice and your motivation during the lesson. I will interact with the other students and ask questions when I don't understand. I will welcome you at the entrance of the school and walk you to your seat in the classroom. I will continue to sit next to you in all lessons and gather all the school resources we will need. By gently rubbing your back, I will also continue to support your sitting up straight in your chair.
>
> During the lesson, I explain to you that I will be working on your behalf. I don't explain why, but I tell you that this will prevent you from falling too behind in your schooling. I remind you that we don't expect you to start participating in the inpatient unit school, but I will do this for you. You stay still while I am talking to you. Your face is hidden by your hand. When I ask if you mind my doing the schoolwork for you, you shrug. I understand this response as acceptance of this change. By now, you are indicating a firm "no" with a shake of your head if you don't like something. The new sets of expectations do not seem to frighten you. By the end of the week, through your gentle acceptance of my presence, I assume that you are non-verbally managing to indicate that you are grateful to me. I share this thought with you. You continue to allow me to support you in walking around to the different rooms of the school. This indicates to me that you are coping with the changes that are taking place.

The first time I was introduced to this concept of *identifying with* the student in school and behaving as though I was that non-speaking student now speaking, I found it extremely difficult to believe that this would help the student. I also worried about how the other students in the classroom would react and how this would impact on my role as a teacher in the school. I worried that the other students would lose respect for me as a teacher. Also, it felt very awkward and uncomfortable, as a teacher, to be in the role of a student. In addition, I felt very anxious that my teaching colleagues would start treating me as "the student" rather than as their colleague. As a teaching team, once we managed to discuss our different anxieties about doing this new kind of learning / teaching, I was able to overcome my worries and engage fully in what felt like a role-play. My undertaking the speaking and participating role of non-speaking Tony in class actually enabled Tony to feel more integrated into the classroom learning experiences.

Subsequently, I realised that role-playing "a speaking Tony" took away some of the shame non-speaking Tony might have, by giving him the opportunity of being in the classroom and doing the things we would expect other students to do (Tate, 1993). My role-playing "a speaking Tony" also offered a face-saver for later it would be easier for Tony, once he was ready, to continue the work I had already started, rather than having to start the academic work alone.

Finally Tony could use me, his teacher, to start doing schoolwork without his peers actually noticing such a big change in his behaviour when he began his work alone.

Week 12 and Week 13

> You settle into the new routine in school. You are starting to show some interest during the lessons. The teachers notice that you seat yourself so that you can look at the board and listen during the lessons. Your head is still resting on your hand, but you can look around the room when you choose too. Your hand is not placed directly on your forehead, but more on the side of your face so that your eyes are not covered by your hand as before.
>
> You remain very quietly attentive during the math's lesson and I feel that you might actually be taking in that which the other teaching is describing. It seems that your whole body subtly follows the teacher around the classroom for I can notice you repositioning yourself, depending on where the teacher is standing. The teachers can momentarily catch a glimpse of your eyes. However, you do not allow them to see you watching, and the teachers do not acknowledge that you are looking at the board. Whenever your eyes might meet the teachers', you look down or cover your face a little more with your hand. None of us give you feedback. The teachers praise me for the school-work I am completing on your behalf in your blue notebook.
>
> You start looking around and are becoming aware of the students in the class. I notice this when you seem to think that I am not looking at you. I see you looking through your fingers. Sitting up straight allows you to rotate your body easily. You listen to the classroom discussions and you start to feel interested in the educational tasks accompanying them. When the teacher sets the students a task to work on, you turn your body towards me. It feels to me like you are indicating to me that you actually want me to complete the task for you.
>
> Then one day, Mark, one of the students, asks you a math's question during a lesson. You feel able to look in the book I am completing for you and point to the right answer! In science class, we were asked to copy a diagram of one of the chemistry experiments from the book. You noticed I was drawing the wrong diagram; therefore, you used your hand to stop me. You then pointed to the correct diagram in the book. You then pointed back at the diagram I had started in your exercise book. As your finger went backwards and forwards between both diagrams, I understood you were trying to communicate that I should be drawing a different diagram. As you persisted in this task of gesturing to me, I felt that you did not feel resistant to letting me know that you were aware of the work that needed to be completed. I did not acknowledge this to you, I just proceeded to do the corrected task.
>
> The teachers continue to have no expectations. You allow them to walk you to the entrance of the school. It feels like you are starting to trust more teachers and students in the school. Maybe you are starting to enjoy your time in this environment? You do not seem concerned that the school is closing for school holiday and that your time structure will change in the next two weeks. You feel much stronger now.

Once Tony starts making noticeable progress, it feels more difficult than ever not to praise him. As a teacher it still feels unnatural, and requires me to go against all my professional instincts. It is also a time when as a multidisciplinary team we start to think about who and about when it would be appropriate to describe to Tony and others what we are noticing in school without risking sending Tony into a regressive retreat. Often other students made comments to Tony about his work or even complimented Tony. This enabled me, Tony's teacher, to see his reactions to his classmates and to assess how he was currently affected by a compliment and the acknowledgment that progress was taking place.

Week 16

> You continue to be present in the classroom, not only physically, but also in other ways. We are also becoming fully aware that you are listening, thinking and taking in your surroundings and this does not seem to frighten you. We allow you to make changes at your own pace, whilst not acknowledging them.
>
> It has become noticeable that you are looking at the white board and listening to the teachers and thinking about what they are saying. However, you hide your face and turn around when you feel they are looking at you. You are not ready to expose yourself. You do not want the teachers to see that you are interested in the lessons and therefore in an emotional place where you are ready to move forward in school. Is it perhaps that you are worried that they will expect you to do more than you feel ready or able to do and you want them to remember that you are still very ill?
>
> I continue to pretend that "I am you" and make sure that I allow you to be the student you would like to be by my trying to understand the lessons, taking notes for you and completing your homework. During a reading lesson, when we are reading *The Secret Garden* (Hodgson Burnett, 1911), I place the book we are reading in front of you. I sit next to you and read on your behalf using a different book. You are very quiet during this lesson, and appear to be listening to all of us read in turns. You look at your book and flick through the pages quite rapidly. You are probably frightened that this action will engender a reaction from the group. I interpret this as your possibly feeling ready to start using some of the school resources. I am not sure whether you are so pleased to have your own book or whether you are pleased to be reading because you used to love reading.

Week 17 to Week 22

> Once weekly, at a regular time, you and I find a quiet space to sit together. I talk to you about the things I have observed during the week and the feelings these might have brought up within you. I mention your touching the book we were reading. It must feel very scary to take a step forward. You might be wondering how people around you will react when they see your progress. You are not ready to be seen as someone who is recovering from a serious illness, you still feel very unwell and are not speaking, eating or holding a pencil.
>
> It is difficult to be perceived differently by people who have seen you behaving in a certain way for a long time. I start talking about the things you might like to do if you did not need to worry about others looking at you. I talk about drawing, making a collage of pictures you like, and reading. I use all the things your parents told me that you liked. I suggest you spend some time alone in a room with different resources so that no one can see what you are doing (Tate, 1993). I offer to stay in the room with you so that you do not feel scared and abandoned.

> I hope that through presenting you with different possibilities and discussing them with you, musing over how you might feel, I will be able to have some intuition, through getting a feeling in relation to your facial responses, regarding which step you will feel ready to take. You do not react to any of the suggestions, however you do not look like you are refusing them either. You do not move and look very calm. It seems to me that you are listening and maybe considering those options.
>
> During one of the meetings I say something silly, and I notice a slight smile. This gives me the confidence to try something new and different. I place a book on your lap under the table. The book I chose was *The Amber Spyglass* (Pullman, 2000), one your parents gave me a few weeks ago. You had started reading it before becoming unwell. Phillip Pullman was one of your favourite authors. I do it silently as I do not want you to think there is an expectation and I do not want anyone in the room to notice. You open the book at the first page and appear to start reading. I decide to leave the room as I feel it might be easier for you if I am not around. You stop. Then you start looking at book that I placed in front of you. During the reading lesson, you manage to turn the pages and follow the story. I continue *to be you* in all other lessons.

At this stage Tony is showing signs that he might feel ready to move on a little. He feels safe in a strong bonding relationship with me, his teacher, whom he trusts. However, as Tony behaved in a certain very regressed way for quite a lengthy period of time, it feels very difficult to find the motivation and courage to do something differently. I sense he fears that by doing so, he will attract a lot of attention from his peers, something that he has been avoiding since becoming ill. We can help by giving him a "face-saver", a way that will prevent him from losing his dignity or self-esteem. An example of this was a silent child wanting to become independent around the classroom by being able to move around unaided. So while supporting an extremely regressed, non-speaking child to stand, we made sure there would always be a wall close by for him to lean on so that he could start walking around the room by using the wall without the assistance of the member of staff.

Week 23

> The teachers told me that when I am not in the room, you read the books that I place in front of you. I decided to approach you and ask questions such as whether you would like to do some drawing. You are able to nod. Maybe you felt ready to do a little more than just read. You have taken an important step in reading and I sense that you still feel safe in this school environment to take another.
>
> During the maths lesson, I wonder whether you would like to answer a question set by the teacher, as you are looking more attentive and emotionally stronger. You are sitting in an upright position, and you seem less rigid and still in your posture. You are covering part of your face with your hand; however your hand seems to move in different directions, allowing your eyes to follow what is happening during the lesson. It also feels like the right lesson, as the answers required would be short and in the form of numbers. I grab some scrap paper and a pen, and place them in front of you. I wonder whether you would like to answer the question

> on the piece of paper. You shrug, it seems that you do not feel able to make the decision, and I feel worried about setting too hard an expectation on you; however, I courageously decide to write the question on the piece of scrap paper. You manage to take the pen and answer the question. I do not say anything to you about this, but instead decide to write down another question. I worry about the group commenting to you regarding your new scholastic step. While you solve the math problems, I copy your answers into your book. I ask you whether you would like to write in your notebook directly. You shake your head, so we continue the lesson in the same way. One of the students notices that you are writing and acknowledges it by complimenting you on your lovely handwriting. You do not seem perturbed by this and continue working.
>
> The other teachers and I decided that although you had taken a big step in the learning process I would keep on working alongside you the same way as before and various teachers would continue to address me in the same way as before when the teacher set you a task and asked me to read out the answer. We will set no expectations immediately, just because you have taken a step forward, for quick change is frightening to you. Therefore I will not automatically place the schoolbooks and notebook in front of you at the start of the lesson. At the beginning of the lesson I will first try to sense whether you would like to do some work and if the moment feels right, once the lesson for the others has started, I will fetch what you need to work.
>
> You communicated more with me this week, not through words but gestures. You started pointing to things in a more direct way; you are rotating yourself on the chair more often. Also your shrugs, shakes of the head and nods look more assured and confident. In this way, you helped me to understand the things you felt strong enough to do.

After having worked alongside each other for a couple of months, the relationship between Tony and me, his teacher, feels strong and a source of security. This means that, at this point, I can afford to take some risks by suggesting different activities to him. Tony will not interpret this as an expectation, and, even if he does, I can reassure him that he has a choice regarding what he decides to do. This more cooperative learning phase shows the importance of having built such a trusting relationship with Tony. As a result of his internalising this trusting relationship with me, he is able to use my support to make more academic progress.

Week 24

> As I walked in the classroom I noticed that you had gathered your pen, notebook and a text book required for the lesson. I sat next to you and wondered aloud whether you felt ready to write directly into your notebook. You shook your head; therefore, I continued copying your answers into your notebook for you.
>
> In one of the art lessons, I did not sit beside you. One of the other teachers, a male teacher, introduced the lesson and then helped the students set up the art resources they needed. As the students had seen you working in other lessons, they asked the art teacher what you would be doing. The art teacher acknowledged it was a very good question and placed some art materials in front of you, reassuring you that you did not have to participate should you

not feel able to do so. Once the teacher had taken his attention away from you, you started working independently, and managed to draw some ducks on a pond completely alone.

Later on in the week, I again was absent during one of the lessons. The teacher asked whether you would like him to complete the work on your behalf, for he wondered if it might feel difficult for you to miss out on the lesson. You allowed the teacher to write in your notebook for you, and you felt able to show him the page on which you were working.

We decided to introduce you to a new area used by the school, the garden in which we played games. You felt able to walk around with me, and I described the country garden to you. I spoke to you about the different names of the flowers and their need for sun and water. I also talked about how the flowers were organised to bloom at different times in the flowerbed, and how difficult it might be to plant a seed and imagine how different it would look once it bloomed. I also spoke about the different areas in the garden and how the young people used those to do different activities, such as playing netball, playing in the water, or sitting and relaxing. We then sat and watched the other young people playing netball.

Week 25

I sat next to you whilst completing some geography homework set by the teacher. I waited for you to answer the questions before I copied them into the book. Then, feeling you might be ready to undertake another task, I asked if you felt ready to write the answers directly into your notebook. This time, you nodded. I stayed beside you while by yourself you completed all the questions regarding the characters in *Chariots of Fire* (Wetherby, 1987).

You need a lot of reassurance while working. You were completing some homework set by your Science teacher. You needed to fill in some gaps in a text using specific words. You filled in all the gaps and then placed the book in front of me and pointed to your answers. I understood that you wanted me to check on whether or not your answers were right.

This week you work in many lessons including maths, science, English and art. You also use an increasing variety of gestures while looking at me to communicate your knowledge and what assistance you require from me. You start using hand movements to indicate that you want me to elaborate on something I am helping you to learn. You also use your hands to mime objects you need. I acknowledge your growing interest in learning more in school and I encourage your participation by providing you with more schoolwork. You still hide your face from the teachers for you may still be worried about being engaged in schoolwork that might require too much of you, and also you may be worried about receiving positive responses to your increased participation in school. The teachers therefore ensure that no direct praise is given, but respond by involving you in a thoughtfully planned, slightly more progressive way in each lesson. For example, the teachers organised a geometry lesson that involved all the young people in answering questions on a white board and lifting their boards to show their answers without talking. In this way, you felt included in the task, with us focusing on what you are able to do.

The teachers then sought a way to engage you in working alongside other students without the presence of a staff member. The opportunity presented itself when some students were given the task of painting a garden table. When a teacher suggested to you that you might help them, you agreed by nodding. You were then paired up with another student, rather than being paired with me as usual. You took this in your stride and eventually completed painting the garden table. You were left alone with your partner, who offered to assist in walking you back to the classroom. You refused. I had to come and collect you. You trust the teachers to look after you but are not ready to open up completely to the world of the young people.

Week 26

You are now walking around the school unaided. This enables you to take more initiative in setting up what you need for lessons. You also take charge by collecting the books and writing materials that you need for classes. As you are in charge of preparing yourself for the lessons, you decide to sit on your own rather than next to me.

While looking through your books, I notice that you wrote down your name and the date at which you took responsibility for gathering and writing in your notebook. I understand this as your communicating to me that you no longer need my support in the same way as you have required it previously. As I am not at your side during the lessons, the teachers decide to start addressing you directly and approach you to support and encourage you with your work. You do not seem frightened by this and go on to work independently in all lessons. The teachers are still not giving you feedback on your participation; however, they start to wonder about acknowledging the school work you are doing. Although your communication is still non-verbal, you manage to make yourself understood more fully through more clearly understood, well-defined hand gestures.

Week 27

As you are completing more work independently, you require greater reassurance and feedback from your teachers. Halfway through a lesson, the geography teacher sets some questions relating to his previous teaching. You wrote down the answer to the first question, then raised your hand so that he would come to see you. You pointed at your answer, using a hand gesture to ask whether you had done it correctly. As the teacher feels you have taken a step forward in asking for help, he feels confident in giving you praise and guidance on your school work. You accept this and persist in doing your school assignments even when the teachers correct your work. The teachers do not praise your participation in the classroom as you may still feel antagonistic to this type of praise.

In activities requiring teamwork, you participate and work collaboratively with the other students. The students have an understanding of your difficulty in communicating verbally and adapt their behaviour to include you.

As you feel emotionally more confident, the teachers decide to involve you in the gentle physical games the other students play during school hours, with the hope that you will engage with your peers. Taking part in physical activities is a new step for you, as it is a step towards health. You manage to participate a little; however, you isolate yourself from the group and do not interact much with them. You still hide your face with your hand.

Throughout the week, you start doing more activities you enjoy, such as arts and crafts. You independently find all the paper and paints you need to do this. This leads me to understand that you remember their places from many weeks ago when I was describing the garden and the school to you. I believe you were more aware of your surroundings, although you were not able to show this.

I decide to remove myself from the lessons in which you are now taking part, to give you the opportunity to evolve and progress at your own pace and with growing confidence. Your communication, although still non-verbal, is well-defined and clear enough to be understood in all areas of your school life. This reassures me that you can manage without my constant and close support. Your face remains hidden, which I interpret as a sign that you are not quite ready to face every day life as a healthy young person. The teachers and I still continue to have no expectations, and help you with your progress in a way that is both tailored to meet your individual needs and supportive to you.

Conclusion

I will try to summarise the techniques we employed in supporting and teaching non-speaking, non-eating, and initially non-walking Tony. The school teachers in our psychiatric inpatient unit would generally employ similar specifically tailor-made techniques for other non-speaking, severely regressed, withdrawn students, *pervasively retreating from life* (Lask, 2004).

At first, the aim is to make the school a safe place which understands and accepts the young person with his regression and retreat from life. We let go of all expectations a school would normally have for its students. All school requirements are reduced to one single non-negotiable activity which is: at least during some of the school hours, the young person has to be in school.

The teachers make this possible by offering care and nurturing understanding. This is achieved through providing physical comfort and security through the use of a blanket as a covering, cushions in case the young person becomes tired and a specially comfortable chair. Structure and routine become important components, which enable the young person to feel safe as he knows what to expect. Not to overwhelm the young person, only a key-teacher and one classroom is initially presented to him. The teachers understand the non-speaking, pervasively retreating young person. To some extent the teachers understand the non-speaking young person pervasively retreating from life and therefore, initially they will not place any expectations on him to participate in school life. Teachers will also accept that initially the young person may not be in a psychological space where he will feel able to speak to others or to respond other than through hiding his face or making hand gestures. At all times the body posture of the young person serves as a communication of his state of mind, and initially the body suggests that the child is in retreat from everyone in the school.

The schoolteachers try to develop a sensitively thought-out relationship with the non-speaking, withdrawn, regressed young person by choosing one especially sensitive teacher who will develop a significantly helpful relationship with him. Each day this key-teacher is the first point of contact for the young person. The named key-teacher will greet the pervasively retreating, nonspeaking young person at the school entrance in the morning and in the afternoon the teacher will say goodbye to him at the school doorway. The key-teacher will spend most of his time with the young person, describing the school environment, introducing him to the other students and teachers, and sitting beside him in the school. The key-teacher will also develop an ongoing, regularly arranged, collaborative discussion with the young person's parents and the home school. This key-teacher's relationship with significant others who knew the non-speaking, severely regressed student well before he retreated into "his illness" will help the teachers and students to get to know the young person better. The dialogue with parents and former teachers gives information which the key-teacher can later use to reflect upon with the non-speaking, regressed young person in regards to the person he used to be and his relationships within his previous school.

By forming a close collaborative relationship being *identified with* and alongside the young person, listening and potentially learning, the key-teacher forms a stable, trustworthy connection with the non-speaking young person. The growing understanding between the key-teacher and the non-speaking student facilitates the development of more reciprocal exchanges involving the young person's accepting the teacher and lessons, as shown through more open facial, hand and bodily responses. It feels as though when the non-speaking young person feels more secure with the teacher, he is able to engage his mind in thinking, rather than retreating, from learning situations.

The teachers, particularly the key-teacher, will be closely observing the non-speaking young person's sequence of actions in response to classroom events. Alongside close observations of sequences of activity, the teachers will use their intuitive emotional responses to the regressed young person to guide them in both understanding and supporting the young person's step-by-step development. The intuitive timing of the key-teacher's interventions supporting the retreating, non-speaking child's academic interest and progress is of prime importance.

My experiences as a teacher have now enabled me to be patient and to trust the educational process I have described in this chapter. Inevitably the young person slowly moves towards developing a trusting, therapeutic relationship with me, his teacher. When he feels safe, he will let me know how much thinking and working on tasks in the classroom he can manage. Gradually he will start writing, drawing, using words instead of gestures to communicate with me, and will begin to join his fellow students in school tasks.

The pairing between the extremely withdrawn, regressed young person and the key-teacher becomes an important step in helping the young person to take up an active role in the lesson. The teacher becomes a role model for the regressed, non-speaking young person, reassuring him that there is still no setting of expectations for him to learn. This technique enables the young person to take responsibility for his own learning. When *he feels emotionally ready*, he can continue with the bridging academic work that has been started by the teacher on his behalf.

The teacher will always use her empathy and intuitive support for progress as part of her offering an emotionally containing relationship with the non-speaking young person. The regressed, non-speaking young person's trust in the teacher facilitates the development of the young person's sense of himself and sense of self-confidence in growing up in a healthy way, until he is able to take up his appropriate place within his peer group.

CHAPTER TWELVE

"Compelled to die": psychotherapy with a girl who does not talk, walk, or eat

Jeanne Magagna

Emaciated, eyes closed to every object or person, she lay on the hospital bed. She refused food and drink and seemed not to notice anything including urine trickling out of her. With her straight dark hair and smooth oval Modigliani face, she looked like a porcelain doll. She was motionless throughout the day and night. When after some time she began to respond, she treated any nurse's touch or word like a mosquito creating a stinging irritation. She looked as thought the umbilical cord that held her in life had been broken. There seemed to be no emotional point to her existence.

Diagnosis

Yufang was admitted into a hospital in a coma. Her right lung had collapsed completely, her kidneys had stopped functioning, and she needed dextrose transfusions because of hypoglycemia. She was being fed by nasogastric tube and diagnosed as being in a state of depressive stupor. Initially the doctors treated her with psychotropic drugs. Those drugs failed. Yufang was slowly dying for she had lost a wish to live. Yufang was suffering from an extreme example of profound helplessness and hopelessness that underlies many severe eating disorders. Her disorder has been labelled as "pervasive refusal syndrome" by the Eating Disorder Team at Great Ormond Street Hospital (Lask, Britten, Kroll, Magagna, & Tranter, 1991). This name, pervasive refusal, is misleading, for Yufang felt "compelled to die" because she was helpless in the face of overwhelming distress. For this reason, I prefer to say simply that "she did not talk, walk or eat" and note that in the course of therapy, Yufang began to develop varying degrees of volition in relation to the pull towards death as a solution to her overwhelming distress.

Psychotherapeutic work

I shall now describe the way in which I work therapeutically with young people who are not talking, walking or eating and may be in poor physical health. I do not support the idea that such young people who do not speak *should not* be offered a specifically modified form of psychoanalytic psychotherapy, nor do I believe in the notion that one should wait till a child is physically fit in order to have psychotherapy. Although the mind is compromised by severe starvation and the body is suffering from severe physical illness, the young person is terrified to be in this predicament and requires the attentive empathic thoughtfulness and physical care similar to that of a newborn baby. Without the containing presence of a fully equipped psychotherapist, the child may never regain the wish to live. I have known of a child living for 10 years in this condition of feeling "compelled to die" because during those ten years the family was not able to access the appropriate individual and family psychotherapy which she and her family, having to find new ways of helping her, could find useful. Professionals can become intimidated by a non-speaking child and not realise that they can speak, think, and offer compassionate understanding even though the child may be suffering severe psychological and physical distress.

One problem for the clinician is that underneath the symptoms of not talking, not walking, not eating, may lie various different psychopathologies including those present in a more neurotic person with anorexia nervosa or in a more seriously ill person with psychotic depression. Others may suffer from anorexia nervosa, borderline personality disorder, obsessive compulsive disorder, various phobias, or a more serious ill person with incipient schizophrenia. A combination of specifically tailored family psychotherapy, individual psychotherapy and specialised medical and nursing care for a particular child *pervasively retreating from life* can result in long-term recovery, but someone with incipient schizophrenia will need years of ongoing psychotherapy to develop and maintain a reasonable life. I have been involved in providing psychoanalytic psychotherapy or psychotherapy supervision for fifteen of these non-speaking young people "compelled to die". I will now describe my way of working with Yufang, which is similar to the way in which I have worked with other young people.

The psychotherapy involves work *in the transference*, looking at the "here and now" relationship through careful observation of the relationship existing between the child and the psychotherapist. It also involves a deep contact with the therapist's *countertransference* experiences which inform understanding of the non-speaking child (Racker, 1953). A psychotherapy training involving infant observation (Bick, 1968) allows the psychotherapist to trace the sequence of non-verbal interaction between the child and the therapist and lend meaning to it, much as a mother does with a non-speaking baby. Most importantly, the focus is on the therapist reaching to the very deepest part of his/her personality to find empathic attunement to the physical and emotional experience of the child. With such a very ill child, initially it is the psychotherapist who needs to make demands on herself to fully understand *the present moment* with the child, rather than expecting anything at all from the child. My experience has led me to believe that the impediments to psychological progress are fourfold. Firstly, the context to which the child will return may not be or be felt by the child to be safe, nurturing, trustworthy, supportive. Secondly, the context (including the milieu and therapies in which the child is participating) may be "too pushy, intrusive, and demanding" of the non-speaking child. Thirdly, family and professionals experience latent aggressivity towards the child who frequently evokes feelings in the *countertransference* of being rejected and feeling impotent. Fourthly, staff may not working sufficiently on their various countertransference experiences in relation to *both* the child and the parents.

The secret is for the multidisciplinary team to remain very patient while compassionately and comprehensively understanding and bearing the child's overwhelming feelings and anxieties about living, while empathically identifying with the family members who are frantic with worry about their very ill child who feels *compelled to die*. It is essential to empathically identify not only with the child, but also with the family, who may easily project their own sense of failure and inadequacy into staff, who can then become hostile to them. Of course, such a non-talking, walking, eating child needs nutrition and bodily care, but no demands should be put on the child to speak. The child will speak when feeling safe, trusting, and more empathically and deeply understood. Therapeutic work involves careful attention to the total contextual milieu and particular attention must be given to the splitting off and projection of undesirable feelings to staff, parents or child. Mutual blaming can occur when all parties involved feel impotent to facilitate significant change immediately. The therapeutic work involves family therapy, parental counselling, and a coordinated multidisciplinary team, including a physiotherapist, teacher and nurse, who meet regularly to think about their collaborative efforts. The parents need to be fully considered as therapeutic agents working alongside the multidisciplinary team to promote a nurturing and facilitating environment for their child.

This chapter illustrates the powerful impact on the environment of a profoundly ill girl in a near catatonic state, depressive stupor, or a profound "conservation withdrawal reaction" (Spitz, 1965). Yufang's physical deterioration was fortunately capable of being gradually transformed. What was problematic was Yufang's not talking and not thinking which led to extreme reactions of wanting to "do something" to get her to talk. Being tugged into "talking" left her moving into further withdrawal. It took time to persuade the team to let me work with Yufang, and only gradually did the multidisciplinary group and the parents develop trust in my work as a psychoanalytic psychotherapist. Medication and electro-convulsive shock treatment were initially preferred, but they stopped both when they were found to be only briefly effective. I personally am completely against ECT as a treatment with young people, for it doesn't actually help the young person develop the capacity to think about emotional experiences and resolve conflicts on the basis of thoughtful processing of interpersonal events.

Presentation

Yufang is a seventeen-year-old girl, the middle one of three children from a middle-class Chinese family who recently settled in London. She had passed music exams in China and had been accepted for admission to a prestigious London music academy, where she would be studying the cello. Her older brother, aged nineteen, had been left behind in China, where he was studying engineering. Her younger sister, aged eleven, had come with the family to London. Her father was a successful businessman, and her mother had been a housewife for most of her adult life. Yufang was admitted to our hospital three months after her family arrived in London. Neither Yufang nor her mother spoke English very well, and for this reason Yufang had been studying English during the first three months in this country. It wasn't clear when Yufang listened to a conversation whether she was simply not-thinking or not-understanding my English, or both. A Chinese psychiatrist had been asked to see her before her condition had deteriorated to such an extent that she required hospitalisation. At that time, he said that Yufang had a lack of self-worth, suicidal ideation, and a strong sense of having done something wrong. She had a psychotic depression according to him, but within the first month of administration of psychotropic drugs, her condition worsened. It was then that she stopped walking, talking, and eating. She did not signal to get help with toileting. It was necessary to tube-feed Yufang. By the end of this early stage of her admission, Yufang was completely mute, lying motionless in bed. I felt the medication had not been helpful, but rather had dissolved her coping ego capacities even further so that she retreated into muteness and motionless, lying in bed. Yufang was so pale and lifeless she seemed nearly dead.

History of the presenting illness

The family was unable to give a detailed picture of Yufang's developmental history. Perhaps her grandmother, with whom the parents lived in China before moving to London, might have had a better sense of Yufang as a child. The maternal grandmother had been the primary caregiver and Yufang felt closer to her than her own depressed mother. Apparently Yufang's developmental milestones were normal. Her parents described her at age 16 as being hardworking and popular, with a wide circle of friends. She was close to her older brother who had been very ill with diabetes throughout his life. This had absorbed much of the mother's anxiety and attention. The father had left the family home to work in Russia for twenty months prior to the family coming to this country to live. This had left the mother feeling very unsupported. When the family moved to London, Yufang met a French boy in her English-language school and she became very fond of him. This was her first boyfriend, and when both he and her parents simultaneously made separate trips away from London, Yufang became ill.

One could hypothesise a series of factors which may have contributed to the severity of Yufang's illness. These included loss of her familiar culture, her grandmother, her brother, her friends, her native language when she didn't know the English language well, residing with a bullying father and depressed mother. It is also not clear what unmet infantile longings permeated her relationship with her boyfriend leaving her bereft when both he and her parents left her temporarily. Accompanying these external factors was Yufang's psychological incapacity for mentalization, her use of denial and her incapacity to acknowledge hostility, which she often dealt with by projecting it into others. During the separation from her grandmother in China, her parents, her brother and her friends, Yufang began to imagine hearing her father's voice saying, "I have had an accident." Around the same time, Yufang complained that the doll she kept on her bed had eyes that haunted her and she was afraid of it. She was afraid to go to sleep for fear of being attacked by it. At this time, she began writing to herself, saying she was stupid and selfish. Simultaneously, she began to stop eating, drinking and talking. Her body developed a waxy "flexibilitas", which meant that she didn't move her body and it stayed in the same position in which her mother put her for long periods of time. She did not even open her eyes to look at anyone.

In desperation, the psychiatrists gave her ECT which momentarily "awakened her", and then twelve days later she went back into her closed-off state. I suggested that I, a psychoanalytic psychotherapist, see her for six days a week for supportive psychotherapy and requested that the psychiatrists hold off ECT until we saw whether or not a relationship with a therapist would enable Yufang to find a way of living without having to have ECT. I was given six weeks to "trial" supportive psychoanalytic psychotherapy. At this time, there was a popular notion in British child psychiatry that psychoanalytic psychotherapy should be given only after a child regains her normal weight, for a notion existed that psychotherapy disturbs and pesters a "very ill" or severely depressed, emaciated child rather than helping her. The current child psychiatry texts also referred to psychoanalytic psychotherapy as being suitable mainly for children who have the capacity to express themselves verbally, to use symbolic thought, and who do not have too much difficulty in forming interpersonal relationships (Graham, 1986). Obviously, I hold a radically different point of view, and such statements as these prompted me to compile this book on "*the silent child's communication without words*". Every child has a right to a thoughtful, regular presence accompanying her during a terrifying journey through mental illness, regardless of whether or not she can speak, think, or experience being physically healthy. During the initial part of our work together, Yufang had her eyes closed, did not speak, barely spoke English and if she spoke at all certainly did not show a wish for a personal relationship. I was having to struggle to convince the professional network that psychoanalytic psychotherapy lends understanding to the sane part of a non-speaking child pervasively retreating from life. With the support of Herbert Rosenfeld, a psychoanalyst working with people suffering from psychotic anxieties, I felt I could "trust the method" of providing appropriately attuned psychoanalytic psychotherapy for Yufang.

Milieu treatment

I became involved four weeks after Yufang was admitted to hospital, a time when all medication had stopped and when ECT treatment had failed. She was referred to an adolescent psychiatric inpatient unit, but there was no vacancy there for four months. For this reason, psychotherapeutic work began in the paediatric unit. The one advantage of this is that Yufang was able to be with her mother each day and this supported her through the anxieties of being so very ill. I visited the paediatric unit daily, except Sundays, physically helping Yufang to hobble with my physical support into the charge nurse's office on the ward for half an hour, six days a week. I then walked her back to the paediatric unit where she remained for most of the time in bed in an open ward with other young people.

Each day I would meet the nurses to discuss Yufang. They felt totally bewildered by a young person whom they experienced as unresponsive and later, hostile to any gesture of concern or practical care that they offered her. She made them feel impotent in using their usual nursing skills and this prompted some lack of warmth on their part. I encouraged the nurses to understand that, although she wasn't speaking to them or responding warmly to them, that didn't mean that she wouldn't appreciate being understood and nurtured in a non-intrusive way by them. She wouldn't eat, but she *might listen* if they played soothing music to her for she was a musician after all. She didn't open her eyes much, but she *could listen* to stories that they might tell her from a book or from experiences of the day. I suggested that I was not really indicating that they were to do something strange, and reminded them of the fact that a mother generally spends twelve months with her young baby, speaking to the baby without expecting that the baby respond to the mother through speaking. The mother and baby are learning to understand one another. I warned the nurses though that their task would be made more difficult if they expected a response from Yufang, because that would be experienced as "pushing her" rather than understanding and supporting her in this state of severe regression and retreat from something overwhelming in life.

Gradually, after they had time to share some of their frustrations and sense of rejection by Yufang, the nurses became interested in the task of nurturing her with their thoughts, their singing, the music, their words, until she developed sufficient hope again to respond to people. I encouraged them to feel what it must be like to be her in order to stay attuned to her. I also encouraged the nurses to talk with her about not too personal thoughts about the day on the ward, and the outdoors which you could see from the window. I also suggested that the nurses think of creating a dialogue between what they put into words and feelings, and Yufang's response to what they offered her. I gave them examples of how they might comment on how she was moving away from them with a flinch or moving towards them with a quick glance. The nurses were encouraged to use their intuition to describe the different meanings of Yufang moving towards them or pulling away from them. For example, they might say, "you are looking at me, trying to find out just what kind of person I am", or "I seem to be frightening you" or "I seem to be making you annoyed with me". I encouraged Yufang's mother to approach Yufang similarly while sharing news from home and news from Yufang's brother and grandmother.

I encouraged the nurses to stop talking "about Yufang". Instead, I suggested that they carefully observe her and their emotional responses to her. I asked them to strive to understand her deeply and think about how they and she were developing a relationship in which she spoke through her facial expressions and bodily gestures and they responded with empathic feeling, identifying with her, and then giving her and themselves meaningful comments on her emotional state. The discussion was now on how *both the nurses and Yufang* were relating and how the nurses were developing their skills of understanding their emotional responses to her and her emotional responses to them. For example, a nurse reported she said, "Yufang, I've brought a book for you I thought you might like." Noticing her immobility, the nurse would open the book, talk about some of the pictures in the book, and then noticing Yufang's continued lack of response, the nurse would say, "You don't seem to feel that I have brought you something of any interest to you". On another occasion, a nurse said, "I'd like to read you a little bit of a story about leaving one's country of origin", and then seeing Yufang look up momentarily, the nurse said, "You seem to like my talking about people who have left their country". The nurses no longer felt impotent, rather they felt challenged by this idea of creatively relating to Yufang as a mother would to a young infant, interpreting the child's non-verbal relationship with her. Unfortunately, so much of the time, there was a painful contrast between other children on the ward who were friendly and responsive and unresponsive Yufang, who was often regressed and in "her own world".

I had to spend a lot of time helping the nurses to think they were nurturing a little hope in Yufang, but it would take a long time to see any visible sign of what was growing inside her. I reminded them of planting a seed in the ground and how there was a lot of growing underneath the soil before a green shoot emerged. I also suggested that Yufang's non-responsiveness could also possibly be a protection against disappointment. If she hoped for something, she might be hurt and disappointed. If no one and no act mattered, then she would never feel disappointed, never feel pain again. In this way, I tried to help the nurses realise that they would need to support each other by acknowledging that they felt very disappointed in Yufang not accepting all their offers of help. I tried to encourage them to believe that they should not feel they were useless in their attempt to foster her wish to be alive.

I also lightly mentioned that being rejected by a young person can stir up other feelings of rejection from their own lives and result in resentment and hostility to Yufang. They must remember that all that they felt might not be directly the result of Yufang's rejection of them. The nurses and I gradually shared a perception that Yufang could receive their concern, their understanding without showing if she had accepted it or felt it to be helpful. We talked about the defensive part of Yufang, but also kept focusing on how their might be a hidden child in Yufang perceiving, listening, knowing, receiving, feeling grateful to be understood. I shared with the nurses my sense that we were working towards understanding Yufang. That was her only hope of survival! I said we had no reason to believe that Yufang would not gradually respond to their nurturing, empathic understanding. I beckoned them to hold onto patience and hope for a better relationship with Yufang in the future. As much as possible, I was talking about developing a relationship with Yufang, observing her responses to them through her eyes, hands, mouth, body posture, and understanding their particular feelings in their relationship with Yufang rather than focusing on "what Yufang was doing". The focus was on empathically observing a process of interaction and discovering its meaning for both Yufang and the nurses.

Creating a therapeutic space in which to work

As I reflected on this first period of Yufang's hospitalisation, I began questioning my aims as a psychotherapist. Why was it that I felt so determined to rescue Yufang? I was struck by the readiness with which I became angry or critical of the psychiatrists, the mother, the nurses. It was much easier to be critical than to face my own incapacities and lack of understanding in this formidable task. It was also much easier to split off and project my own aggression, my own violent phantasies, into the ECT and the two psychiatrists recommending it, while owning my own loving, caring feelings towards Yufang. It also seemed to bring a kind of inner psychological relief to locate aggression in others rather than in Yufang, a hopeless, ill and potentially dying young person.

Splitting of love and hate, *projection* of aggression into others, seemed to be an accompaniment to the multidisciplinary team's work with Yufang. We needed to own and integrate these feelings within ourselves to be able to deeply understand who Yufang was and the nature of our relationship with her. For Yufang, I was part of a clinic team, partnered with the family therapist, and the psychiatrist managing the treatment. When Yufang met me, she rubbed her hands, looked at the black-and-blue marks on them and fostered my temptation to become cocooned with her against the hostile external world that had given her pre-treatment medication marks linked with the ECT. In this frame of mind, I became too protective, too maternal. The tone of my voice was too soothing. It lacked sufficient strength and thoughtfulness. In order for me to find the appropriate therapeutic relationship with Yufang, it was necessary for me to acknowledge that I had been part of the therapeutic team that had permitted ECT to take place. This was working in the *total transference* espoused by psychoanalyst Betty Joseph (1985) and described in my paper on psychotherapy in an inpatient unit (Magagna, 1998). I also had to accept that I could not evade disquiet and guilt regarding my own aggression by evacuating it into external figures. I knew that it was essential to be linked in a collaborative way with the psychiatrists and others in order to maintain a therapeutic space for thinking about the team and family dynamics surrounding Yufang's individual psychotherapy. It would be confusing for all concerned if we did not have a "joined-up" approach, and the continuation of the psychotherapy and development of my capacity as a psychotherapist were dependent on reintegrating my hostile projections and helping the team contain projections surrounding work with Yufang.

As the weeks passed, the nurses and I became aware of how much we *expected some response* from Yufang. We felt this despite *rationally knowing* we should be simply providing deeply compassionate understanding to our interactions with her. Each day I listened to the nurses and shared comments relating to the slightest responsiveness from Yufang. "She looked interested in the music!" "She cried!" "She looked at me today!" When there were days on end when Yufang simply lay in bed not moving, it was easy to feel irritation or even anger with her for "not trying" as though she were completely competent to challenge her regressed pathological condition. Then we had to step back and mentor our own interactions with Yufang; what did we do which fostered an appreciative look and what did we do which pushed her back into retreat? For example, on one occasion the music teacher managed to get Yufang to sit in a chair with a cello between her legs. Although interest in her cello beckoned her to get out of her bed, playing it was obviously far too advanced for her for she could barely walk unassisted. When the teacher felt disappointed with Yufang's failure to lift her hand to the cello, the music teacher immediately became a persecutory figure from whom she turned completely away. The cello became "a bad object", although she had loved music dearly since she began playing music at the age of five. We learned not to take independent moves without checking out with each other whether or not we were "moving too fast forward". Slow, steady progress, with tiny steps indicated through Yufang's emotional stance, were more likely to lead to her wishing to engage in her life with others again. Achievmant rather than emotional maturity had been the story of her life. Now we had to find ways of taking care of Yufang's "before words" preverbal baby-self who had greeted a depressed, unresponsive mother and was beckoning for us to heal the inner trauma.

We clarified our therapeutic aims for the team: our task was to create a therapeutic space for thinking about how Yufang felt in her relationships with us each day. We needed a structure to the day, a regular rhythm of carers and some idea of what she could expect hourly in the way of nurturing experiences for her, offers of music, stories, conversation and thinking about how she interacted with us. We were not to create expectations of her, for if we did she perceived us as horrible demanding figures. We could think of minimal structured progressions in the structure of activities provided for Yufang and we needed to think together about the ways in which we encouraged her development. Our responses to Yufang, our countertransference, had to be carefully monitored and discussed. Yufang's withdrawn state could leave us feeling hurt and deprived by her! Yufang's role as a young person in hospital was in danger of being compressed into the gratification of our need to feel helpful and not destructive in our roles as nurses and therapists. We felt frustrated and impotent. The result was that we could detect in many of our comments a sense of superiority, barely perceptible, but present, as we professionals searched for weaknesses in Yufang's family. A tone of blame and irritation in our comments about the family concealed the team members' annoyance with each other's differing points of view about how to proceed and about what was being experienced by Yufang. Our comments included many hypotheses about the damage that may have been done to Yufang by her family and by her boyfriend.

Present in the team dynamics seemed to be a thwarted wish to be angry with someone: the father, the family, the doctor, the referring psychiatrist. The theme of "who is to blame" seemed to permeate the team's informal discussions. Scorn was barely concealed; Why had the doctor let things go on so badly for so long? Why did he let her get so emaciated before referring her? Why did he pump her with chloropromazine, whose side-effect made her considerably more stuporous? This attempt to place blame somewhere was shared by the family. They were impatient with our lack of progress and lack of certainty about a healthy future for Yufang. Why hadn't we given her the right medication? We didn't seem to be making her better, rather, they felt we were hurting her for she was beginning to cry, something which she had rarely done before in her entire life! To make very critical remarks amongst ourselves and about each other seemed an easy, common outlet for our ignorance and impotence - both experiences shared by the treatment team and the family. Blaming also defended us against experiencing Yufang's deep despair and our despair in being unable to readily relieve her of her psychic pain. Blaming also interfered with a deeper exploration of our own internal psychological states and the team dynamics involving old revived sibling rivalries regarding who knew best, who had the best relationship with Yufang, who was most helpful to the family and so on. All these issues could only be understood, not through textbooks but through patient curiousity in our exploration of loving and hating feelings in Yufang, the family and the multidisciplinary team working together with the family.

In retrospect, I realised that blaming the family was preventing us from looking at the hostility present in Yufang's relationships with her family and us. The professional network was in fact unwittingly re-enacting an unconscious process, not yet understood, within the family dynamics (Britton, 1981). It was more difficult to create "a containing treatment framework" for bearing paranoid anxieties and living with Yufang's despair and hidden hostility felt inside us. Blaming had a certain energy but what we needed was courage to sustain the painful hope that if we could nurture Yufang with our understanding of her feelings, she might be drawn to life, to a figure who understands and provides hope for life. We worried that sustaining hope would be futile, for Yufang seemed very attached to a "death-wish", very committed to her internal propaganda that there was "no point in living".

The family met weekly with a psychotherapist to assist in the task of supporting Yufang and developing insight into the family interactions that might interfere with or support her progress. When Yufang was able to sit in a chair, she joined the family meetings, even though she was mute and withdrawn. During these sessions, the family members each shared worries about Yufang and what they felt it was like "to be in her shoes". The family tried to find ways of supporting Yufang and each other during this family crisis. They also talked about their deep sense of loss of the grandmother, their son, their home, their Chinese customs, language and food. Everything was so different for each of them. The mother described how she also worried about the life of their oldest boy, aged nineteen, who suffered from a severe diabetic condition with which he sometimes went into a coma. The entire family was sad about separation from all that was familiar in their own country and a source of comfort, security, and happiness in their lives.

Yufang seemed to hold the extreme version of the family's reluctance to take in, feel, and accept the sadness and resentment about separation from all things loved and familiar. The family had borne the separation from father for eighteen months and had little control over father's unilateral decision that the family was moving to London. Each family member, particularly the mother, felt the need to passively accept the transition to London in order not to lose the father on a more permanent basis. The father and mother were unable to take into account the adverse emotional aspects of moving to London without the English language to smoothe their entry. Work with the family helped contain their anxieties; they became more able to allow themselves to own their sad and conflictual feelings previously projected into Yufang, and to support Yufang in attending her individual psychotherapy. It is a matter of some controversy, but as demonstrated in Yufang's family, *the symptom-bearer* may be holding shared family defences against psychic pain, and thus the family may require family therapy and/or parental counselling accompanying the individual psychotherapy for one child. Personally, I see that family therapy is essential in ensuring the child's ongoing therapeutic progress beyond hospitalisation, for it is the parents who will be responsible in helping their child sustain the therapeutic progress made in hospital.

Individual psychotherapy and accompanying therapeutic work

In my opinion, any child - whether speaking or not-speaking, borderline or neurotic, intelligent or not very intelligent, physically well or physically ill - should be considered a suitable candidate for psychotherapy at any stage of his or her illness, as long as there is the appropriate inpatient or outpatient network of professionals and parents who jointly support the treatment effort. What is crucial, though, is that the therapist be suitably willing and able to undertake *the particular form* of psychotherapy which the child requires, making the necessary modifications of techniques to suit the child's psychological and physical requirements. Perhaps most important is the therapist's capacity to bear psychic pain, alongside a willingness to have an empathic identification with the child and the ability to provide enlivening company, as described by Alvarez in her book *Live Company* (1992).

My task in working with Yufang was similar in many respects to that of the parents and other members of the multidisciplinary team. I needed to be attuned to my emotional and physical experience of being with Yufang in *the present moment* of the session in order to give meaning to her communications, which involved many feelings being projected onto me and transmitted in a non-verbal, bodily way. This work is similar to that described by Schore (2002a). For instance, I could physically feel tired in an instant when some silent hostility was present. It was as though my mind/body was being attacked by her thinking, "there is no point in this encounter, there is no point in living". I could also feel physically enlivened when she gave a flicker of interest in what was being said, as though her acceptance of what I gave her was a generous gift of life to me! Confusion and lack of integration in Yufang could be linked with a mismatch in communication in her primary experience with her parents. For this reason, she needed me to consider her primitive experiences in her regressed state, including sensations and the movement or stillness of her body, before she could symbolise these experiences via her dreams, drawings or words. An integration of her body and psychological self could then occur.

To remain focused in the depths of the encounter between Yufang and myself, I held in mind the words of Murray Cox, who said:

> Shared silence interspersed and punctuated by gaze and gesture may be far more eloquent and reach the young persons at a depth impenetrable to words. The therapist may gently and quietly need to follow the young person until he reaches a point where he is invited into that area of experience sealed off in which the psyche has sought refuge from an intolerable reality.
>
> (1988, p. 21)

These words made me recognise that it would take time for Yufang to emerge and feel safe enough to find words for her experiences. Deep inside, Yufang was hungry for us to comprehend her, even though initially she seemed cocooned with *mouth closed* to food, *eyes shut* to people, *words absent* to share feelings. Walking in the world was given up in favour of residing in some form of womb-like claustrum (Meltzer, 1992) where "no-thinking" was present.

I would like now to describe some particularly difficult aspects of my dialogue with Yufang in which I used my countertransference as cues to the meaning of her non-verbalised messages. My countertransference experience was the base of my communication with her. Initially Yufang seemed to have little awareness of many fragmented parts of her personality which were isolated, lonely and out of communication with everyone including herself. There was very little sense of a Self present. Following the technique recommended by Rosenfeld (1986) who supervised my work, I began the psychotherapy for half-hour periods six days per week. He suggested that missing two days on a weekend was too much for such an ill girl. Because she really wasn't walking much at all and required physical support to do so, I met Yufang in a nearby nurse's office on the paediatric ward for four months. As an illustration of how I worked with Yufang, I shall draw on sequential selections from our sessions during the psychotherapy. As I joined with the hospital team, supporting the nurses and talking with the psychiatrists, I was able to share many feelings with them. It helped to verbalise my experiences rather than simply keep them mutely residing inside me. Meanwhile Yufang remained mute, immobile, with an incredibly sad, vacant look on her face. It was difficult to bear Yufang's retreat from our offers to help and this made both me and the nurses feel useless or annoying as well as unfortunately, sometimes annoyed. It was important that we acknowledged whatever feelings we had to each other so they didn't permeate our relationship with Yufang!

The following session is from the second week of Yufang's therapy and it is typical of the early sessions.

> Yufang does not acknowledge me and her eyes remain faced downwards when I greet her with a friendly hello and feel my "hello" falling flat to the ground. She holds onto my arm with much of her weight upon me as she slowly walks with her feet barely lifting into the room. Yufang closes her eyes completely as she sits down, but I can tell that she is listening to the sound of the radiator which seems irregular. Yufang begins to show tension and fear in her face. Opening her eyes she searches for the door. I say "This room doesn't feel good. The sounds are disturbing. You don't like them. You want to get out. You don't like my speaking." I say this while not looking directly at Yufang, fearing I will be experienced as too intrusive, but when I do look at her briefly, she looks into my eyes for a second. I think she felt understood by me. As Yufang glances down at her feet again she struggles unsuccessfully to mouth the word, "Go". I speak as though I am Yufang saying in a frightened but insistent tone, "Let me go. I don't want to be here!" After a few moments Yufang almost imperceptibly nods in agreement. I talk then about how she is so uncertain about what any sound means. She isn't certain if I can be trusted to keep her safe in this room which isn't at all her usual space. Her usual space is in bed.

I realise that making changes is frightening to Yufang. Leaving her bed seems to leave her feeling thrust out into a dangerous, hostile world in which anything can happen. I realise that Yufang was not only disturbed by the new space, by the sound of a broken heater making light banging noises, she also wanted to get out of my room, out of my presence. Yufang seemed in "a shell', like children Spitz (1965) described, or like the Jewish refugee orphans who, having no emotional link with someone, give themselves up to death. At times, she viewed me as a dangerous enemy threatening to break into her protective shell of non-feeling, of depersonalisation, of disintegration, of non-thinking. However, for a moment, Yufang was able to meet me with a fleeting acknowledgement that I existed and an acknowledgement that I understood how frightened she felt. She had come alive to her feeling of fear and that was better than being in a state of "not-knowing" what she felt.

It was only much later that Yufang let me know that there was often a malevolent force, a voice in her head condemning her to starve and to die. This sense of being a passive victim of imposed cruelty is a major problem in regressed young people not speaking, not eating, not walking. Nine months into therapy, Yufang told me about the beginning of her illness: "When I was ill I had to starve myself. *I had to die. I didn't want to die, but I had to.* I starved and became unconscious. I felt I was dead." Yufang also explained some of the pressure towards retreating even further into a shell of "not-knowing":

> When I was ill, I could not look in a mirror. I could not look in a mirror because I did not know who I saw. I could not see myself. I saw another girl. I thought I was someone else. I felt I was a girl, my friend, who had difficulties with her parents. I felt strange when I couldn't see myself in the mirror. I worried about other people looking at me, because I was afraid that they could see through me.
>
> In these descriptions, Yufang suggested that she had lost a sense of her *self.*

She did not feel her ordinary self, but was depersonalised. She was passively experiencing herself as under instructions from a malevolent, destructive part of her personality which she did not experience as part of herself. This split-off destructive part dictated how she must treat her *self,* and she felt she had no *self* available to struggle with "the dictator". Yufang movingly said, "I didn't *want* to die, but I *had* to."

Helplessness

It has been pointed out that a sense of helplessness (Garber & Seligman, 1980) leads to a picture characteristic of post-traumatic stress disorder (PTSD). The features illustrated include numbing of responsiveness, reduced involvement with the external world, pervasively diminished interest in the normal activities of daily life, and severely constricted emotions. Those are followed by exaggerated startle responses. These symptoms, shared by young people with PTSD, prompted our psychiatric team to assume with virtual certainty that such a global avoidant response must certainly be linked with a traumatic event such as physical, sexual or emotional abuse, more specifically the witnessing of threats, violence and mental illness at home.

In this working context, it was very difficult to maintain a psychoanalytic stance of "not-knowing" (Bion, 1962) and being curious about who Yufang was and what her internal and external experiences were. In particular, it was difficult to remain open to those emotions in Yufang which might have been different from those of a helpless, frightened child, a victim. Ken Nunn's work (Nunn & Thompson, 1996) suggests a more complicated understanding of what he calls "pervasive refusal syndrome", which I prefer to call a pervasive retreat from life, involving regression and not thinking, talking, walking and eating. He maintains that separation anxiety is a prominent feature. This is accompanied by social withdrawal and depression. The young person feels, and may be actually experiencing, that it is impossible to control situations relating to health, safety, and happiness within the family. He suggests that hopelessness occurs in these situations and prompts the emergence of the regression to not talking, walking or eating in certain young people. As our psychiatric team was so influenced by those ways of interpreting Yufang's regression, as I said before, it was very difficult to maintain an open mind necessary for psychoanalytic psychotherapy, to just use my countertransference to discover clues to Yufang's *unique* personality and particular personal narrative.

Denial of destructiveness

Because Yufang looked so weak, helpless and vulnerable, it was difficult to imagine or even notice Yufang having any destructive, jealous, contemptuous, omnipotent impulses that could contribute to the causation or perpetuation of her depression and regression. Intellectually, I was aware that it was impossible to facilitate Yufang's development without ridding myself of the notion of her being a "helpless victim of hostile external events". I knew that I needed to experience *all of her;* yet even when the supervisor suggested to me that Yufang's giggle might be contemptuous, I still found it difficult to accept this. Yufang's central psychic defence was a massive denial of conflictual feelings accompanied by projecion of her aggression onto others. This was accompanied by intense fears of real or phantasied persecutory fears of aggression from the external world.

How could I even *dare to think* that she had some destructiveness within her? If she did, would it be cruel and damaging to talk about it? There was also a deeper task, which was to recognise that both in her and in me there might be personal responsibility for evoking these responses of contempt. In other words, I needed to ask what in me, and my personal narrative and my actions might have caused her to be contemptuous of me? It was difficult as a therapist to see contempt in Yufang's giggle, but even more arduous to realise that I might have provoked a contemptuous reaction to my words. For example, my being repetitive in my interpretations, speaking too patiently, too kindly, without much depth of feeling, could provoke disdain for the lack of personal strength I showed and it might also provoke disdain for the meaning of what I was saying, even if what I was saying was correct. I also needed to ask myself, if in her silence or "don't know" she was erecting an omnipotent defence against being understood and opening herself to overwhelming feelings? (Rosenfeld, 1987).

Silence as deprivation or communion

There are other issues to which I would like to refer when talking about this phase of the work. I did not think it was helpful for Yufang to come into the room and sit in a motionless, severely depressed silence for more than five minutes. My impression was that if I did stay silent, she felt I had invited her to be in a room to be deprived by me, deprived of my attempts to nurture her through sharing my thoughts and feelings with her. I thought doing this would be like a mother not talking to her infant, not treating her infant as a baby with a mind. At other times there existed between Yufang and me a prevailing desire for a static space devoid of feelings, because feelings were so disturbing to her. Members of the hospital staff had tried asking questions but Yufang had remained with her lips shut most of the time. My own questions took the form of being curious while speaking aloud to myself in Yufang's presence. I sometimes talked to a stuffed animal which I had in the room, describing my experience with Yufang aloud to the animal. I used various ways of thinking aloud, also using dolls talking to one another, for very easily questions and thoughts about Yufang, which were directly spoken to Yufang, could be experienced as intrusive and demanding.

What seemed most important was my talking about Yufang's experience at that moment in the room and generating in her an interest in her emotional life. I tried to identify with Yufang, using her physical posture, glance of her eye, expression of her mouth and hands, to describe what she was feeling and how she was responding to what I said. At times I spoke in first person as though I were Yufang in various developmental stages. I would "be Yufang" as a younger child and then talk to Yufang the older child about this "younger regressed person". Often, I described things as I would with a baby or very young child, talking about what Yufang and those around her had been doing during the day, talking about how she responded to her mother coming and staying on the paediatric ward and going away from her. Then I would think in more detail about the experiences that Yufang had. She lacked capacity to observe herself but observations were provided by the staff's daily descriptions of their mutual interactions with Yufang. These observations of how Yufang greeted a particular staff member, how she responded to the staff member talking to her, reading to her, leaving her were all part of the ongoing dialogue with Yufang.

Meanwhile, the focus of my thinking was on the developing relationship present at that moment between "the-little-child" in Yufang and me. I described a mood that I felt in the room on each given day: good to be here together, suspicious of me, curious about what I will say, pushing me away. I might comment on how she greeted me when I first met her that day. Each non-verbal response that Yufang made became a possible opportunity for another dialogue. For example, I would say: "You looked up when I came into the room. You have been looking into my eyes listening with interest some of the time I have been speaking. Now, when you are leaving, I know you can nod goodbye, but you have chosen not to." Yufang giggled when I said this. I then said, "You giggled as though you agreed that you could have nodded goodbye. Perhaps I should experience 'the goodbye'." My aim was to meet Yufang's most immediate emotions present in the therapy. This involved "listening to her mood" as one listens to music. I thought if she were playing her cello for me, her music would go where her words were not able to go, and then I might understand more, but that was for later. Now, as Yufang remained immobile, I had to allow her mood to enter me and then name it. My idea was that internal change in Yufang could best be facilitated through comments that met her feelings and anxieties *in the immediate present* in our encounter. When Yufang subsequently used words, I would rely on her to talk about whatever was on her mind, as I would with any other person in psychotherapy.

In the initial phase, however, Yufang was primarily lifeless, mute, and as there was no verbal conversation, it seemed necessary for me to use my heart, my body, my soul to help her gather her *whole being* together "to be emotionally present" in the room. I sometimes experienced an image of a turtle gradually peeping out of an impermeable shell and disappearing back inside the darkness. My feeling emotionally present and using words of understanding were vital in evoking Yufang to leave the dark world of "not-thinking" and use her apparently disintegrated emotional and mental functioning again.

Using dolls for stories of the child's experiences in the family or ward

I sometimes brought out a set of dolls and told stories to Yufang about her relationships with different members in her family, including her absent grandmother and older brother. For example, I used the dolls to dramatise the story of how Yufang's mother came to visit her daughter, Yufang, and how for a moment they greeted each other, looking at one another. I described and how her mother fed her soup. (Although Yufang still had the nasogastric tube, she had begun accepting being fed by spoon, but only by her mother.) Initially, I told the story in the third person, more emotionally distant, sitting slightly to the side of Yufang. I was deliberately leaving her free to ignore all that I was saying. I would then say that if Yufang looked at or touched one of the family dolls that she wanted me to think about, I would say something about that person, telling her about what I know about her relationship with that member of her family. I would tell her about that person. Although she was actually 17, when Yufang was more regressed it was easier to use toy animals, rather than little dolls initially, to tell stories about her. At this point I might use animals for any age of child or adult, for animal figures can feel less troubling when a person is feeling so overwhelmed. I think the faces on the dolls were too human and they disturbed her wish to remain "without people". I talked about the frightened rabbit, very alert to sound, closing her eyes, wanting to run away from everyone and everything that touched her heart.

Later on in therapy, however, I spoke more directly to Yufang; for example, when she touched the father doll, I said, "You seem very frightened of your father." "He's 'the boss' of the family and sometimes he became very angry, and you didn't know what in the world to do then." Yufang was quiet, and subsequently tears rolled down her face as she silently cried. She made no effort to wipe them away. At another time, when she touched the mother doll, I said, "Your mother seems so loving to you, but so sad. She also seems frightened of your father and feels she absolutely must obey him." Yufang remained immobile, not looking up. On another occasion, I used the dolls to show the whole family crying. I said, "Your parents, but particularly your mother, are sad about being in this new country with a different language, sad to have left your brother behind in China." Yufang looked at me and I said, "You need the protection of your mother and me in hospital. Now you are beginning to accept us." Within this framework of enacting family issues through play, I was able to comment on my sense of our *transference relationship,* a confusing experience in which Yufang both distrusted me as a frightening figure at times and depended on me as a nurturing figure at other times, one who was curious about her experiences and trying to understand them with her. Part of the success of this therapy was due to our very frequent meetings allowing us to keep the scattered shifting view of me and others in mind within a steady, emotionally containing context.

The young person's transference relationship to the therapist

Psychotherapy in only partly a talking cure, for that which cannot be spoken about or conceptualised by the young person can nevertheless be conveyed emotionally and physically to the therapist. I attempted to create a narrative of Yufang's experiences through describing shared, obvious, external family issues such as the loss of the grandmother, the brother and homeland,

and the frightening anger of father and sadness of mother that left Yufang feeling without a mother at times. I also described some problems she had in relation to the French boyfriend without being clear exactly what had been upsetting about the relationship, apart from his leaving her for two weeks to go to Spain to visit his family. My real task though was to help Yufang note her present emotional experiences with me and lend thought to them in order that they would not be so overwhelming to her. Now illustrations from the sessions will illustrate how I attempted to use Yufang's communications to elucidate her relationship to the internal parental figures as represented by me in the transference relationship. It was through a detailed experience of the transference that I was able to assist Yufang in deepening her understanding of the conflicts in her relationships with internalised parents and siblings. I was also able to gain a more comprehensive picture of internal and external factors contributing to Yufang's depression and regression. Lending thought to feelings somehow enabled Yufang to develop an internal psychic structure to bear the stresses of her external life. Through this more developed internal psychic structure she found the courage to move from her regressed state of not talking, walking or eating.

Illustrations from the sessions

The following excerpts from eight sessions illustrate how Yufang and I worked together; some elucidating comments regarding technique and interpretation are also given. I have selected a small number of sessions which illustrate some particular changes in her states of mind.

A second-week session

Yufang is not speaking, but her fingers are picking away at the skin of her thumb in a very aggressive way. She stops moving her hands, becomes completely motionless apart from her eyes, which guard my eyes attentively. I suggest, "You look at me wondering what I am thinking about your picking. Can I accept your picking?" In the following session of the same week, Yufang's eyelids begin to flicker as she initiates a tumultuous, unrelenting sobbing. It feels like a convulsion of sadness erupting from her.

A fifth-week session

Yufang sways precariously from foot to foot as she wanders to the session. She cannot seem to find her balance and appears like a toddler requiring support as she is beginning to walk. I know Yufang is not under the effect of any "drugs" or medication, but her giggling makes it look as if she is drunk without much of a thinking-self present. After she has collected herself in the chair for about 15 minutes of the session, Yufang says, "Dream about brother." She then begins sobbing with a very painful grimace. She says no more, but she is reluctant to leave. I say, "I am needed to hold your sobbing self. You don't want to go out and be without me." In a session later that week, she says, "Brother dead', "Must die". I suggest, "Your brother feels dead. You don't see him. You feel now you must die." (I think she is implying that she must die because she has killed her brother in her dream and she isn't sure if it is a dream from her internal reality or a fact from external reality.)

A sixth-week session

In the fifth week of therapy, Yufang began walking without holding onto me, but she spent this whole week with a pain in her leg, with no apparent underlying physical difficulty. It is as though she did not feel emotionally ready "to walk alone" last week. She is virtually unable to walk to the session, but with much encouragement and help she comes. I say, "Poor leg. It is feeling so much pain. It is suffering hurt from somewhere." As I speak, Yufang's still statue-like face unfolds from being expressionless to being contorted with pain, with her eyelids flickering rapidly as tears flow down her face. Her nose is also dripping. As usual, she makes no effort to wipe her nose or her face, both of which are covered in tears. I offer her a tissue, which she does not acknowledge or accept. Instead, Yufang bites her lip, then looks into my eyes and opens her mouth, but no sounds emerge. She turns her head away from me. I say, "You want me to know something important that makes you cry. You are not allowed or you do not dare to tell me." When it is time to leave the room, Yufang hangs on to my arm, and she will not let go when I leave her at her bedside. It takes some moments of saying, "I will come back to see you, but it is very hard to say goodbye. It is hard to be left with all these feelings you want me to help you with." The day after this session, Yufang is playing her cello for the first time since she became ill. I heard her playing. The music continued for five hours; it was monotonous, not melodic, not reflective of any of Yufang's previous considerable musical skills. It was more like sawing out one or two tones in a grating way. Her lips had not opened but now Yufang was allowed some way of expressing the discordant, irritating feelings present with me and during the separation from me. Yufang could not bear to tear herself away from the cello either and the nurses had to struggle with her to leave it aside and rest.

A seventh-week session

For the first time ever, Yufang arrives looking somewhat cheerful as though the sun has come out after flooding rain. She doesn't speak. She appears bored with me and she yawns while I am talking with her. In fact, Yufang appears to be completely out of touch with the fact that I am in the room with her. After I have spoken for some time, Yufang silently mouths some words, yawns, goes blank. This is very disconcerting, for she is emotionally present, then mentally absent. I speak a little more about how she seems to just want to go to sleep, cover her mind, not let me touch her, but then she joins me and leaves me. Yufang moves her lips again without looking at me and begins to cough several times. When she leaves, she seems to almost fall backwards. When I put my arm out to hold her, she leans back on me as though she is going to collapse completely. After this session, Yufang virtually stopped drinking and eating for four days. She also did not utter a word to anyone, including her mother.

Comments on the second to seventh weeks

The narrative of Yufang's inner life experiences was beginning to be repeated in her transference relationship to me. In the second session, when Yufang picked her finger, I commented that she was punishing herself, or someone in her mind, perhaps me. I felt that the picking of her finger was linked with an attack on an internalised figure. Later, when her fingers were very red from her scratching skin off them, I would describe what she was doing, and Yufang would categorically deny that she was picking. She was not able to accept any responsibility or any angry or destructive impulses. During the fifth week, although she said she didn't remember dreams, she was able to remember a dream of an important relationship with her brother. In the dream, he was dead. It felt premature to interpret my sense that her developing closeness to her mother and me meant that she wanted to push her brother out of her mind. I could, however, interpret that as she grew more trusting of me, she wanted to push the other young people out of my mind. Her punishment was that she should die in identification with the "dead internal brother" represented by the other young people whom I saw for psychotherapy. Separations were difficult in themselves, but each separation evoked unworked-through feelings about previous separations, which included feeling left by her mother as she remained depressed and preoccupied by the unstable diabetic problems of her older brother who remained in China; separation from her grandmother in China who had replaced her mother as her prime caregiver; separation from the French-language school boyfriend whose unknown relationship with her and his departure might have precipitated her breakdown into her psychotic depression, not talking, walking, and eating. Yufang's growing wish to possess her mother more completely for herself and her growing trust in me left her feeling overwhelmed with possessive jealousy.

In the second and sixth week of psychotherapy, Yufang goes deep within herself to experience a multitude of different emotions erupting in a convulsion of tears. In the sixth week, she attempts to give these emotions words to share with me, but is biting her lip, holding it shut, as though she feels worried to open herself to knowing her inner experiences more fully. Her feelings are too overwhelming, and there is a fear they will take over. I wonder also if she is "forbidden to speak" by a part of herself, or maybe even by others. Yufang's primitive protections against knowing her own overwhelming painful feelings include picking and creating physical pain, which is less intense than emotional pain, becoming mentally blank and entering a dissociated state, somatising through yawning, coughing, pain in her leg, losing muscle control of her body and not being able to walk, not drinking, eating, or talking for days. She used her cello-playing to "hold herself together" emotionally through non-stop playing until the nurses stopped her. She may also have found some relief in pouring out "sounds of feelings" expressed through the grinding monotonous music. Within seven weeks, the narrative of her inner life revealed dependence, pain of loss, anger about loss, and persecutory anxiety followed by an unconscious somatic and emotional retreat into a cocoon of not living "in her external world" through talking, walking, or eating.

Gathering the transference to the therapist is an important aspect of psychoanalytic psychotherapy, and my task was to consider the evolving nature of Yufang's relationship with me as a reiteration of her internal conflicts. In the initial sessions, I felt I was to be present to *simply experience and contain within myself* a flow of Yufang's undifferentiated feelings and sensations.

By the fifth week, there was a *splitting process* developing in her transference relationship with me. On the one hand, she was able to dream, remember, and share two words of this, which suggests a developing trust in me and a growing faith in the emotionally containing, thinking process that therapy provided. On the other hand, her growing dependence upon me aroused a protective, distrustful part of her opposed to talking with me, so she bit her lip that had been trying to talk with me. There is an *oscillation* between two different physical/ emotional responses. Yufang cries, coughs, lets mucous run from her nose as though trying to let out some noxious substances and experiences, in these situations *she is aware* of something "not good", "not pleasant" needing to erupt from her body. States of boredom, going blank and yawning reflect massive *denial* and when she giggles it seems there is an increase in the force within her against sharing her experiences and thinking about them with me (Rosenfeld, 1987). *Massive denial* leaves her cut off from experiencing distress of any sort.

Attacks on her actual skin on her fingers, the biting of her lips, and then the somatisation of pain and aggression to her legs (and later her heart and chest during the Christmas break) suggest that her rage goes underground to the *internalised objects* of her internal world and thus protects the external figures, her parents and me, from her rage (J. Symington, 2000). But the question remains; what developmental level is being experienced by Yufang? I had the distinct impression that we were experiencing together her very earliest infantile anxieties of being attached to the protective, nurturing mother and feeling that she was falling into an abyss when separating. If, in the earliest stages of development, a baby is devoid of caregivers who fully understand her psychobiological needs the baby is prone to what is know as a *basic fault* in the personality (Balint, 1968). Later in life such a person is then prone to regression to certain kinds of illnesses (See chapter 13 for a more detailed description of the basic fault).

By the fifth week, Yufang seemed to be losing her balance so that I had to prevent her from falling. Her reluctance to leave the session suggested to me that she now had become attached to the "thinking space" with me. Being left by me at the end of the session and between the sessions left her feeling "dropped by me". The falling is a dramatisation of how "the child in her" feels dropped. If I do not hold her in mind all the time she falls down repeatedly, letting the bits of her mind fall apart. If Yufang experiences any dependence on me it feels overwhelming, like the extreme dependence of a newborn baby. In this state of massive dependence, when there is a separation from me, both her mind and body seem to regress. She cannot walk and she is clingy. I talked directly with Yufang about feeling like I dropped her, while I wondered to myself if her leg pains were linked with her anger with my parting. I felt that Yufang's denied anger became unconsciously directed to the internal object: she attacked my legs walking away from her and *identified with* me and my damaged legs. By the sixth week, she was hanging onto my arm, not wanting to separate at all lest in our separation she would begin to fragment and fall apart entirely.

An eighth-week session

It is the last session before the Christmas holidays. Yufang does not speak. She yawns but seems to be in a manic excited state. After she has given me a wrapped tin of cherry tea, I again discuss my Christmas break, which will last for ten days. Immediately, Yufang seems to see something dancing before her eyes. She begins to giggle. I feel that she is in a dizzy, confused state which makes the impact of what I am saying minimal. Later she turns to me and makes some very ugly smiling-monster faces, three or four times, and then laughs. I suggest that I am to feel scared by a "bad cruel monster" as I witness her shockingly frightening and grotesque faces. When I take out the family dolls and describe how she will be going home for a few hours on Christmas day, Yufang says, "My mother is a very, very good cook", adding, "I like my mother's food." I tell Yufang, "Now there is a good, loving mother who feeds you love and good food." When I put the dolls back into their container, for the first time she comments on how the dolls are being flattened. Later in the day, the doctors are called to investigate Yufang's severe chest pains, discovering them to be without a physical basis. When the doctors examine her, she becomes sexually excited and temporarily manic. I feel that Yufang is again dramatically feeling, in her body, her emotional experiences of "being flattened" by my departure, my putting her away. The sexual excitement seems to be created by the doctors' touch and she is then pulled from a flattened "low state" into a manic state.

Comments on the eighth-week session

I described to Yufang how there was a sense of happy, dancing figures cruelly looking down at the "child-Yufang" who was feeling the separation from me. Initially it seemed Yufang was hallucinating cruel faces. She identified with these cruel figures, imitating their faces, while I was to be the terrified child facing monstrous faces. In contrast to this, there existed a very good mother who made good meals and stayed with "the little girl Yufang", looking after her, not going away at Christmas time like me. I thought Yufang was showing off this "good providing mother" to foster jealousy in me, but I was relieved that now she had a sense of something good. Experiences were no longer "all bad". When we parted for the Christmas break, I realised Yufang had given me a gift to show her appreciation, but I recalled feeling flat inside as we were nearing the end of the session. I interpreted my leaving as squashing her, making her feel the life was being squashed out of her, as she had shown by her squashing the dolls back into the box. The pain in Yufang's chest/heart suggested once again that the therapist inside is being attacked for being uncaring and leaving her. I wondered if it was Yufang identifying with the damaged therapist which left her feeling pain in her heart.

A ninth-week session

When I return from the Christmas Break Yufang cries profusely and then feels her stomach. I say, "I feel your tears." She replies, "Not crying." Then she is silent. I suggest that she is crying but does not want to be close to the pain. After a long pause Yufang queries, "What is the difference between belief and trust?" She then cries more profusely. I wonder aloud, "Can you trust me enough to tell me what you are feeling?" Her lip trembles with incredible sadness and tears flow down her cheeks. I say, "You may have been very sad while I was away." She mumbles some inaudible words. I say, "You are relieved that I have come back. You weren't sure I would." After a long while Yufang says, with a hint of pleasure, "My brother is coming in the spring." Being projected into me is a feeling of being unimportant, a feeling that perhaps Yufang herself has had when I left her. Simultaneously I realise that Yufang is beginning to hold unto some hope of having good experiences in the future and having me return was in itself a good experience for her.

Assisting the nurses and mother in working therapeutically

While offering Yufang six times a week psychotherapy, I also engaged the nurses and Yufang's mother in containing Yufang's emotional experiences. Initially they had talked about her feeling in a "not good, not safe" new place. Later, they began talking about her need to find a safe place in hospital with them. Then they were able to describe *split emotions*: being curled up in bed felt good, but outside bed felt bad. Gradually, more positive experiences were able to be described to her: the nurses were able to say that Yufang was pleased when her mother was with her, pleased when the nurse was present. She looked forward to her mother's return and her favorite nurses being on a shift. The nurses and mother were encouraged to inform Yufang about when they would be away and when they would be returning. They then were encouraged to describe in detail to her when she felt distressed or angry because they were late, were away, were talking to others, or had misunderstood what she experienced. The nurses and her mother were also encouraged to comment upon when Yufang liked an experience and when she was annoyed by silence or too much talk. The nurse's and mother's giving words to her experiences gradually enabled Yufang to find her own voice and speak about her own feelings.

An eighteenth-week session

When finally a vacancy on the inpatient psychiatric unit became available Yufang's medical condition had improved so much that Yufang, her parents and the consultant psychiatrist decided that she was well enough to be cared for at home. Yufang seemed less paralysed by physical symptoms now that she had a trusted psychotherapist to tolerate some of her mental pain. She was walking, talking, and thinking about some of her emotional difficulties, eating, and regaining her physical health. The decision for outpatient treatment was based partly on the fact that the consultant psychiatrist felt that Yufang was making good use of six-times-per-week psychotherapy and agreed for her to have outpatient psychotherapy three times per week, and begin two cello lessons per week, in order to put some structure into her days. Yufang misses the first outpatient appointment, because her mother was unable to bring her. On the second appointment, she arrives wearing a new white long-sleeved blouse, looking as elegant as a woman in *Vogue* magazine. She apologises for missing the first appointment and says that since she couldn't come, she decided to write for the first time in eighteen weeks and put some thoughts in a notebook. During the four days we have not met, she has written haiku-style poems, which she reads dramatically, following each word with a pause:

> Night star, moon wind
> noise, light, shine, whisper

sound, a hint a code
Be fragrant, silent
warmth, asleep
The moment of silence
hanging in the air.

She has also drawn a cartoon-style picture of her beloved grandmother who is in China. On the next page is an aeroplane which she draws to represent a film which she has seen on the day she missed her session. At my request she describes the film saying: "A plane was searching for a man who fell near Mt. McKinley. Someone was calling out from the mountain, 'Naomi, Naomi'. The man died near the foot of the mountain."

Yufang then reads out the words on the last page of her notebook:

If I had a scoop of melon,
the world will be all right.
If all the houses are upset
but tree won't move other place.
Space is all round, round and round.

I can hear the voice from other space.
I have to do something, my mind go fast.
I broke the window.
That is mad but not mad.

There is an empty white space on the sheet beside the poem, and Yufang tells me it is "a glass window". She says, "I wanted to break through the glass window and throw myself out of the window. I wanted to do that when I was ill."

Comments on the eighteenth-week session

The move from inpatient to outpatient psychotherapy was an important transition, and it was accompanied by Yufang missing the first session. What was impressive was that Yufang could be an active partipant in gathering together and trying to make sense of the multitude of emotions racing through her mind. I strove for simplicity in the session because too many feelings were threatening to deluge her.

Gradually, I let her know that she had missed the session which was very unusual for her. She felt the silence of the missed session, felt very lost. When we didn't meet, she had begun to try to find some ways of taking care of herself. She found a notebook, writing down her thoughts and her dream. I also described how terrible it felt inside when she risked letting these feelings get too big and take her over. I was aware of, but did not comment on, the fact that today she had slipped into the identity of "a fashionable mother" in her silk blouse, in an attempt to "hold herself together" and she was continuing to do so. At this point, what was important was that she was making attempts to contain her emotions in whatever ways she could, rather than to deny them. This was a very significant step forward for such an ill young person.

A session in the twenty-second week

Yufang arrives with a little straw nest holding three tiny toy bluebirds. Some feathers are scattered around the nest. She tells me this dream:

> Military officers from two countries were hiding behind trees. It was midnight, the men were shooting at me. I was a boy. I was standing there questioning, "What was the best way to die?" I thought to myself, "Fast firing guns are better than dying slowly." There were many children with families in the dream.

When I asked Yufang for associations to the dream, she replied, "In primary school there were three children who were angry with me and I didn't know why. When I was in China I was angry with my mother."

Comments on the twenty-second-week session

In this session, Yufang seemed to be expressing her conscious wish to preserve the babies of the mother represented by the three birds in the nest. I sensed that there was a hint of compassion, suggesting the development of a good, loving, sensitive aspect of herself - necessary for reparation of *internal damaged family* figures. However, Yufang also seemed to be aware that there was a destructive force inside her from which "these families with children" required protection. Yufang describes herself as feeling anger to "the mother". In her dream, there is shooting representing on some level her own "shooting feelings". A boy is being shot. Yufang describes herself as feeling anger and jealousy towards "the mother" with her own babies. In her dream, there is shooting representing on some level her own "shooting feelings". A boy is being shot. This leads to an incredibly violent, punitive guilt, represented by the military men killing her. She seems fascinated by the killing; "Slow or fast killing?" she asks herself.

In her therapy with me now, Yufang was starting to find an emotional space to symbolize her inner conflicts. These inner conflicts augmented the weight of any external trauma she may have experienced. The external trauma included an aggressive father whom she split off and projected her own aggression and a massive sense of loss. The over-use of denial of all these internal and external conflicts contributed significantly to her regressed state of "near-death".

Yufang's three-times-weekly psychotherapy continued for three years until sadly it was stopped by her parents. They felt that there was no reason for her to continue therapy when ostensibly she was so much better. I felt she needed more time in psychotherapy to consolidate her inner psychological development, but the parents did not agree. Yufang felt she had no choice but to go along with her parents' decision for she was successfully enrolled in a music academy and they were paying for her therapy.

Just what had happened in the therapy? Yufang had initially retreated from the outer world, not talking, walking, or eating. She had nearly died. Her terror of "feeling mad" internally had led her to withdraw into a "non-thinking" state. Through my presence, commenting on her non-verbal expressions of feeling, and through my "story-making", I had patiently encouraged Yufang to share the experience of thinking about her inner and outer experiences. Initially, she had projected all her hostile feelings onto her aggressive father and everyone who had left her, in particular her parents and her boyfriend. Then she was persecuted by "poison food", the frightening external world, and she had retreated completely from it. I worked with her in her physically ill state, being present with whatever suffering she felt. Through working through her experiences of separation and loss of my understanding or my presence in the therapy, I had enabled her to find ways of feeling pain rather than somatising it. Gradually, Yufang was able to move from a state of persecution by bad, attacking internal and external figures to a reintegration of her hostile feelings. She began to feel more secure internally as she introjected my capacity to think about her emotions, as is shown by her writing in her diary when she had a missed session. Although she had a greater inner capacity to tolerate psychic pain, I realised that, without therapy, a developmental crisis might overwhelm her fragile capacities.

It is true that through psychotherapy Yufang had developed more capacity to stay with a feeling, lend thought to it, and make decisions accordingly. *Projecting* feelings into others had diminished considerably, and I felt she was more able to *introjectively identify* with "the good internal mother" rather than just slip into her shoes in an imitative fashion suggestive of *intrusive identification*. Yufang was very successful in her new cello studies at an excellent music academy, and felt pleasure in describing to me how she loved her music and was playing with more feeling than ever before. With some shyness, but with much enjoyment, she was socialising with both British and Chinese friends. Despite all this, I still felt Yufang had a very fragile state without sufficient emotional depth to lend thought to and *contain* her extremely passionate feelings. I heard later that she very successfully graduated from the musical academy, had regained her capacity to remember, and she was modulating her emotions through thinking more about her emotional conflicts.

Further considerations regarding treatment

There is a question of technique when faced with a child severely traumatised by internal and/or external destructive events. George E. Gray (1983, pp. 319–322), writing about his own severe depression, says, "The results of a session should be carefully assessed. If it makes the patient feel worse rather than better, further sessions should be suspended. A patient should be allowed to sit quietly in the corner for as long as he wants or needs to." I have heard quite a few psychiatrists say, "Let the patient be, don't intrude with psychotherapy. Such a severely depressed patient's ability to think and concentrate is dramatically impaired. Therapy will only make her worse." I know there is research on this subject; however, as far as my own philosophy is concerned, I shall try to remain true to what I have learned from my own clinical experience of working with these severely regressed, physically ill young people who do not speak, walk or eat and initially avoid thinking about emotional experiences. I know that out of the fifteen not talking, not walking not eating severely regressed young people whom I have seen in long term psychotherapy, Yufang has made the most progress, in the briefest period, in integrating with her family and peers and resuming her music studies successfully. Not separating from parents during the illness and intensive six times a week psychotherapy seemed particularly beneficial to her during her inpatient admission. During her hospitalisation, she was encouraged to think about what she wanted to do with her time. This element of choice was important as long as it was compatible with a structure of living her days that we felt would be good for her. She received physical and emotional "nursing" undertaken daily by her mother and a few hours of hospital schooling with other young people. The paediatric nurses supported the mother and fostered her having a more emotionally attuned relationship with Yufang. Family therapy was concurrent during the acute phase of Yufang's illness.

During Yufang's six half-hour sessions a week, I tried to avoid creating a situation where she would be traumatised or invaded by overwhelming feelings. It did happen that she did cry profusely at times without any obvious prompt on my part. During the therapy, I tried to provide and open up the space for her to acknowledge and eventually think about both her loving and her negative feelings and thoughts. My desire to offer psychotherapy to subsequent young non-speaking young people *pervasively retreating from life* like Yufang is based on Yufang's remark: "I didn't *want* to die, but *I had* to." The implication of this remark is that, regardless of whether or not there has been an external traumatising factor, the healthy part of the regressed not talking, walking, eating young person is overwhelmed by helplessness in the face of an impulse to die and get out of the inner and external experiences with which she is faced. At times death may feel a good alternative to feeling severely mentally disturbed! In this context, it seemed callous not to help Yufang struggle with the cruel internal forces that attacked hope and almost succeeded in propelling her into death.

One serious treatment difficulty is when I am perceived in the *transference* as the embodiment of the destructive tormentor (from external or internal reality). I found it extremely difficult to convey to the staff that *working in the transference* involves gathering all the negative feelings to the therapist so that the child's external world is freed of conflicts of "the inner infantile part of the personality, the inner child". I had to bear and work with the staff's belief that I might be taking the young person into the room to torment her with psychotherapy. Being experienced as "the witch" during some of the psychotherapy sessions inevitably occurs because it is inextricably paired with "gathering the transference" (Meltzer, 1967), which means being the receptacle for the bad, painful, emerging negative transference of young people not talking and not eating. Feeling angry or even humiliated about being rejected is also something one has to be working on within oneself if one is the psychotherapist. During this phase of psychotherapy, the therapist needs to search to see if there is any sign that the young person may be experiencing relief as well as the inevitable pain that mainly derives from the unfreezing of feelings and the facing of hitherto denied, unnameable, dreaded feelings. The hands a child uses to wheel herself into therapy, or the child's legs that walk the child into therapy, can hold split-off positive feelings towards the therapy. To have a therapist take "the brunt of emotional pain" is a relief for the young person.

When confronted with anxiety about slow progress resulting in a worry that the therapy is useless, I hold on for dear life to a former non-talking, walking, eating regressed young person's written words: "Even if I don't talk, it doesn't mean that therapy doesn't help." I would now add that even when she did not talk, it did not mean that Yufang was not communicating. When the young person has virtually given up life or is rigidly protecting herself through silence, psychotherapy is essential to help a young person to reassemble her sense of self. My words and emotional acceptance of Yufang's non-verbally communicated states of mind seemed vital to evoke and gather together her disintegrated emotional and mental life. Yufang deserved the experience of being deeply understood as well as the experience of being given gentle encouragement to participate with *her very own choice of tiny steps* into the ordinary activities of life. The pleasure and relief in being understood created the trust, hope and the possibility of growing physically and developing psychologically. Yufang's development in this regard was facilitated by various therapeutic endeavours of the multidisciplinary team. I think frequent but shortened individual psychotherapy sessions accompanied by her mother's supportive, nurturing protective daily presence and the gradually introduced company of the other young people as well as the predictable, consistent nursing care all contributed to the best recovery plan possible.

Theoretical conclusions regarding psychotherapy with a regressed, not talking, walking, eating young person

I have subsequently worked with or supervised work with fifteen other regressed young people, aged nine to nineteen years, who arrived in hospital not talking, walking, or eating. They had become unresponsive to any social stimuli and failed to indicate pain. As they became slightly better, they began to withdraw when spoken to or touched. A psychodynamic view of this regressed state involves taking into consideration the external situations of the child through family work, as well as the child's inner world through individual psychotherapy. The inner world of the child is peopled by aspects of figures first loved and hated in life and also contains aspects of the child herself. These inner figures exist in phantasy and are experienced "as real, or even more real and actual to the child in his unconscious feelings than external events" (Riviere, 1952, pp. 346–369). Internal figures are not exact replicas of the external world but are always coloured by the infant's and child's phantasy and projections of feelings (Segal, 1981).

The external world of the regressed young person who is not talking and eating and thinking is characterised by separation anxiety, social withdrawal and depression. The young person feels no control over the external events and this might often incur a sense of hopelessness. Uncontrollable events may include family relocation, including migration from another culture, the loss of loved ones, severe illness, often a viral illness, mental illness and unreliability of the parents. Abuse, whether it be physical, sexual or emotional, as a form of inescapable trauma may be another contributory factor. These uncontrollable events may occur against a background of parental overprotectiveness, but, more importantly, of parental helplessness and hopelessness. To an outside observer such as a teacher, the premorbid young person may ostensibly be achieving both academically and socially while internally the child is failing to meet personal developmental expectations (Nunn & Thompson, 1996). The external family of these children often have had weakened psychic structures, too weak to contain the child's intense feelings of love, fear and hate and anger. There is a marked tendency to use denial of psychologically painful experiences and denial of aggression on a day-to-day basis. In some families, this may then lead to explosions of hostility, which can take the form of parents shouting, hitting, throwing pots and pans, resorting to sleep as a flight from anxiety, sobbing uncontrollably, and relinquishing parental responsibilities. Sometimes in these situations, the child's hostility is denied and unconsciously directed to internal family figures. This may protect the child's relationships with the parents, but it leads to destruction and the breakdown of the child's already fragile psychic structure, coupled with depression and persecutory guilt due to the damage of the internal family figures. For example, Yufang thought that she had "killed her brother", and she was convinced that her father had "died in an accident". Her dreams conveyed a feeling of the whole internal world being destroyed by an earthquake. It is notable that, prior to the onset of their illness, the other fifteen non-speaking young people *pervasively retreating from life* whom I have seen for individual psychotherapy denied conflict and were unable to express any hatred or anger directly towards their parents. In some families, this was understandable since one of the parents was feared as a potential retaliator if a family rule was broken. This fear was partly evoked by the fiery temper of one parent, but it was also linked in other situations with a fragile mother and the child's projection of her own aggressive, hostile feelings towards one or both parents, making the child experience the "good-enough" parents as feared parents.

Lacking an inner psychic structure for dealing with the pressure of emotional stimuli arising from internal and external sources, the child retreats from the external world and all stimuli emanating from it. The young person is in a kind of "claustrum" (Meltzer, 1992). Some young people have reported afterwards that they could gradually begin to hear and understand when in this state but were initially very confused. They said they felt that they *could not speak,* even though sentences or phrases might be forming in their mind in response to what was being said to them.

When the young person ceases having any emotional link with anyone and gives himself/herself up to death, not eating, talking, or walking, hospitalisation is then required. The separation of the regressed child from the parents is extremely traumatic because the child lacks an "internal parental figure" for protection to help with living independently of the external parents. For this reason, keeping the parent by the child's side may be a preferable mode of treatment initially. The child feels that it is essential to cling for dear life to the external parents and feels deeply hurt and rejected by them when the hospital requires the parents to leave the hospital. After an initial phase of crying for the parents to stay, many children give up crying and break the loving emotional link with them in a way similar to very young children described by the Robertsons (1971). Although the parents are simply following hospital instructions to leave the child in the care of the hospital unit, the parents are perceived by the child as bad and abandoning for they are filled with projections of the child's hostility regarding abandonment to the nurses.

Nurses may approach the child, but they, being transference figures for the parents are now perceived as hostile enemies and are ignored. The child does not want, or is not able to take in, anything from them. All have become persecutory figures containing projections of the child's violent rage about separation. Because of the regressed child's life-threatening physical state, the child causes deep concern and confusion in the paediatric ward. The child's emotional needs are often overlooked because the child is persecuted and retreating from staff and her bodily needs are so great. Staff often overreact with either passivity, or avoidance, or impersonal invasive over-activity. The staff's countertransference to the child is often linked with the child's transference feelings towards them, representing the child's persecutory internal parents filled with child's hostility. It is extremely difficult and demanding, but absolutely essential, to hold in mind the child's and the family's total emotional situation and needs, and to sustain an empathic, cooperative, understanding psychological intervention. A consultant to the staff often has to contain the staff's anxieties and negativity to the parents by asking them to identify with parents fearing their child will die. Parents' anger to staff is often their first way of projecting their own guilt regarding having such a very ill child. The not talking, not walking, not eating, regressed child is overwhelmed with a sense helplessness and passive surrender. The child attains self-preservation through mentally removing the *self* from the external world into "an inner claustrum" (Meltzer, 1992). The name "pervasive refusal syndrome" implies a sense of agency which such a child does not have initially, and is better stated as *pervasively retreating from life*. In my experience, characteristically such a regressed child goes through the following emotional phases initially:

1. *Overwhelming sobbing*: This feels as though it will never end. One can experience in the child's sobbing a panic about the traumatic nature of the intense feelings and anxieties which can be psychotic in their severity. At times the feelings are multiplied by the separation from, and loss of, parents while in hospital.
2. *A sense of being persecuted*: The child may hit out at people as though they have become bad, terrifying monsters if they approach, touch, or offer nurturance which feels an intrusion.
3. *Hallucinating a monstrous "male figure" or having an inner sense of a primitive protector not allowing contact with the nurses, the therapist, or others*: During this stage, the child may be more aware that others have something helpful to offer, but this inner figure functions as a kind of concentration-camp prison guard. It promises protection to the child as long as the child obeys it by withdrawing from any kind of human contact. When the child attempts to eat or talk and therefore to depend on the nurturing figures in the form of nurses or therapists, the hallucinatory figure or split-off inner voice threatens punishment. This is the work of the destructive omnipotent part of the personality against life, hope and dependency. The monstrous "part of the self" is at times turned to as one's "ruler" or "companion" (Rosenfeld, 1987).

The psychological trauma that these children have experienced varies from child to child. Garland (1999) reminds us that it is the interaction between internal states of mind and external situations which creates the intensity of inner trauma. In the present emotional climate, where sexual and physical abuse are more prominent causes of disturbance, clinicians feel tempted to investigate abuse as a matter of course. My own feeling is that, unless the child has first established a trusting relationship with a nurse, therapist, or family member, investigation of trauma can itself be traumatic. In the throes of a severe breakdown of the personality resulting in severe regression, not talking, walking, or eating, the mentally regressed child cannot bear more emotionally intense issues.

The first step is not to talk about more trauma, but to build an emotional bridge to the child. This empathic connection to the child will give the child the necessary protection to become re-acquainted with the trauma, both inner and external, that prompted a regression into not talking, walking, and eating.

Steps forward often made by a regressed child who is not talking, walking, or eating

In individual psychotherapy, there is often a sequence of emotional developments that occur within the child. In the most severely ill children, the child is at first almost completely immobile, as though the cord holding the child in life has been broken. The child's eyes are closed and the body has a kind of waxy flexibility as though there is no *self* owning the body. The child may be suffering from a painful physical illness such as Crohn's disease which causes extreme pain in the gut, but the crying out in pain normally accompanying an illness of this kind does not occur. The child gives no suggestion that physical pain is present. There is no response to stimuli, as though the *self* has vacated the body.

When the child begins to flinch, hit out, or moan to avoid a persecutory situation, the child is again beginning to have a perceptive mental apparatus able to struggle against something perceived as negative or destructive. Occasionally, the child has retreated in a phobic way from intimate relations with people in the external world, but there may indeed be other relationships taking place: the child may be involved in listening to or seeing hallucinatory figures.

Gradually, if the environment is sufficiently emotionally containing, the child begins to secretly glance towards and listen to people, but will retreat immediately if anyone notices. Sometimes, the child prefers turning to peers rather than adults. Subsequently, the child may regain a relationship with the self when "deeply touched" emotionally. The emotional response of the child is then uncontained and overwhelming, taking the form of copious crying, uncontrolled hitting, or manic states of mind. Any "uncomfortable" experience suggesting emotional pain or conflict in relationships can be followed by a massive withdrawal, sometimes through immediate sleep. In time, however, there is clear evidence of the child being able to regain a mind and enjoy pleasurable activities. This heralds the beginning of a possibility of intimate relationships, as long as they are relatively conflict-free. The child begins to signal through more overt mindful gestures, to draw, to tell dreams, or write thoughts in a private diary before discussing difficult issues with a therapist or keyworker. Conversations may ensue if they are not about the child or not filled with too much emotional intensity. The child might make sparse replies such as "no", "yes", "good", "feeling left out". Finally, the child may begin to be curious about inner emotional states and external events, and begin to discuss conflictual events that may have contributed to his or her difficulties. It is in this latter state of therapy that the child can describe "how paralysed" around speaking or eating he or she felt initially even though gradually being able to make sense of what was being said.

This therapeutic work with such a pervasively retreating child is important, for it presents an extreme version of the child's withdrawal from the intimacy of human relationships and food and drink and understanding its necessary for life itself. Withdrawal into a "claustrum" (Meltzer, 1992) can be seen as a *life-protective* mechanism saving the Self from further encounters with more traumatically adverse emotional experiences. Such withdrawal is similar to the predicament of the foetus when totally helpless, unaware of the self and of feelings. The regressed child when moving forward may sometimes comment on missing the "old experience" when all needs were met through the naso-gastric tube-feeding and total nursing care and he or she didn't have *to do* anything.

If the psychotherapist provides an emotional experience that is enlivening, interesting, nurturing, and pertinent to the child's *present emotional life*, the child may begin to turn to the therapist to journey through an exploration of his or her inner life. The introjection of the therapist's goodness, emotional courage, and understanding will gradually facilitate the child's growth and hope to live again in the world outside the hospital.

CHAPTER THIRTEEN

Countertransference in the psychoanalysis of a silent adolescent boy

Nancy L. Bakalar

In this chapter, I shall discuss the case of a late adolescent boy who became almost completely silent for four months within the first year of analysis. As any therapist might, I struggled as to how best to help the boy overcome his anger and resistance, while struggling with my own negative feelings about the stand-off. Only after I was able to relax and allow myself to fall into a more profound countertransference experience and have an unsettling dream about the young man was I able to find a way into his silence so that our work could continue in a more classical analytic fashion. The situation required that I enter into phantasy and share my thoughts with him, much as a child analyst might do with children in play therapy. As his analysis unfolded, the many dynamic meanings of his silence were revealed and worked through. I then discuss thoughts about different countertransference experiences and my dream about the young man, which I used to better understand him and to help him to understand himself more fully and to move forward developmentally. I end with a discussion about training experiences which contribute to working more deeply in the countertransference.

Brief background on theory and technique of treating the silent patient

From the time psychoanalysis began, the silent patient has baffled and bewildered analysts. Freud required that the patient obey the fundamental rule, and say whatever came to mind without editing thoughts. If the patient were unable to comply, Freud believed the resistance was due to transference around sexual conflicts related to the analyst; in the case of male patients due to homosexual longing and its attendant anxiety, and in the case of female patients, a desire to be overtaken and seduced by the male analyst. The anxiety around the sexual conflict then served as a resistance to whatever issue the patient was trying to avoid (Freud, 1914).

Psychoanalytic theory and technique were not sufficiently advanced during the first few decades of this new science to help psychoanalysts manage these transference problems, so when an analyst was confronted by silence, he may have been moved to anger, experiencing the patient as defiant, stubborn, resistant and therefore, not analysable. In early psychoanalytic papers on the topic, much of the language gives the impression that analysts felt under attack when patients fell silent, and that they had to "confront" the resistance. If the analyst "accused" the patient of sexual or other motives, the analysis often became stalemated and ended because the patient could not bear the external attack coupled with her own attacking internal object relations.

Since the publication of Breuer's and Freud's *Studies in Hysteria* (1893), a rich literature on the theory, technique, and challenges of treating the silent patient, has evolved. Ferenczi (1919) recommended that after educating the silent patient as to the purpose of free association, "… the analyst should oppose the patient's silence with his own (silence)" (Calogeras citing Ferenczi, 1967, p. 538). Many analysts held on to this advice for too many decades. Glover (1927) suggested that while analysts should not "counter-attack" patients with silence, sometimes the analyst's silence is appropriate and necessary:

> To meet silence invariably with silence is to court a sort of silent combat, which confirms (to the) obstinate or aggressive type of patient in his view that analysis is a kind of psychological pugilistic encounter to be settled by the gaining of points. On the other hand, this is precisely the type of patient to whom it is necessary to demonstrate that (the patient) is attempting to convert analysis into a fight …
>
> (Glover, 1927, p. 513)

We now understand that an individual's silence can have various dynamic meanings and may occur for reasons out of the person's awareness; or, the silence may be conscious, but the person inhibits verbalisation to defend against guilt, shame, or embarrassment; or, silence may develop out of fear of verbally attacking or trying to seduce the analyst. Some patients with more concrete, primitive thinking styles cannot distinguish the difference between words conveying ideas about anger or seduction from the actual behaviours, so they resist verbalising those thoughts to the analyst. Segal (1981) named this kind of thinking *symbolic equation,* meaning that in the patient's mind, the words for a thing are experienced as equivalent to the thing itself, and so language expressing aggression and seduction may not be spoken. Silence also may represent a kind of mental carapace, reminiscent of observed infants who form a kind of *body-shell* by flexing their musculature when anxious or frightened. For the silent patient, the mental carapace of silence shields the patient when in a paranoid-schizoid state from feeling under attack or feeling about to fall to pieces or collapse when besieged by emotions. A different kind of "silence" occurs when the child talks incessantly without apparent meaning, destroying meaning, and blocking awareness of emotional life, as a way to block her own thinking and that of the analyst.

All patients communicate by unconscious as well as conscious mechanisms during analytic sessions. Besides speaking, patients also emanate a mood or tone directed toward the analyst by what they do or don't do. They may glare or show no eye contact; pick at the analyst's furniture; pick at themselves and drop pieces of skin, nails, hair or mucus. They communicate by breathing patterns, facial expressions, and bodily movements, sounds or odors to which the analyst attunes herself as a way to understand the patient. The silent person may use such bodily sounds and gestures more profoundly and the analyst will likely be more attuned to, and affected by, these communications because of the absence of language.

Alternately or in addition, the patient may use projective identification, an unconscious to unconscious communication with the analyst, because he is unable or unwilling to use words. The patient attributes thoughts and feelings to the analyst and then "treats" the analyst as if those strong affects reside in her instead of in himself (Ogden, 1982). The analyst may feel taken over from within by strong emotions, may at first feel attacked or baited, and may be pulled into enactments. This is a transference/countertransference phenomenon, and requires that the analyst understand what is going on inside herself affectively as a way to understand what is going on between herself and the patient, and what the individual is attempting to communicate about his own internal state. Once the analyst understands these projections, she has a better chance of making an interpretation that will be helpful to the patient.

Balint (1958) put forward his theory about *three areas of the mind* correlating to a one-, two-, and three-person psychology. The one- and two-person psychologies are particularly relevant to working with silent patients. Before I discuss that, a brief overview will be helpful: the three-person psychology relates to the *Oedipal situation* in which the individual and two others are present. The individual competes with one of the triad for the love and attention of the third. The period is characterised by conflict and competition, and can be understood and worked through with language. For this reason these patients are less likely to fall into long-lasting silences in the course of treatment.

The two-person psychology pertains to what Balint (1958) termed the *basic fault*, referred to by others as the pre-Oedipal or pre-verbal period of development. Balint elaborated that in the pre-verbal weeks and months, all that matters to the baby is that he gets his needs met. If there is a good-enough fit between what any one particular infant needs and what his mother can provide, the baby experiences the world as good enough, develops trust, and experiences love. However, if the baby's needs are too great either because of physical illness or his temperament, or if his mother cannot provide basic good-enough caretaking, where there is a deficiency of attention, attunement, or satisfactory physical care, then the baby suffers immensely from primitive rage, anxiety, fear of falling apart or collapsing.

Patients who suffer with deficits related to the *basic fault* feel as if they are broken, psychologically fragile, and as if something were missing. The feeling states don't lend themselves to verbal expression because the assault or damage to the infant occurred in the pre-verbal years. These individuals generate strong feelings in the analyst and communicate an intensity of emotion when slighted, which appears in excess of the injury. When these individuals experience ordinary frustrations of life, Balint noted that:

> They cannot accept that there exists any other cause for a frustration of their desires than malice, evil intention, or at least, criminal negligence ... Remarkably, all this is simply accepted as a painful fact and it is most surprising how little anger, still less a willingness to fight, is mobilized by it ... Though feelings of emptiness and deadness may be very strong, behind them there is usually an earnest, quiet determination to see things through. This queer mixture of profound suffering, absence of cheap pugnacity, and an unshakeable determination to get on makes these patients truly appealing - an important diagnostic sign that the (analytic) work has reached the level of the *basic fault*.
>
> (1968, pp. 19–20)

Children and adults who suffer in the arena of the *basic fault* and who cannot put into words the feelings surrounding a deficit in maternal love, emotional understanding, and physical care, and who have ill-formed feelings of anger around the deficit experiences are more likely to go into extended periods of silence during treatment. At such times, it is important for the analyst to think about what it was and still is like for the patient to be that helpless and dependent infant, to have had experiences of not being thought about, not cared for, perhaps experiencing the mother's resentment or even hatred for having to be cared for. The analyst can put into words for the individual what it must have been like, so that the patient can begin to work symbolically and consciously with what he experienced in his pre-verbal months and years.

Balint's one-person psychology is difficult to observe and study because it occurs inside the patient himself, not in relation to others, and can be an area of creativity, or in my view, also terror, when the person is in the throes of psychotic thinking. In considering a silent patient in the analytic situation, Balint (1958) points out that the silent individual may be running away from something (resistance) or may be running towards something creatively. Balint elaborates that this is:

> ... a state in which (the patient) feels relatively safe and can do something about the problem bothering or tormenting him. The something that he will eventually produce and then present to (the analyst) is a kind of "creation" - not necessarily honest, sincere, profound or artistic - but nonetheless a product of his creativity. True, we cannot be with him during the actual work of creation, but we can be with him in moments just before and immediately after, and, in addition, we can watch him from the outside during his actual work. Perhaps if we can change our own approach - from considering the silence as a symptom of resistance to studying it as a possible source of information - we may learn something about this area of the mind.
>
> (1958, p. 338)

Balint is alerting us to the possibility that the silent individual may be withdrawing into a paranoid-schizoid state of the *basic fault* or into a creative state which only can be observed and not entered into directly with him until the child re-emerges and begins to talk about it. As analysts we need to think about both possibilities when in the presence of the silent person so that we can proceed empathically as much as we are able. Winnicott (1958) brought to our attention that silence in a child need not indicate resistance, withdrawal, control nor fear. He pointed out that silence in the presence of the analyst may indicate a sign of achievement or maturity. Winnicott discovered that children who are calmly attached are able to play independently in the presence of the mother, neither being clingy nor avoidant. This is a necessary step on the way to achieving mature, independent, separate play and to be creative. An insufficiency of this experience with mother prevents the development of the capacity to be alone. Such a child or adult would then have difficulties in attachments to others, perhaps being unable to function when alone, or even being frightened in the presence of another for fear the other would go missing. So, when we as analysts encounter a silent child, we must consider whether the silence represents a withdrawal or avoidance, or a capacity to be alone in the presence of the other and as a period of internal thought and creativity.

Numerous other authors in the latter half of the last century wrote about the importance when treating silent individuals of being more flexible with the fundamental rule of free association. Among those were Khan (1963), Nacht (1963), and Zeligs as reported by Waldhorn (1959). Calogeras (1967) allowed for "a parameter", which released Mrs. W from the obligation of the fundamental rule so that she could remain silent which "initiate(d) a noble change in the whole affective tone of the... analysis and (took) tremendous pressure off her", which Calogeras then reported greatly diminished her silent periods.

Emphasising countertransference experiences to understand the silent patient

Many authors have written about the necessity of suspending the fundamental rule when working with silent patients, and of understanding the silence itself as embodying the kernel where the analytic work needs to unfold. Extended silence is a communication in itself and carries the dynamic of the patient's difficulties. In most cases, this dynamic represents a deficit with respect to the relationship with the primary caretaker, experienced in infancy or young childhood, which gave rise to a *basic fault*, as just discussed (Balint, 1958). The working through of the silence, being mentally present for the patient during his silence, and giving words to the experience, *is* the work of the repair of the *basic fault*, after which more traditional conflict analysis can take place.

Two authors particularly have captured the quality and challenges of working at the level of the *basic fault* with adult patients: Khan (1963) and Nacht (1963). Khan analysed an eighteen-year-old boy named Peter who had withdrawn from life, declined to attend university, and occupied himself alone in his room listening to classical music and reading novels. The boy's mother had suffered a depression when Peter was three; the source of Peter's own depression and withdrawal. Peter's previous therapist had discontinued his treatment because she could not bear his silence.Khan (1963) wrote about how he struggled against his wish "to somehow rattle (Peter) into aliveness", or to reassure Peter as he lay silent and deadened. Khan felt the urge literally to nudge Peter or to "act on him with verbal interpretations". Khan interpreted to Peter that his silence was an attack on Khan, but these interpretations left Peter more morose, sullen, and withdrawn, "a collapsed heap of a boy on the couch". Khan came to understand that his role as Peter's analyst was to bear the pain of futility and hopelessness that Peter had experienced as a toddler in relation to his depressed mother. Khan described that at times in the analysis he experienced himself as that toddler with a depressed mother. At other times, Khan reported that Peter re-lived the experiences of being his depressed-toddler self, while Khan felt like the depressed mother in the countertransference. Khan concluded that "... (it) was the judicious withholding of therapeutic intervention, either through excessive interpretation or reassurance, that enabled (Peter) to communicate his real inner conflicts and predicaments" (p. 300); "My role and function during those silences was to provide a sentient, concentrated, alert attention. This attention had to be more than merely listening. It is listening with one's mind *and body* ..." (emphasis mine, p. 306).

Nacht (1963) approached his silent patient similarly to Khan, but his theoretical understanding was more like Balint's. Nacht pointed out that speech separates two individuals, each an object of the subjective self, while silence joins two people together in a union, or possibly fusion. There is a tension in the human condition between wanting to be separate and differentiated from the other, versus wanting to be close to or even united with the other. Language and conversation demarcate and differentiate one person from the other as each expresses individual thoughts and affect through words, intonation, inflection, loudness, and cadence. In contrast, non-verbal communication, such as nearness or touching, breathing, murmuring, or gazing into the other's eyes, unites, lessens, or perhaps even obliterates boundaries between self and other, similar to the experience of the infant nursing at the mother's breast, both in reverie.

Nacht (1963) elucidates that many patients come to analysis needing to re-experience union with another for repair of the self (the *basic fault*), and elaborated that this cannot occur unless the analyst and the patient are without fear of both silence and closeness. The patient is seeking an experience where "He feels himself secure in the non-verbal to non-verbal, unconscious to unconscious relationship" (p. 337). If the analyst is uneasy about the silence, he must first analyse his own anxiety in relation to the patient. Little by little, as the analyst is able to sit with the silent individual, he will communicate non-verbally his own calm, an openness and availability, an interest in the patient, whether he speaks or not. Nacht described the analyst's attitude as one of "authentic benevolence" (p. 337) or "as a gratifying presence, in which the patient perceives a deep-down attitude of availability and hearty attentiveness" (p. 338). In these cases, at certain times, and in limited ways, Nacht recommended *not* preserving the rules of neutrality and *not* withholding all gratification, by positively responding to small requests, such as a change in time or by extending a session by a minute or two, so that the patient might have an experience of his analyst as someone who need not be feared, who is benevolent, and who does respond to real requests.

In Nacht's (1963), Khan's (1963), Balint's (1958), and others' papers on working with the silent patient, all make clear that it is imperative not to excessively gratify the patient, or to allow the patient to get pulled into a regressed, dependent transference which could not be analysed or worked through successfully, and which could result in a failed analysis. In general, these therapists utilised the techniques and goals of classical analysis: abstinence, not gratifying the patient, ameliorating the harshness of the superego, and strengthening the ego. What they have recommended in the work with the silent patient is a modification of classic technique so that earlier, really more primitive injury to the psyche, can be repaired or at least strengthened.

I now would like to return to Nacht's (1963) ideas about what he termed a "deep understanding attitude" with silent patients which constitutes a special "presence" of the analyst.

Khan (1963) demonstrated those attributes in his work with Peter. It seems to me that Nacht is talking about the analyst's willingness *and* desire to *Know* the patient in the sense that Bion elaborated in *Learning from Experience* (1962), *The Elements of Psychoanalysis* (1963), and other works. Bion (1962) said that "an emotional experience cannot be conceived of in isolation from a relationship" (p. 42). That is, that *Knowing* the patient has to do with having a real, lived experience with the patient. Bion believed that these basic emotions in relation to others could be reduced to only three feeling states and their opposites: *Love, Hate,* and *Knowing* signified by *L, H,* and *K,* and their opposites signified by *-L, -H,* and *-K.* Balint, Khan, Nacht, and others each described the quality the analyst must possess is the desire to *Know* the patient, in order to treat patients with problems in the arena of the *basic fault.* It is the analyst's capacity to sit with the patient, to mentally take in the child's confusions, distress, thoughts, and unbearably painful feelings, to attempt to understand and sort them out, and then to speak to the patient about them, that constitutes Bion's notion of *containment.* Through the active process of mental *containment,* the analyst comes to *Know* the patient and the patient experiences being *Known.* It is Nacht's "authentic benevolence, gratifying presence or attitude of availability or hearty attentiveness" that relates to Bion's *K, Knowing* the other. It is the desire to be interested in and learn about the patient, and to be willing to suffer the "pain, frustration and loneliness" (Symington & Symington, 1996, p. 28) that getting to *Know* someone requires. It is not dissimilar from that quality parents have for their newborn infant, or lovers for one another, wanting to *Know* the other through sight, sound, taste, touch, smell; through time and over time to create a history, so that a past, present, and future-to-be can be held in mind and memory, *Known,* which then forms the basis of deep and permanent connection - the basis of a meaningful life.

Willingness and desire to *Know* the patient has nothing to do with *Love,* and certainly nothing to do with *Hate.* In fact, *Love* and *Hate* contaminate "getting-to-*Know*" and *Knowing* the other (Bion, 1962). When strong feelings emerge between the patient and the analyst in the treatment setting, the analyst must work to understand her countertransference feelings and set them aside, awaiting the moment when they can inform the analysis and perhaps be used to formulate a response to the patient. Below, I present the case of Michael, who developed a strong erotic transference early in his analysis, in response to which I developed a set of disturbing countertransference feelings. These had to be thought about, mentally metabolised, and understood. Bion (1962) termed this process *alpha function*; it constitutes what Bion saw as mental *containment* of the patient's unbearable and not understood emotional distress. Once worked through, I used my understanding to help Michael to move forward in his analysis and development.

Case presentation

When I first met Michael, he was nearly sixteen years old. His family lived in a rural area where there are few mental health care providers. His parents brought him for evaluation upon the recommendation of a church elder. Michael suffered from severe obsessive compulsive anxiety symptoms, especially in the areas of doing homework and in helping his father in the family business. He stayed up until the early morning hours doing school assignments, reworking math or science problems, feeling unable to get the answers correct or the notebook paper neat enough, which left him distraught, depressed, and intermittently suicidal.

His parents own a small food distribution business, and it was his task before and after school to fill orders. He worried about getting all the orders packed correctly and had fears that he had cheated customers by omitting an item or cheated his father by including something in an order that did not belong there. He repeatedly asked his father to check his work and reassure him that he hadn't made mistakes in the inventory. This left his father weary and irritated.

Michael was born into a devout fundamentally religious family and is the fifth of nine children, consisting of three boys and six girls. The family lives in a close-knit, religious community. All the children are about two years apart, and he is flanked by both older and younger sisters. His parents said he was a quiet boy, who took his faith seriously and often expressed worry about being condemned for minor wrong-doings.

He was a strikingly handsome boy with an angelic face. He skin was clear and his cheeks rosy. He wore his clothes tidily and tucked in. He spoke softly and showed glancing eye contact. He told me that he worried about stealing; that once he had borrowed a pencil from a school chum and felt that he had to repay his friend with a candy bar because he had "stolen" some of the pencil lead and eraser. He agonised over "stealing" a clean piece of paper from his brother's notebook. He felt guilty about masturbating, worried that he would be condemned to hell.

Michael accepted twice-weekly psychotherapy. Early sessions were filled with long, circuitous, obsessive ruminations, spoken in a monotone. His thinking was convoluted, tortuous, and torturing, which reflected his internal confusion and chaos. He used words and facts like concrete bits and arrived at faulty conclusions. I struggled to understand him and several times reflected that his concern about details seemed to hide his feelings from himself. He was unable to use my observation.

Sessions left me bored and sleepy, or frustrated and baffled as to how I might help him. After a couple of weeks, I told him that I was sorry that I didn't understand what he was saying and felt confused. My statement surprised him, as if it never had occurred to him that he was not making sense, as if no matter what he said or how he said it, I should understand, like a mother who would ideally understand exactly what was going on with her infant. He said that he really did want me to understand, and so he slowed down, and began to pause between ideas, glancing at me and checking in with me to see if I were following his meaning. So, rather than being "talked at", his stories came to involve both of us; they became relational. As he worked to help me understand what he was struggling with, it appeared he also began to listen to himself.

Michael proved to be motivated, curious, and thoughtful. Sexual concerns were prominent, and he had many questions about sexuality. Further exploration revealed moderate physical masochism in his masturbatory practices. He also was too severe with his younger siblings, and treated the family pets harshly. He developed minimally disguised maternal and Oedipal longings for me which rapidly evolved into an eroticised transference. His father asked that I also evaluate a depressed brother and Michael strongly objected, explaining that he wanted me exclusively for himself. He was very sensitive about time boundaries, feeling "brushed aside like a fly" when I announced the end of sessions. Most times he simply stood up, walked out, angry and hurt, without saying anything. A year into therapy, when I was more aware of the depth and manifestations of his difficulties, I recommended he enter into psychoanalysis, which I felt offered a greater likelihood of securing relief for this young man. He and his parents readily agreed.

Beginning psychoanalysis

At the first session, I told Michael that I would be speaking less than I had during his therapy so that he would have more time to explore his own thoughts. He experienced this as rejection and withholding myself from him. He was unsure how to use the analytic couch, uneasy lying either on his back or his stomach for fear that I would see his "hips" or an erection, so he never lay down. Because of his discomfort and young age, I conducted his analysis face to face, several feet apart, five days per week.

One of Michael's early concerns was that I would terminate his treatment before he was ready, despite the fact that we had just increased his number of sessions from two to five per week. The ends of sessions and weekends were very painful for him. Acutely aware of when sessions began and ended, he challenged me if he felt like I had ended sessions even seconds early. He tortured himself believing that I tried to get rid of him or couldn't stand him if sessions were a bit short; and if a bit long, he convinced himself I must love him as much as he loved me, and pressured me to verify his beliefs.

Separations between daily sessions and weekends left him feeling as though he would die. Indeed, he experienced very painful psychic falling apart, which he was able to manage only because he returned to his large family and usual routine. Near the end of the hour of the last session before my first winter break, he said poignantly, "It's not that I am going to miss you; it's that I *need* you!" Tears silently rolled down his cheeks. I was shaken and deeply moved. Michael was letting me know about his painful experiences from early childhood; about how he was frightened and felt as though he would fall to pieces if he lost connection with his mother/ analyst.

Seeing him five times weekly, the maternal/erotic transference quickly intensified. Michael found a magazine in the waiting room with an alternate business address; smiling victoriously and sadistically, he told me that he knew where I lived. He said he had looked up the address on MapQuest and now knew how to get to my house. He tried to figure out which car in the parking lot was mine, and when he saw me there, tried to figure out where I had been by what I was carrying. These incidents left me uneasy, as if he actually would stalk me.

In sessions, he asked me personal questions such as who was in my family and what I did when I was out of the office, with the aim of confirming his ideas about my personal life. When I declined to answer his questions or interpreted his longings, he became livid. His attitude was one of "How dare you not give me what I want!" He made it crystal clear: he did not want to be in analysis; he wanted a *real* relationship with me instead!

For weeks, Michael talked about my body explicitly, saying he wanted to be held on my lap and breast-fed, or that he wanted to have intercourse. He wished he could see me without clothes. He wondered what intercourse was like for me. He scrutinised my movements and supposed that I must need to use the bathroom because I moved my legs. Michael's remarks left me squirming internally, and I became self-conscious and felt pressured to stay motionless.

He asked questions about sex to watch my response, later guiltily admitting not only that he wanted the information, but also that he wanted to see what he could glean about my sexual life by voyeuristically watching my reactions to his questions. Michael's analysis later revealed that he experienced these conversations as an actual sexual exchange. As stated above, Segal (1981) referred to this style of thinking as *symbolic equation*, one in which a person experiences his thoughts as being identical to the thing or activity itself.

Michael responded to my comments to help clarify his own thoughts by playing "cat and mouse" with me, smiling sheepishly and flirtatiously, avoiding answering and instead turning questions back on me, so that I could see how it felt to be the one analysed. He hated the asymmetry of our relationship, that I was the analyst and he the patient, instead of our being two people attracted to each other who might develop a real-life romantic relationship.

In the countertransference, I was awash in feelings of being attacked by exciting seductions and demands for attention. Because of Michael's sensitivity to feeling rejected, feeling crushed even by my ending sessions, I felt powerless and in a quandary as to how to intervene so that Michael and I might get some thinking space, a transitional space to play with ideas and fantasies. I felt controlled by Michael. Within several weeks, I had a dream about him:

> I am walking from the waiting room into my office proper. Just inside the office door I see Michael. As I step into my office, he moves towards me. He appears much taller and broader than in real life. He comes closer to me and crosses into my body-space comfort zone. I tell him to stop and move back, but he doesn't. I feel and see his arms and legs undulating around me like an octopus suspended in water. It feels sexual and aggressive. I have faith and hope that he won't hurt me, but I am not certain of it. I wake up anxious and angry.

Michael had really gotten into me. I was disturbed by the dream and the case, and consulted a colleague. The dream allowed me to experience more consciously Michael's behaviour as aggressive and to see how invaded, threatened, and powerless I felt. I also understood that this was an unconscious transference communication through *projective identification* from Michael, that he was under attack by his old experiences of desperately wanting and needing his mother and, at the same time, feeling rejected by her. Fairbairn (1952) described these emotional states as experiences of the *need-exciting* and *need-rejecting internalised bad objects.*

Fairbairn (1952) theorised that infants are *object-seeking* from birth and that they seek a relationship with mother as a person towards whom to direct love, hatred, anxiety, and fear. When the infant has a painful experience with his mother, when she excites his desire for her excessively, or rejects him when he really needs her, the baby feels emotional pain and anger, which must be repressed into his unconscious. The memory trace of his painful experiences tied to the image and experience of the mother, forms the *internalised exciting* or *rejecting bad objects.* Because Michael was filled with these old experiences, these memory traces, this internal bad object set which he enacted towards me, he was powerless to move forward in his development.

The dream and consultation deepened my understanding of what was happening between us, so that I then was able to find my own position, my own psychological footing, to make an effective intervention with Michael. Neville Symington (1983) described moments when the analyst realises that she has been under the pressure to think and act in a certain, constricted way, brought about by the patient's desire to control the analyst, and communicated to the analyst by the patient's behaviours, thoughts, and tone of voice. The mechanism of asserting control over the analyst is by *projective identification* (Ogden, 1982, and others). Neville Symington (1983) saw the analyst's *realisation* of being under the patient's control and then mentally throwing off the oppression inside herself as an *act of freedom*, and named it the *x-phenomenon*. Once the analyst has had such a moment of *freedom* internally, the analyst can then take an independent stance or action *vis-à-vis* the patient. I describe several instances of the *x-phenomenon* below.

At the next session, when Michael began to make pointed remarks about my body, I told him that I had been giving a lot of thought to what he had been saying, and that his remarks felt "too personal." He was shocked, confused and hurt. He thought I had been enjoying this talk as much as he had. He was sad. He said that he did not want to hurt me, signifying early oscillations into the depressive state which I saw as a hopeful sign of growth. His remorse was blended with suffering from persecutory guilt, worried that he may have damaged me, or worried about what he might do to me, or what I might do to him. And lastly, he felt attacked, rejected, and angry over my bringing to his attention that his sexual comments, really vaguely disguised sexual advances, were unwanted. Over the next few sessions, Michael earnestly apologised several more times. He was suffering internally, from shame, from rejection by what felt to him like an admonishment from me and from the concern that he had hurt me. Then he became nearly silent. The tangled, dry, confusing, boring, obsessive ruminations vanished; there were no more questions about my personal life, nor comments about my body.

Retrospectively, I understand that the initial relative silence was Michael's way to protect me from further attack, to protect himself from acting out inappropriately and from being "attacked" by me in return. Nevertheless, it felt as though we now had a two-person relationship, that he was able to experience me as a separate, whole other person (a subjective other), instead of as an inanimate being or *part-object* towards whom he had directed his dry, obsessive ruminations and his sexual phantasies by speaking them. So, now there was a transitional space where we could share ideas, feelings and phantasy as a way to explore and understand his internal world.

Period of silence

Within a week, Michael became almost totally silent for four months. This followed the vignettes described above and several short absences when I had to be away. He had been very angry that I wouldn't tell him where I was going and what I was doing. He concluded that I must not love him, and in fact, must be trying to get away from him, thus leaving him feeling rejected. In the transference, I was shifting from his exciting and rejecting bad objects (Fairbairn, 1952) to a severely rejecting bad object. Michael reacted to my refusal to give him personal information by taking a day off from analysis himself, declining to tell me why, as a reason to "get even" with me and to "show" me what it felt like to be left and not know why.

Months of painful silence followed. We sat in sessions, facing each other only a few feet apart. I kept my mental focus on him for the most part, glanced at him occasionally, but did not stare. Occasionally, I asked him what he was thinking; he gave me glancing eye contact and either said nothing, or echoed back my question. He sat deathly still, sometimes dozing off into a light sleep. Other times, I looked up and was startled to find him intently staring at me. I oscillated between feeling helpless, frustrated, anxious and angry, and feeling maternal towards him. Sometimes I felt especially angry with him for wasting his parents' scarce financial resources and wasting my time. I kept silent myself during those times, but he noticed my frustration. I wondered if the silent period would ever end and if his analytic treatment would have to be aborted. I cringed at that thought, knowing how such an outcome would be a repetition, leaving him feeling dropped, rejected, unlovable, and as if he had killed off his loved and hated mother/analyst. I also didn't know how long I could bear the silence.

In consultation with my colleague, I decided to spend sessions with Michael crocheting an afghan. Choosing to do handwork occurs rarely and is generally discouraged, but it was necessary for me so as to bear Michael's deadening silence and so I would not have to prematurely terminate his treatment. It allowed me to fend off boredom and sleepiness, defences against my own anger and frustration and allowed me to be more peacefully present for him as we struggled together. This gave him an opportunity to use me as he needed, in a way that I could manage. It took the pressure off him to speak; we could spend our time "just being together", which he needed and craved.

The first day I began crocheting Michael asked, "Why are you doing that?!" It was as if the crocheting were a separate object that Michael felt in competition with, or a separate part of my self (my desire to feel alive) that enraged him. I explained that I needed to do something in order to stay more present for him. He was furious. His cheeks and neck flushed. Although he spoke softly, he said it was my responsibility to sit with his silence no matter what; that I should be completely at his disposal whether he spoke or not. Klein (1975) described the infant's and young child's phantasy of omnipotent control of the other as a manic defence against helplessness and loss. Michael related to me from that belief, as though he had the right to expect me to be available for him in just the way he wanted and to satisfy his needs. I realised how angry Michael was that I had taken an independent action which showed him that he didn't have control over me, and that I would go on living and being, regardless of what I came to experience as his trying to torture me with silence and emotional rejection, what he had experienced as a baby when his mother was absent and he felt abandoned. Although I believe Michael felt that I was abandoning him by the handwork, in reality the crocheting allowed me to provide to him my present, experiencing and thinking mind.

Several days later,

> I find myself thinking about the time in my early twenties, just after I was married. I had wanted a son who looked like my husband—a little boy with blond hair who would be about Michael's age now. I am feeling sad that I never gave birth to such a child. Then I notice Michael staring at me. He is sitting at the end of the sofa, his hand and forearm laying across a thick, rounded sofa pillow, as if it were mother's breast. Near the end of the session, Michael asks if I remember his birth date.

In the countertransference, Michael became the son I never had, and in the transference, he asks the mother/analyst if she remembers when he was born, perhaps even that he was born. This let me know that Michael had the experience of feeling as though he had not been kept consistently in his mother's mind. It linked up with his feeling frantic, tormented, and desperate during separations. It explained his death-like stillness during the silence, the baby, not crying or moving, but listening and waiting for mother's return, while at the same time seething with rage at having been left alone, terrified that his mother had forgotten him. I told Michael that I did remember his birth date. He appeared satisfied and relieved, a confirmation that he had not vanished from the mother's/analyst's mind.

The next day, Michael entered the office with a couple of magazines in hand, smiling sheepishly and teasingly. At first, I didn't know what he was up to. He sat down on the sofa, promptly opened the magazine, and pretended to read while I crocheted. I was amused and smiled. He smiled back. Several days later, the following happened:

> As I crochet, Michael lifts the magazine in front of his face so that I am blocked out. I am amused and impressed by his creativity, as if we are enacting a play. I say, "It feels like we are an old married couple, you the dad, reading the newspaper at the breakfast table, and I the mom, sewing." He smiles warmly. The afghan takes me back to happy memories of making baby blankets for my daughter and nephews. I had been feeling maternal towards Michael, keeping him safe, watching over him in my office. Now, I am thinking about him as a husband and dad. I ask what Michael is reading. He says he wants to see my afghan, in a tone of, "I'll show you mine if you show me yours." Then he motions with his outstretched arm to spread the afghan over the sofa. Michael has the phantasy of our snuggling under the blanket.

In the silence, we communicate about maternal–infant and male–female couples. I think of baby blankets and a married couple at the breakfast table. He thinks of a married couple under the afghan. There is a tension between us of not giving in without getting something. So, attempts at mutual seduction continue: I trying to seduce him into a more standard analytic process of verbalising his thoughts, and he trying to seduce me sexually.

Several weeks later, tired of sitting in silence and being confronted with Michael's "cat-and-mouse" tactics, accused of not trying to help him emerge from his silence, I began to "think out loud" in his presence about him. I say, "I can think about what you might be thinking or feeling, but there is really no way for me to know for sure. Sometimes I might be right, and sometimes I might be totally off base. The only way I can really know for sure is if you tell me." He looked at me quizzically. This was a new experience for him to see how I was thinking about him, myself, and both of us in relation to each other. My speaking in this way allowed Michael to see that I *was* thinking about him, *how* I was thinking about him, and *how* I thought about *his and our predicament* of the silence. I doubt that he had ever had the opportunity to hear another person think about him, nor do I think he had a conception that *another* would or could have thoughts about his own thoughts and feelings in her mind. I was showing him how I was relating to him intersubjectively; that is, I was showing him how I was thinking about and experiencing him inside myself as a separate self, a person who had his own internal thoughts and experiences. Intersubjectivity is a modern psychoanalytic concept originated by Stolorow et al. (1978) and elaborated by Benjamin (1988, 1990, and 1992), Stern (1985), Fonagy (1991), Ogden (1986, 1989, and 1994), Natterson (1991), and Natterson and Friedman (1995). These references were drawn from Aron (1996), who summarised these authors' contributions.

When a young person has the experience of the other thinking about him by trying to understand the workings of his mind, even when the therapist doesn't "get it right", the young person usually feels supported and understood because he sees that the other is interested in and motivated to understand him, *to Know him*. This usually soothes and reassures the young person, if not immediately, then over time, as the analysis progresses and the child builds up experience of being in the presence of the analyst who is trying to think about what he may be experiencing and is trying to understand. My telling Michael that I could better understand him if he told me what he was thinking freed Michael to begin to speak once again, explaining months later that he really did want to get better and had seen that he needed to speak to me to do so. He also revealed later that he began speaking because he had been feeling guilty about wasting his father's money.

Resolution of the erotic transference and countertransference neuroses

Ever since the session in the first year of analysis when I told Michael that I thought his comments were too personal, Michael had treated me with concern, even though he still had wishes and phantasies about having a personal relationship. Then, whenever these issues came up in the analysis, he phrased his concerns gently, in a non-penetrating way. It felt as if his comments were directed into the transitional space between us where they could be thought about, played with, named and understood, rather than shot into me like bullets. I was grateful for this shift. I no longer dreaded his sessions and had become quite fond of him.

Approximately one year later, Michael again raised the issue of how attached he felt and that he did not want to think of the day when he would have to say goodbye, a herald of termination. He still worried that I might end his treatment before he was ready. One day he gently told me that he still loved me and longed for that personal relationship. I thought I had responded to him appropriately by sharing my understanding of what he had said and was experiencing. Retrospectively, I now see that I was moved again by his re-expression of love, and that I also pulled back from my own stirred-up affectionate feelings, not wanting to get caught up in the countertransference neurosis once again. Whatever I said that day must have felt very impersonal to him, because at the next session, he was really angry. He said, "Yesterday I told you that I loved you, and you didn't seem to care. It seems that what I said didn't carry the meaning that I wanted it to..." On one level, but to a lesser degree than before, he wanted to engage me once again in the erotic transference-neurotic countertransference in a controlling way ("... it didn't carry the meaning that I wanted it to", meaning "It didn't have the effect on you that I had intended"), and was angry that I had emotionally distanced myself. On another level, he was longing for a real, personal response from me, and so the way I responded to him, in tone and by what I said, didn't carry the affection he longed for.

On the surface, he was angry about how I responded. In the countertransference, I experienced his hopelessness about ever having the close connection to a woman that he so desperately desired. I felt sad for him. I associated to my experience of observing infants, and how newborns communicate with and feel connected to their mothers through sensory modalities of sight, tone of voice, smell, taste, and especially skin-to-skin touching. Then, I was pulled to speak to Michael from a deeply personal place. I said, "Words limit you. Words of love and affection cannot carry the meaning that can be expressed through the body by actual touching and physical closeness. So, try as you may to tell me how you feel, the only complete way to express it would be through touch for which you deeply long and which we cannot have. We are separated by decades, roles, geography, and cultures. So, this is a huge loss for you." I was feeling a huge loss as well; it stirred my own sadness about lost youth, lost possibility, lost opportunity, and limited time.

Over the next week, I found myself thinking about Michael more, excitedly looking forward to his sessions. Then Michael said, "I'm thinking about wanting to start dating a girl in my church." I felt betrayed and blurted out in an embarrassing enactment, "Oh, Michael, you're breaking my heart!" Michael and I were both surprised by my outburst. Michael said, "Did you mean that?! Or are you teasing me?" Feeling it important to be truthful, I said, "We have spent a lot of time together. You have touched me by your gentleness, love and concern. Of course I have positive feelings for you." This intervention helped lessen Michael's eroticised feelings of longing, which he had temporarily transferred to me.

Over the next fortnight, I worked through my countertransference crush of affection for Michael, a projection of his love for me blended with the gratitude I felt to him for allowing me into his personal world and for all that he had taught me. For several more sessions, Michael questioned my feelings for him, then spoke again about dating. He reassured me, "Just because I start dating doesn't mean that I don't love you." Touched by his tender concern, my eyes glistened, and I held back tears; I felt gratified that he was able to mourn, hold a depressive state with respect to his affection for me, and feel ready and desiring to move forward in life to find a more suitable love object.

The meanings of Michael's silence

As his analysis progressed, numerous underlying dynamic determinants of Michael's silence became apparent. It developed following several of my brief absences and after he realised that I had experienced his questions and comments about sexuality as intrusive and attacking. Most importantly, Michael's silence occurred because he felt rebuked and rejected by me when I said his sexual comments felt "too personal." He withdrew out of anger towards me in reality and towards the mother/loved analyst in the transference. His silence protected him from internally attacking and psychically destroying the good object/mother/analyst whom he both loved and hated. The silence afforded a quiet, safe place for him to be in my presence as the longed-for mother/analyst and served as a powerful communication to me of what it was like for him to feel ignored, dropped and forgotten as a baby. Michael used his silence as a kind of game to try to control me. He liked to see if he could make me speak first, and when I did, he smiled victoriously. The game was motivated by his infantile wish to control (M. Klein, 1975) the comings and goings of his mother, perhaps a game he had used in phantasy when he truly could not get mother's attention and longed for her presence as a baby.

Michael felt abandoned between sessions, sometimes mentally collapsing on weekends, so that when I missed a day or two, he became severely distraught. Absences signified that I disliked him and was trying to get away. He sensed his excessive neediness, and feared that he would destroy me by draining me of my internal resources if I met his greedy needs. Lest he push me away further by these aggressive, needy attacks, perhaps to the point of truly abandoning him, he dampened down his demands by withdrawing into silence. So his silence protected him from the guilt of aggressive attacks on me and feared retribution by me, and protected me from his attacks in reality. In the silence, even though he didn't get everything he wanted, he still could sit with me and feel partially consoled.

The part of Michael that compelled him to sit in silence added to his anger, frustration, and longing for a stronger emotional connection to me, but these feelings were locked inside him; he was unable to express them or to tell me how he even more desperately needed to feel close to me and to feel that I cared about him. In her chapter on difficult to reach patients, Joseph (1975) described a split in the ego where a part of the patient wants to be cooperative and in relationship with the analyst, and another part jealously or enviously attacks the relationship or withholds part of the *true self* (Winnicott, 1960). Splitting off parts of his ego, characteristic of Michael's way of relating, had to be kept in mind and interpreted throughout his analysis.

By projective identification, Michael induced in me his feelings of helplessness, hopelessness, frustration, anxiety, and anger, so that I might understand him better. His silence signified his anger for not getting what he wanted, a personal relationship and complete access to details about my life. It powerfully communicated what it was like to not have access to the longed-for mother. This was a repetition of his experience in relation to me when I left him in the present and to his internalised mother in early childhood.

Thinking more consciously about the *octopus dream* allowed me to better appreciate Michael's aggression towards me and to appreciate my anxiety and anger towards him in response. Once I worked through these thoughts and feelings, they were detoxified and more manageable. Thus I was more able to work with Michael from a place of calmness and a sense of freedom, feeling much less under Michael's control. Once my negative countertransference feelings diminished, paradoxically I was drawn toward Michael and was able to enjoy his underlying charm and "play house", which we did in phantasy. Later this could be named, spoken about, and worked through in the analysis.

Michael's silence was also a resistance against the difficult analytic work:

> Sometimes I just want to give up. It looks so difficult. I don't want that much pain... I could make myself say everything that came to my mind, but I would be embarrassing myself in front of you. Anyway, why should I have to expose myself when you don't have to tell me what you are thinking?

Ultimately, Michael provided an intimate unconscious communication of playfulness, gentleness, tenderness and love. He tested me to see if I would stay or go. Could he use me ruthlessly, not be abandoned and still have a place inside my mind to help him understand himself?

On the first anniversary of the beginning of his analysis, Michael gave me a letter in which he highlighted how he had experienced his relationship with me, expressing his love and aggression fully, concluding "... to the best and the worst woman in the world. I have been mad enough to chop you into pieces and loved you enough to put you back together again."

Space does not allow for a more comprehensive discussion of the many other aspects of Michael's analysis. Suffice it to say that Michael's depression, obsessive compulsive symptoms and aggression greatly diminished. He became more empathically aware of the impact of his behaviours on others much of the time. He moved into a line of artistic work which he enjoys and has developed a lovely, intimate relationship with a girl whom he intends to marry.

Using the analyst's dream and countertransference to help Michael

It took time to open myself more fully to my countertransference experiences and dream about Michael, and to become more aware of how these would be useful in my work with him. I was bombarded by Michael's aggression and was not able to process all that I was feeling. I had distanced myself from him as a self-protection and as a way not to act out against him, and threaten his analysis. Finally, when I was overloaded with not-identified, not-symbolised, not-thought-about experiences, my dream and awake phantasies fostered a way to begin to understand what was beginning to feel like a therapeutic impasse; what I was up against with Michael in reality, and with my own internal challenges to do the analytic work.

In his chapter "The countertransference neurosis", Racker (1968, pp. 107–108) elaborates the many ways in which an analyst's dynamics can be activated by the patient's transference. The analytic work then is blocked until the analyst becomes aware of what is going on inside himself and works through it. In this case, the consultation with my colleague about the *octopus dream* allowed me to understand more fully Michael's anger and how he was trying to control me. My internal conflict about feeling I must absorb Michael's aggression because he was so vulnerable to feeling rejected then greatly diminished. I found an internal mental space to think about what Michael presented to me.

The mental space I refer to is what Bion (1962) called *containment*, the function of which is to unconsciously take in raw, unidentified, un-thought-about experiences, referred to as *beta elements*, and to apply a process of unconscious thought to them, termed *alpha function*, so that the experiences or feelings are symbolised with words, can be named, at least partially understood, and thereby detoxified. The idea for and the act of crocheting was possible only after I experienced the internal mental freedom to take an independent stance as described by Neville Symington (1983). The crocheting, my independent gesture, let Michael know that I would not be paralysed by his silence and desire to control and this allowed me to be more available, rather than pulling away emotionally from Michael as protection.

In considering the idea of bringing in handwork, I had the phantasy that I would be like a grandmother sitting in a rocking chair in the evening, sewing by candlelight or on a front porch at dusk, available to children and grandchildren, to hear their dreams, stories, questions and problems. With Michael, moving my hands kept me alert, but not having to concentrate on the repetitive stitch of the handwork allowed me to relax into my own *reverie* to see where my phantasies would take me as a way to better understand what was going on emotionally with Michael. The concept of *reverie* was first explicated by Bion (1962), and elaborated by Ogden (2005). In *This Art of Psychoanalysis*, Ogden states:

> ... in the notion of reverie all of the meanderings of the psychesoma of the analyst including the most quotidian, unobtrusive, thoughts and feelings, ruminations and daydreams, bodily sensations ... usually feel utterly unrelated to what the patient is saying or doing at that moment. Reveries are not the product of the psychesoma of the analyst alone but of the combined unconscious of patient and analyst.
>
> (2005, p. 124)

So, I allowed my mind to wander; sometimes I had thoughts and phantasies about Michael, as I indicated in the case material; and other times my mind wandered to aspects of my own life. Even when my thoughts did not seem to be related directly to Michael, upon analysing my countertransference associations, I made connections to and found relevant meaning in Michael's situation which aided my understanding of him.

My crocheting kept me at a bit of a mental distance from Michael so that I was not intrusive. It kept me occupied while he used me consciously and unconsciously. The change in my mood alone must have felt lighter to Michael too, reassuring him that he could be present with me without torturing me. Because I was relaxed and enjoying being present with him, he relaxed too. This is what Winnicott (1958) described about the need and achievement of being alone in the presence of the other. Much of what Michael needed from me early in his analysis was simply my presence and having access to my mind to help repair or mitigate the effects of his *basic fault* (Balint, 1958). Now, instead of dreading Michael's silent, humourless, or aggressive sessions, I looked forward to them, as now the sessions felt more restful and creative for us both.

Though initially it left him angry, my decision to take the independent action of bringing in the handwork reassured both of us that he would not destroy me or his analysis. Furthermore, the crocheting of three strands of yarn at once symbolised my attempts to understand him, to take the strands of his conflicts and communications, and to weave them into formed ideas to share with him; so the afghan became a symbol of our work together, co-creating his analysis, which allowed for insight and lessening of his suffering.

The importance of truth in analysis

Bion's ideas about the human mind, its development, and motivations departed from those of Freud (1920) who believed that the *pleasure principle* and avoidance of pain were the basis of human motivation. In contrast, Bion (1965) believed that humans sought truth, even if it were painful, so that emotional growth could be achieved. He said that "... healthy mental growth seems to depend on truth as the living organism depends on food. If it is lacking or deficient the personality deteriorates" (p. 38).

Bion likened deprivation of truth on the personality as analogous to physical starvation on the body (1962). If the young person is willing and able to handle truths about himself, and others, he will experience pain and frustration, but he will also be freed to grow emotionally.

In Michael's analysis, the most useful and powerful *interventions* were those in which I was able to state a truth about a real aspect of our relationship simply, straightforwardly, absent love and hate. Here I use the word truth as a distilled and rather non-contaminated nor complex feeling, close to a pure feeling. I say *interventions*, not interpretations, because a verbal interpretation is not as powerful in helping the individual make links and understand himself as what I describe in Michael's analysis. Interpretations, many times, are logical, verbal explanations for what the analyst understands about the young person, unfortunately some of the time conveying little feeling of the analyst and consisting of logical, factual links instead of affective links. *Intervention*, on the other hand, implies a tone, a lived experience between analyst and patient, more as two people interacting, rather than as one, the analyst, making statements about the other's, the patient's, associations.

Those *interventions* in Michael's analysis were when I told him that:

1. "I could not understand his obsessive-compulsive ruminations that led (appeared to lead) nowhere." Because he so desperately needed me in close relationship to him, he had to begin to communicate in a meaningful way, which then established me as a subjective other in his mind. The requirement moved him out of a kind of autistic-infantile style of relating in which he held the unconscious belief that I should be able to understand him no matter what he said or how he said it, a belief or perhaps even position that he need not make sense. I don't know how he came to have this style of communicating, but believe that it resulted from too little "back and forth" interchanges with his parents when he was very young; and perhaps his parents did not make an effort to understand *him* enough in his preverbal years.
2. "His remarks about my body were too personal." In this situation as well, he hadn't seemed to consciously understand how he was affecting me. He was treating me as a part-object. By telling him that his pointed sexual remarks were affecting me, the phrase "too personal", implying that he was getting too close and that I was uncomfortable and felt under attack, left him furious and feeling rejected. However, my statement constituted an independent act of freedom on my part (Neville Symington, 1983) which "forced" him to see me as a separate, whole other, one who had her own set of feelings, thoughts, and wishes. Over time, he had the experience of my not rejecting him because of his treatment of me, and I believe that opened him up to experience empathy, compassion, and caring for me, the other/mother/analyst, a move from the paranoid-schizoid to the depressive state of mind.
3. During his silence, when he was reading a magazine and I was crocheting, in the midst of a shared phantasy, I said that "I experienced us as a married couple." This pleased him. It acknowledged not just his phantasy and longings, but mine too, and gave him the experience of being understood. He succeeded in communicating to me through his transference and my countertransference. He even indirectly expressed his wish that we snuggle together under the afghan. Although I didn't take that phantasy up with him directly, by my action of only holding the afghan up for him to see, I communicated a boundary that would not be crossed.

Consciously he understood that the boundary wouldn't be crossed, and unconsciously he was not disappointed because what he really wanted and needed was for his longing to be close to me physically, to be recognised and understood, and not acted upon. All of this reinforced the notion that he was safe in being with me while consciously and unconsciously sharing his wishes and longings.

4. During the silent period, I told him that "I could not really *know* for sure what he was thinking. I could only guess, and would not always be accurate." Again, this reinforced that I was a subjective other with a separate mind and that I didn't have magical powers to "read" his mind; and most importantly, that I was curious, wanted to *Know* him. There is probably no other aspect of human relationship that is more motivating for living than to have someone who wants to *Know* you.
5. After he had gently told me that he loved me, and I hadn't responded in kind, the next session he returned angry. I responded, "Words limit you. Words of love and affection cannot carry the meaning that can be expressed through the body by actual touching and physical closeness which you long for, but which we cannot have." My thoughts and feelings arose out of what he had communicated to me in the transference, blended with my own experiences of what I understood about the communication of love between two people, both personally and through my experiences in observing infants with their mothers. Again, by finishing the comment with "which you long for, but which we cannot have" did not anger him, because I understood and spoke to his infantile and adult sexual longings, that is, I acknowledged a truth. My statement again reassured him that nothing would happen between us and he was safe to continue to explore the area of his pain and aggression, his *basic fault.*
6. When he told me that he was thinking about dating, I responded too quickly and from my unconscious, "Oh, Michael! You're breaking my heart!" (said with a bit of sarcasm). Immediately I was horrified that I had blurted out in such a potentially hurtful and embarrassing way. Did this express what I truly felt? Rethinking it now as I write, I realise it was both true and not true. It was true in the sense that I was deeply attached to him, truly felt affection for him, felt like I would lose him not only as a patient - his analysis would come to an end - but that I would lose him to another woman! My jealousy and competition were stirred, and energised me to blurt out without thinking. But his declaration of wanting to date was a gift to me as well, in that he was eager to move forward in life and grow; his analysis was showing a positive result.

However, I also made the remark with a bit of a mocking tone. What was that all about? Well, I suppose it reflected my anger at him for wanting to turn to another woman, but also, I believe it signaled to him that I would not collapse if he sought a more appropriate love interest. My unconscious attitude was one of "Go ahead and date. I will be fine." My tone was tinged with jealousy and anger, but also, I believe provided relief for Michael because it signaled that I really would be fine, and that he should feel free to pursue his intended girlfriend. My remark caught him off guard. He responded, "Did you mean that?! Or were you teasing me?!" I *Knew* that what I had said was mainly true. A super-ego-ish part of me felt guilty about my counter-transference feelings and for having made the inappropriate remark, so I felt compelled to tell him that I was teasing him. How hurtful that would have been, and how much rage it would have engendered if I had told him that I didn't mean it. I was just kidding! This was a moment when it was absolutely imperative for me to be *Truthful* in a way that was neither seductive nor hateful, but rather as a statement of fact in acknowledging a *Truth*. I said, "We have spent a lot of time together. You have touched me by your gentleness and concern. Of course, I have positive feelings for you." I didn't gush out with the countertransference crush of affection I had experienced earlier in his analysis, which was not the truth, but was merely a processing of a set of transference and countertransference feelings. I simply stated my fondness for him as a fact. Michael seemed satisfied with that, and gratified that I told him the *Truth*. Had I not told him the truth about my feelings, there would have been no basis for trust between us, and ultimately the analysis would have failed or would have had to be extended perhaps months in order to get this sorted out and his feelings worked through.

The six interventions elaborated above have several characteristics in common: each one is a *Truthful* statement of how I felt in relation to, and in relationship with Michael. The statements arose inside me, but also inside our relationship, out of Michael's desire to communicate with me and my wishing to understand and *Know* him, even during those instances when Michael was silent, refusing to speak. These *interventions*, these statements to Michael, did *not* arise in me separate from him, as an objective observer commenting on his mind and conflicts. They did not even arise out of what I might call my assessment of my own countertransference responses to Michael. Rather, my statements (*interventions*) were based in genuine feelings that arose out of our shared, lived experiences together.

I am not proposing here that only these kinds of more personal statements (*interventions*) are helpful to a young person. In fact, this type of intervention should be used judiciously, fairly rarely, and requires that the analyst be very clear in her own self what she is feeling in the countertransference. More traditional and classical interpretations serve other legitimate needs patients have to understand themselves and their history so that they can move forward in life. However, in Michael's case, I found the *interventions* I made, which arose from my genuine feelings in relationship to him, were extremely powerful in softening and removing defences, and in ameliorating the torment associated with Michael's *basic fault*.

Struggling with and strengthening one's capacity to work in the countertransference

Working analytically in the countertransference is challenging; the analyst suffers the pain of uncomfortable thoughts and feelings, just as the young person does, and sometimes is caught off guard with *beta elements* that she cannot *contain* and *symbolise* immediately. Perhaps it becomes easier over time, as one gets more experience with being confronted with the *not-yet-symbolised* and with disturbing countertransference feelings. There are several ways to enhance one's skill in working with young adults where these powerful feelings are evoked: by one's own analysis; by dreaming and paying attention to daytime phantasies as a way to understand and analytically make use of one's countertransferences; and by studying what others have said about the use of countertransference.

I also have found these skills were strengthened in my training at the International Psychotherapy Institute in Chevy Chase, Maryland, where we learn together using the Group Affective Model (GAM) as developed by Jill and David Scharff (2000). Finally, another powerful learning experience is to do infant observation and to learn together in a seminar group where observations are read, discussed, and worked through experientially (D. Scharff, 2005). The observer role requires that the student not interact with the baby or mother, nor give advice, but only observe and take in what she sees, hears, smells, and otherwise senses, which then powerfully concentrates the countertransference for understanding.

Conclusion

In this chapter, I have given a brief overview of some of the theory and technique in the analyses of silent individuals. I then presented the case of a late adolescent boy who developed an eroticised transference and became silent for approximately four months. Utilising information gained from paying close attention to countertransference thoughts, dreams, and feelings, a technique of working with the patient was put forward which involved a kind of direct honesty with the patient about what I was thinking and feeling in relation to him. I labeled this as an *intervention* to distinguish it from what is traditionally called an *interpretation.*

I processed these thoughts and feelings by dreaming, thinking and in consultation, so that love and hate were metabolised, and what was presented to the patient was, from my perspective, a statement of *Truth.* These *Truths* were far more powerful in assisting the patient resolve his symptoms and to grow emotionally, compared to *interpretations* which in many cases are statements of facts and historical connections. I emphasised the use of and working through the countertransference before making such interventions; the importance of not acting out love or hate towards the patient; and to working with the young person directly about *Truths* derived from the transference/countertransference experience. I finished with recommendations about how we as therapists and analysts can enhance our training to use the countertransference more effectively in treating our patients, young and old.

Acknowledgements

I wish to thank David Scharff for thinking with me about Michael over several years and for providing encouragement and insight. I am grateful to Stanley Tsigounis for reviewing an early draft of this chapter and directing my attention to other authors whose ideas were useful in understanding and then elaborating this case. Jill Scharff, M.D., Sheila Hill, LCSW and Richard Simons, M.D. also reviewed drafts and provided comments which stimulated additional thought and understanding. I am indebted especially to Jeanne Magagna, from whom I have learned so much about infants and young children, and who invited me to write up this case, and then provided invaluable guidance and encouragement through the process. Finally, I wish to thank my husband, daughter, extended family, and good friends who were patient with my absences during work on this chapter.

CHAPTER FOURTEEN

A journey through family therapy with a non-speaking child

Cynthia Rousso

> There are accents in the eye which are not on the tongue, and more tales come from pale lips than can enter an ear. It is both the grandeur and the pain of the remoter moods that they avoid the pathway of sound.
>
> —Thomas Hardy (2003, p. 175)

The retreat from thinking and / or speaking on the part of the referred young person should not be seen as a deterrent to family therapy but instead should be understood as a powerful reflection of family dynamics. The aim of family therapy is to understand communication within the family, not just verbal communication, but communication through gestures, facial expressions, play, actions and interactions. In this chapter, I will look at the way the style of not-speaking in the patient was generalised and ultimately understood as a family style of communication. I will use clinical examples from family therapy with a family in which the fifteen-year-old son, Barry, had stopped talking, walking, eating, drinking, or caring for himself. It is my hope that some of the ways of understanding this family and their structure, patterns, and boundaries may be applicable to many families with a non-speaking child.

Meeting the referred young person

Each morning there was an inpatient psychiatric unit community meeting in which staff and young people would individually share their views on what was helpful and unhelpful from the previous day. I arrived at the meeting on a Thursday morning to discover that a new young person, Barry, aged 15, had arrived. He did not speak or walk or hold his own head up. He was fed with a naso-gastric tube and I was told he spent virtually all his time on the unit crying or sleeping. He had a tremor along his right side and if his hands were not restrained in some way he would continually pinch himself.

I was totally unprepared for my response to Barry. As the meeting commenced and the young people began to speak, Barry's constant moaning turned into louder crying. It was a distressing, disturbing cry which evoked so much feeling in me that I almost felt like I could not make it through the meeting. I was concerned about how the other young people would react and found it difficult to concentrate myself. The cry was similar to that of an infant who desperately needed attention. I found the cry so disturbing and distracting that by the end of the 30 minute meeting, I felt like crying myself.

Given my strong countertransference reaction it was with some trepidation that I consented to work with Barry and his family. My initial feeling was one of inadequacy and worry. How could I possibly help his family if Barry felt unable to speak? Many professionals had been involved with Barry previously and making a diagnosis was difficult, for there were a variety of complicated symptoms creating numerous diagnostic possibilities including brain tumor, anorexia nervosa, post-traumatic stress disorder, chronic fatigue syndrome and most recently, pervasive refusal disorder. While many physical investigations were carried out, no physical cause for Barry's illness had been identified. Was I meeting in Barry someone who had turned his back on the trauma of life and who could not be reached? This was certainly how it appeared, but then I wondered about his moaning and I had a sense that somewhere he still held onto a belief that someone would be able to hear and understand his plight.

This led to my thinking about the role of family therapy. Is there more to communication than speech? Why did I feel that what I usually offered families was not enough in this case? Was Barry's crying any different to an "acting out" of another young person? Waddell (2002) describes how the function of acting out is to reduce internal conflict through the replacement of thought with action. Barry's not-speaking and his crying were actions and I felt that if I could understand the internal conflict, perhaps the actions could be transformed into thoughts about the intolerable feelings and internal conflicts that led to these actions. Clearly, I did not know why Barry was presenting in this way but tolerating "not understanding" when with a particular family is the position from which each family therapist initially begins.

Beginning treatment

> Innocence always calls mutely for protection …
>
> (Graham Greene, 2004, p. 29)

Role of the therapist

As a family therapist I have often mused about my theoretical identity. While initially drawn to the systems approaches of Ackerman, Satir and Minuchin, I then became interested in the psychoanalytic ideas of Freud, Klein, and Bion, among others. The former traditionally worked with families and the latter with individuals, although the families-in-the-child's mind and the family in the external world were often involved to some extent. Bion's *Experience in Groups* (1961) describes small group behaviour and the basic defence mechanisms preventing thinking from taking place. Bion describes the defence mechanisms such as pairing between siblings, fleeing from the subject, arguing to avoid psychic pain, and getting excited about sexual subjects to avoid thinking about some other serious matters. All of which are certainly relevant to family group functioning. I raise this because it will be evident from the work below that I have at times interspersed psychoanalytic thinking with systemic practice. I believe that concepts arising from different arenas of thinking can be used creatively and effectively in the consulting room.

Working with a new family means taking on the role of both observer and participant. As an observer I can listen to the stories of the family and reflect on their strengths and difficulties. As a participant, I want to open up space for the not-yet-said. I want to create a place for symptoms to be understood and emotions to be held, considered and given meaning. Box (1994a) describes the family therapy session as a "space for thinking" (p. 3). This space to think is predicated on a belief that the way individual family members experience themselves is intricately related to the internal state of other family members. Thus, troubled aspects of the family group can find expression in individual members and troubled aspects of the individual can find expression in the family group.

The "space to think" is facilitated by careful attention to myself, the session and the family. While I could not offer them a magic cure for an illness which had ravaged Barry's family for over two years, I could offer a setting with a frame of regularity and continuity. They were desperate for "knowns" about their son and I offered a known space, time and setting in which we could engage in a joint effort of understanding. Winnicott (1953) describes the "good-enough mother" who meets the emotional needs of her infant in part by helping her child process the distressing feelings. In a similar way, the family therapist is seeking to understand and process the communications of all family members, whatever form those communications may take. The family therapy session can serve as a model of thinking together, helping the parents to be available to their children on an emotional level.

Assessment

Inevitably the family entering the consulting room for the first time brings with it a wealth of feelings. Often, the whole prospect of a family meeting suggests to family members that they are to blame in some way for the young person's difficulties. I try to meet these feelings with an atmosphere of empathy, warmth and attunement. By attunement, I mean being where the family is, attempting to understand things from their perspective. Each family member is going through a developmental process, and the family therapy is aimed at improving family functioning and promoting growth and differentiation. I explain that we are not here to blame but to understand the way in which the family fosters but also hinders the development of individual members. I note that a child's feeling, for instance sadness, might be evidence of sadness in the entire family group.

I started, as I usually do in families, thinking about how Barry's difficulties might provide clues to family difficulties. Barry's not-speaking indicated that family communication styles would be crucial to understanding his difficulties. He was also extremely helpless, dependent, and vulnerable. Rice (1969) describes the primary task of a family with an adolescent as helping him to individuate and form a sense of identity, which enables him to eventually live separately from his family. Given Barry's apparent retreat from life outside the family I was particularly interested in each family member's capacity for functioning outside the family context. Also I wondered: How did each family member respond to differences and disagreements? How tolerant were individual family members to different ideas and feelings? Were they able to be supportive to the child's developmental achievements or were they often more attentive to the child's difficulties?

While there are numerous family assessment tools and extensive guidelines for helping practitioners make a biopsychosocial assessment of families, my goal in the first few family therapy sessions is to get to know the family and begin to understand their family structure, patterns and boundaries. I was particularly conscious with Barry's family of striking a balance between gentle inquiry and leaving room for spontaneous thoughts and communication. Given Barry's "no-entry" stance, (Williams, 1997b), I did not feel that it would be initially helpful to question him, apart from asking if he could give an eye or hand signal to show his agreement or disagreement to what was being said.

First, in engaging with the family, I am interested in helping the family tell their version of the problems as they see them and describe how they are each affected by the problems they perceive. As the family members describe their perceptions of difficulties, I would also suggest they try to answer the question: "What do you think your brother would say to your ideas now if he joined in the conversation?" I would also use some circular questioning to develop thoughts about other members of the family. For example, I might ask, "What do you think your mother understands about your brother when he is crying like that?".

Fairly early on, I find constructing a genogram to be a useful way of obtaining important information about the family's strengths to cope with this difficult situation, and I would also involve all family members in describing various aspects of the members in the extended family. The shared task of completing the genogram emphasises a focus on the entire family, not just the referred young person. It highlights the importance of a transgenerational picture which allows the family to view their development as part of a transgenerational narrative. I am interested in how the parents' lives reflect their upbringing and in what way their experience with their own parents has impacted on their relationships with their own children. The genogram is often a non-threatening way for the family to get a sense of the therapist's interest in their reflections, relationships and culture. Simple observations such as who is seated next to whom, who appears engaged, who appears reluctant, often prove useful in illustrating alliances and splits to family members and therapist.

As I met Barry's family for the first time, his parents entered together and a nurse followed pushing Barry in a wheelchair. Immediately noticeable was the fact that when his parents were present Barry stopped his often perpetual crying. Barry was not speaking, but this formed a very clear, strong communication and it confirmed that Barry certainly had a sense of what was going on around him. His behaviour also highlighted his attachment to his parents and his desperate desire to be in their presence. Bowlby (1969) looked at attachment behaviour and suggested that in potentially dangerous situations children seek proximity to their attachment figures. Barry's obvious perception of the treatment centre as dangerous led me to wonder about his internal vulnerability, his feelings of danger within himself and his family. Barry did not make eye contact and stared at his lap. It was as if he felt so overwhelmed that he had to stay locked up within himself. While the treatment team was saying "You need to be here for inpatient treatment", his behaviour was indicating that the separation from his family was traumatic, and his not-speaking suggested there were things that were unspeakable or being silenced by the family's style of interacting.

History

The parents began to describe the history of the illness as well as the history of their family. Barry was the third child in a family of five children. He had two older sisters, Jaimie, nineteen, and Lucy, sixteen, and two younger brothers, Paul, aged eight, and Peter, aged six. Mother worked as a physiotherapist in the local hospital, and father was working as a car salesman. The family lived near the centre of Birmingham.

Mother and father were a close couple who liked to keep to themselves. They married when they were twenty and twenty-eight, respectively. Mother's five pregnancies were planned by both of them despite busy working lives and tight finances. They talked about how, when he was twelve, Barry had a large number of physical complaints like colds and headaches. This coincided with the onset of puberty, which was earlier than that of his closest peers. He was noted for his academic achievements and was integrated within a group of school friends.

Then, when he was fourteen, Barry's health began to deteriorate, meaning he spent a fair amount of time at home, followed by his actively refusing to attend school or participate in home tuition. When his parents had to work, Barry was sleeping as much as fifteen hours a day, eating very little, and feeling unable to walk more than a few steps. While medical professionals were involved at this point, there was a misconception that Barry was stubborn and did not want to get better. Doctors were considering diagnostic possibilities such as chronic fatigue syndrome. Numerous behavioural plans were put into place to encourage Barry to eat, walk, talk, and do things for himself. When a tremor started on Barry's right side, he was reluctant to go into hospital. There was a realization that Barry, feeling helplessly overwhelmed, was pervasively retreating from life and he was admitted to an outpatient unit for a year.

As the parents described Barry's life during the first meeting, I was looking at the demeanour of the family members. I was particularly interested in the process of their communication, not simply the content. I was thinking about how they related to me and to each other. Interestingly, as the parents spoke, Barry began to slide down in his wheelchair until he was almost falling out of it. Father would move behind him to sit him up, only to have him slip down again. This led the parents to speculate on how we might address this problem. Perhaps a strap could be placed between his legs, or we could move him to the large bean bag he used at other times of day; maybe the chair was too slippery. There was an immediate inclination to find a practical solution. I wanted to draw the parents' attention away from the external practicalities and to focus on the meaning of Barry's behaviour. What was Barry feeling as I spoke with his parents? What was he trying to communicate through his way of existing, his body postures and his facial expressions? At first, the parents found it hard to think in this way. In their view, that *was* the problem, he was not communicating. His slipping was out of his control, he could not help himself, and his muscles were not working.

I acknowledged that, although it was true that he was not speaking, he was telling them things through his non-verbal expressions of feeling. I wondered if there were ways to understand Barry's behaviour. I also noted that when we discussed Barry's illness, he did not slip down in his chair, but as the conversation turned to other siblings and life at home, Barry provided a distraction that required that we stop the conversation and readjust his position on the wheelchair before we could carry on. In my view, he was saying, "You need to think about me, I can't bear it if you focus on anyone else. Barry usually reacted quite strongly when he felt he was slipping out of the conversation, out of sight. His actions felt like a request that his own feelings needed to be "thought about".

As I thought about this, I wondered about his internal psychic structure. Did Barry leave school rather than face the anxiety school expectations raised? Was conflict-avoidance a family style? Barry was clearly reluctant to come to the inpatient unit. I wondered if this was similar to his reluctance to go to school. Was there a fear of what might happen if he engaged with me, the treatment team, his peers, his school? As Barry averted his gaze and stared at his lap, I was reminded of some of Melanie Klein's (1952) views on transference; she said, "... the child is bound to deal with his conflicts and anxieties re-experienced towards the analyst by the same methods he used in the past. That is to say, he turns away from the analyst as he attempted to turn away from his primal objects" (M. Klein, 1952, p. 55).

Understanding Barry's total transference (Joseph, 1985) to the institution meant understanding how threatening treatment would be to Barry and his family. In the therapy sessions, I came to represent the entire persecuting team, for being on the unit created the sense that the multidisciplinary team would gradually deal with situations in a manner that was different from Barry and his family. A feeling of differences can create anxiety in the family. Being in the therapeutic milieu of the unit involved opening up, examining, and understanding the anxiety-provoking symptoms with which Barry was presenting. That meant that I needed to provide a way of being emotionally present and trustworthy for Barry and his family. My being trustworthy would permit Barry to feel sufficiently secure to relinquish his current way of coping, which was to look down, close up, and cut off from those around him.

Family myths and scripts

As I gradually became acquainted with Barry's family, a number of family myths and scripts revealed themselves. Byng-Hall (1995, p. 4) defines family scripts as the "family's shared expectations of how family roles are to be performed within various contexts". One of the family's beliefs was that a "black cloud" hung over the family. The "black cloud" myth was regularly called upon to explain family difficulties such as father's drinking, sibling rivalry, and difficulties with mother's employers. This myth meant family members followed a particular script in which they felt they could no longer bear taking responsibility for their actions, leaving them feeling less guilty about difficulties but at the same time impotent and powerless. This brings to mind Seligman's (1975) theory of "learned helplessness" in which a person gives up when they do not have the power to change their situation. I wondered if Barry was communicating that he had given up, for he felt helpless to manage the turmoil that he was having to bear inside himself and perhaps outside himself as well.

If the family didn't blame the "black cloud", they often enacted a family script involving projecting parts of the self into other family members, thus leaving each family member holding an assigned and unchangeable role. For example, some members represented loving feelings, others sad feelings, and others angry feelings. Barry's feelings were consistently portrayed as warm and loving, even when his actions suggested otherwise. When he fell down in his wheelchair, hit or pinched his leg, or dropped items, the family had a hard time connecting these actions to Barry's feelings of anger or aggression about feeling left out. In the family's mind, Barry's oldest sister, Jaimie, nineteen, was all things malevolent. As she became the focus of all family negativity, her actions of separating herself from the family and going travelling through Europe, while developmentally appropriate, was conceived as hostile and negative. Mother was perceived as strong and capable, like her own mother, while father was perceived as passive and weak, like his mother.

In other words, family anxieties motivated family members to place people into metaphorical boxes in an effort to make feelings more manageable. Box (1994b) describes the process of projective identification in which unconsciously shared elements which cannot be tolerated by one or more of the family members are reallocated inside or outside the family in an attempt to avoid the experience of internal conflict. This type of splitting undermines the family's ability to understand the people behind the labels and makes it difficult for them to think reflectively and comprehensively about their actions.

Zinner and Shapiro (1972) use the term *delineation* to describe a process in which parental behaviour conveys to a child the parent's image of him. If this behaviour is determined more by the parent's defensive needs than by the realistic attributes of the child, this is termed a *defensive delineation*. Projective identification is a particular form of defensive delineation and functions as a bridge between individual family members and the family group. The excerpt below is taken from the first family session, as parents were describing Barry.

> Mother said, "Barry has always been a homebody. From the moment he started school, it was obvious he wanted to stay at home and be with us. We always did such fun things together: doing woodwork activities, painting the house, playing music together. Honestly, sometimes we did more interesting things at home than they ever did at school."
>
> Father said, "Barry said he had friends at school but he never invited them home. It was as if he kept home and school very separate."
>
> Mother said, "There was even a time just after he started secondary when he would come home from school, hide his uniform so he wouldn't have to look at it and then shower.

> I thought it was a type of passing phase. We're all kind of like that. We prefer being together at home to doing anything else!"
>
> Father remarked, "I didn't think it was too strange as I often felt like showering after work. Wash off the stress of the day and then start fresh at home."

The interaction exemplifies mother's delineation of her son, Barry, aged fifteen, as someone who prefers home to all else, and father's delineation that he understands Barry because they are very similar. While at the time it was not clear if parental descriptions reflected Barry's realistic attributes or not, as I began to know the family better it seemed that parents needed to view Barry in this way to defend against their own anxiety about themselves as a "happy couple". The outside world, filled with the parents' hostile projections, became viewed as very harsh while home life became viewed by the family as a type of sanctuary.

As Barry entered adolescence and his ego capacities matured, he was particularly vulnerable to the conflicting delineations he was getting from his parents. On the one hand, they were suggesting it was Barry's task to grow up, achieve, and join in activities his peers. On the other hand, the family group was characterised by disturbances if individual family members showed independent functioning in social life outside the family. The family script that suggested, "We are a fun-loving family who just want to be together all the time" left little room for family members to share feelings that were not "happy", or to separate and individuate from the family as they matured. Another latent message was that family members should keep uncomfortable, worrying, sad, or difficult feelings to themselves. Worries seemed unbearable to the family's psychic structure. Barry's not-speaking suggested that he had taken this message to the extreme.

Family life cycle stage

Like many organisms, families fear change and seek to maintain a state of homeostasis to ward off the anxieties that accompany change and separation from the family. There is a fear about the fact that ultimately the couple will be left alone without the children. Unaware of the way earlier coping mechanisms are no longer useful, the family seeks to uphold their usual organisation and function, even when the results of this *status quo* appear to be dysfunctional. The "happy family", and the "we just want to have fun together as a family", leave little room for the various life-cycle developmental changes necessary for family members. Mother described her joy when the children were under eleven years old. She painted a warm picture of a big, happy family who only needed each other for fun. Eight years later, with two older daughters, a fifteen-year-old son in hospital, and eight-year-old and six-year-old sons, the needs of individual family members were dramatically different.

Carter and McGoldrick (1989) describe adolescence as marking "a new definition of the children within the family and of the parents' roles in relation to their children". With the exception of infancy, adolescence is the most radical of all developmental periods. Waddell (2002) describes the demanding psychic agenda for adolescents as they strive to find the capacity to manage separation, loss, choice, and independence. While chronologically Barry was an adolescent, as his illness progressed, he became more and more like an infant requiring constant physical and psychological care. This required family members to stay home with him while keeping him a primary focus of their attention.

Adolescence requires that the young person rely on the internalisation of parental capacities. In primary school, which was geographically close to the family home, Barry managed fine. The difficulties arose when he required inner resilience to function independently from his family within his peer group and face the psychosexual developmental changes brought on by adolescence. He felt unable to negotiate his wish to be top both socially and academically, and experienced intense rivalry with his peers in his large secondary school, far from the family home. He had liked a girl at school who was not interested in him, so that fostered further difficulties for him. I wondered if these external difficulties might have exacerbated his fears around internal conflict, within himself and within the family home.

Identifying strengths in the family

Barry's family had many strengths. His parents seemed clearly committed to understanding what was causing distress within the family. His siblings seemed interested in one another and, with the exception of Barry, could verbally describe their views of family difficulties. Family members seemed to enjoy being together and had a history of happy memories. Barry getting better was a purportedly shared goal for all family members, and this became the rallying point for change.

Identifying difficulties in the family

During the assessment process, the family was very clear that their biggest difficulty was Barry's illness. In my view, this illness was a symptom of other family difficulties that included: an inability to acknowledge feelings and the use of primitive defence mechanisms in lieu of internal containment of anxieties. By leaving feelings unacknowledged, Barry and his family were following the family scripts, leaving no room for family members to differentiate themselves from one another, develop, achieve, and leave home with the family's blessing.

Internal containment of emotions

The concept of containment originates in Bion's (1962) model of container/contained. This model describes the process whereby the mother tolerates the infant's frustrations as well as her own and then relays them back to him in a way that is bearable. As the infant repeatedly experiences this, he is able to learn from this experience and develop an internal container that will help him self-modulate and mentalize. Without this adequate internal container, it is difficult to be open to new experience without being disrupted by it. In the excerpt below, we see mother move to silence father's expressions of his internal state. Father's expressions challenge her definitions of herself and the family, and she does not feel emotionally capable of either understanding or containing father's worries. They feel too much for her. In fact, father generally uses talking of nothing too important or conflictual as a form of self-protection.

Father: I sometimes find it difficult to speak to my wife because she is a different kind of person than me. When she is faced with difficulties, she springs into action and starts finding practical solutions. I tend to shut down and feel overwhelmed. I don't like to talk to my wife because I know my worries will be too much of a burden to her.

Mother: I find it very difficult to know what to do or say to him. I don't want to make him feel worse, but I am very worried myself. I thought we were a team. Maybe we need to go to marriage guidance because obviously he cannot talk to me. We're not really partners. He is closer to Barry and I am closer to Lucy.

Father: This is why I don't share worries because she always takes everything as a statement that SHE is doing something wrong. Just because I'm worried doesn't mean it is her fault!

Mother: What I'm worried about is that you won't speak to me about things and then you'll have a nervous breakdown like your mother did. I thought now that you were successful at work you would feel better about things.

Becoming aware of the family's defence mechanisms

Primitive defence mechanisms are essentially defences employed against anxiety. Klein (1946) gave them special significance as characterising the earliest phases of development, and she included the defenses of projection, splitting, and denial. Barry and his family, because of their lack of inner psychological capacities to bear anxiety, resorted to the use of primitive defence mechanisms when confronted with new or unfamiliar experiences such as a change in school, employment, or life cycle. They were able to disown the undesirable aspects of themselves through splitting and projecting them into external figures or institutions. This allowed them to maintain a sense of goodness about themselves while putting their "badness" into external objects. It is easier for the family to imagine, through the use of splitting and projecting in others, that they are warm and loving and the outside world is harsh and dangerous.

Parallels between the difficulties of the presenting child and those of family members

Barry's emotional conflicts diminished his capacity to think in the same way that unacknowledged family conflicts diminished the thinking and coping mechanisms of individual members. For example, his parents felt paralysed and unable to speak directly with the older sister, Jaimie, when she began to be promiscuous. They feared speaking might make matters worse. Again, the parents seemed drawn to a belief that not talking about difficult issues was the optimal mode of operating.

Middle phase of treatment

Having started to get to know the family through the assessment process, the middle phase of treatment is an opportunity to work on the identified difficulties. Barry appeared to be unable to achieve the adolescent tasks of separation/individuation because of his unconscious fear about the anxiety these normal developmental changes would produce in the family group.

His anxiety appeared to come from his unconscious assumptions that the parents could not survive as a couple if he made this move away from the family, as it would threaten the family script of perpetually wanting to be together all of the time. This left Barry feeling helpless, dependent, and vulnerable. These were feelings both parents, because of their own difficult histories, defended against in their own current lives. Similarly, the symptom of "not-talking" is a symptom not just of Barry's illness, but of the entire family with respect to communicating about conflict, change, and differentiation. Barry's use of his body to express emotional distress and his somatising when stressed was similar to something father did when his work unhappiness was expressed through migraines, which gradually declined during the family therapy.

Role of the therapist

The role of the therapist in the middle phase of treatment is to provide a containing function, to help the family develop a narrative of their experience, and to continue to provide a safe place for the acknowledgement of feelings and anxieties. Like the parent who helps the infant to contain his unbearable feelings, so the therapist helps the family to modify rather than evade their own frustrations or anxieties. As I met with Barry and his family week after week, with little tangible change in Barry, the family began to doubt that Barry would ever recover. I also wondered to myself if our work would be sufficient for Barry to leave the inpatient unit. My role was to tolerate and hold this doubt until it could be relayed back to the family in a form that I felt could be assimilated by them. I was reassured by the team, who said it was necessary to be patient; stable inner development would necessitate slow external signs of progress for a boy as ill as Barry. During this phase of treatment, I feel it is especially important to leave room for all feelings to surface. This begins the moment the family enter the consulting room while I wait for them to begin. The example below from our ninth session shows the way I attempt to understand the latent content of the family's communication.

Mother: How was your weekend? Wasn't it gorgeous? We just loved walking through the countryside near the inpatient unit and hearing the sheep. Were you in town or did you go away?

Therapist: You have a lot of questions about what I did this weekend. I guess you are wondering what I am like as a person, what I enjoy. I wonder do you also have questions about what's happening in here, about our work together?

Mother: We actually like coming here to see you. We think you're great. And we're so grateful!

Father: Yes, we really appreciate everything everyone is doing for Barry.

Therapist: I wonder if there are other feelings? Feelings of the sort that perhaps aren't so positive.

Mother: What do you mean? No, I always say if you don't have a positive attitude positive things won't happen.

Father: We like coming here but we hated going to the other family therapy team at home.

Mother: Yeah, they made us feel like crap parents. They were just looking for things that are wrong.

Here, we see the parents' efforts to split the treatment into the good/inpatient, bad/home team. They are not speaking about difficult emotional experiences residing inside the family, and they attribute difficulties to external sources, mainly because they must defend against an anxiety that they are to blame because they have such an ill son. There is a pervasive mutism about states of mind, but a plethora of evidence about outside trouble-makers. As I think about the total transference, I sense they feel it is extremely dangerous to share anything other than positive feelings about our work, and they are afraid of looking at difficulties, for if any were mentioned, they could feel criticised and feel like bad parents.

Not speaking as a style of interaction

It became clear quite quickly that not speaking about important matters was the entire family's style of interaction. It is not that they did not speak, for their words filled the therapy session, it was that they did not have the emotional capacity to create a narrative regarding their internal difficulties. By ignoring or covering up difficulties through endless positively toned conversation or externalising difficulties, the family maintained a sense of security obtained from their "happy family" belief. For example, father's migraines and drinking were attributed to problems with his colleague at work. The six-year-old son's bedwetting and nightmares were attributed to Barry's illness. Barry's illness was attributed to physical causes. Not speaking about their internal feelings, particularly negative and painful ones, and externalising the difficulties, was the family members' only way of protecting themselves and others from anxiety.

Barry's non-speaking stance mirrored the family style in many ways. While family members spoke so much it was often hard for me to find a space in which I could speak at all, they had a great deal of anxiety about seeing and speaking to one another truthfully and directly about conflictual issues. What started to become apparent was that in the family process of communication, all conflict was denied, because they lacked the sturdy, resilient mentalizing structure to bear conflict. In the absence of this containing inner psychic structure, the family members' unwanted parts were projected, leaving various members very stuck in their positions.

As we started to work together, I provided a thoughtful presence to bear anxiety, helped the family become aware of what they were doing, and illustrated other ways of dealing with anxiety through my style of interacting with them. Family members were able to acknowledge their feelings to themselves and eventually to other family members. This led to the capacity to think and creatively resolve some of the difficulties. Internalising the beginnings of another way to deal with difficulties, by thinking about them, also led to lessening of the family's somatic difficulties such as bedwetting, nightmares, migraines, and father's drinking too much. Prior to this, family members would defend against thinking about a deeper issue by moving away, talking over another person, or even leaving the room.

In the excerpt below, we initially see Barry try to distract his older sister, Lucy, sixteen, from speaking about her feelings:

Lucy: [Older, sixteen-year-old sister.] This unit does not seem as stifling and depressing as it did the first time I was here. The atmosphere seems happier and Barry seems much better. He is making eye contact and he seems interested in our conversations.

Therapist: It must have been very difficult at home with Barry being so ill.

Lucy: I guess I would have to say I felt sad, angry, and also a bit guilty. Initially, I didn't really understand Barry's illness and I felt really cross when he refused to do what the doctors were saying. You know, advice about eating, sleeping, and walking. I also felt like my parents were only thinking about him and spending money on him and this left me feeling really jealous.

Therapist: I wonder what happened to your feelings? Did they just disappear?

Barry begins to cry loudly, bringing everyone's attention to him.

Mother: I think perhaps Barry also feels guilty about his illness.

Lucy: He was so different before. Do you remember? He was so funny and loud and his laugh. It felt really contagious.

Mother: We all loved it!

Lucy: I thought when Barry was fifteen, he'd be able to come with me with my boyfriend and we'd be able to do all kinds of things together - go to coffee shops, to parties. It's like this illness has robbed us of all that.

Again, Barry begins to cry loudly and deliberately.

Mother: I think Barry also feels disappointed that he cannot do these things.

Barry stops crying and appears to listen.

Mother: The thing is that Barry is quite good at showing his feelings, even if he does not explicitly describe them.

Lucy: All in all, I would say we're a fun family.

As the session continues, we see mother literally and figuratively turn away from reflections she perceives as critical:

Therapist: I wonder if there are other feelings too?

Father: I don't think there is often room for the other feelings.

Lucy: I like to do things in my own time and not be nagged.

Mother: I can usually tell when something is bothering Lucy, but she will often deny it if I say anything.

Lucy: That's because I'm an independent kind of person. Barry is more of a homebody. Mum and I place great importance on getting things done but Dad, he likes to dwell on the difficulties more. I'm not a sympathetic person like my mother.

Father: I think your mother has a certain amount of sympathy and that's that.

Mother: I feel like I am sympathetic.

Father: You are, but you're not afraid to give someone a kick up the backside if necessary.

Mother's face fell and she turned away from the family and looked out of the window.

Father began to fidget in his chair.

Not-speaking

Therapist: Let's stop for a moment. What's happening here?

No one speaks.

Therapist: Let's look at what has happened between you. Father was expressing his opinion, mother got offended, and father appeared to shut down. Let's see if we can replay it in slow motion.

Father: I don't feel like I was saying anything negative, but I think my wife took it that way.

Mother: I basically hold this family together and it's like a slap in the face to be called unsympathetic.

Father: I feel like I shouldn't say anything anymore because my wife will take it the wrong way.

Lucy: It's true, mother always feels criticised by even the tiniest comment.

Mother: I guess in a way I don't want to be overly sympathetic. Not like my brother who would take a week off work for a small sniffle. My mother just "doesn't do illness" which is why she just keeps moving along at eighty.

Lucy: I think my parents are different because my father moves quickly to get everything done while my mother cooks but lets my father do the household chores. He likes jogging and keeping fit instead.

Discovering shared family symptoms

As the treatment continued, a complicated web began to surface. It seemed Barry's illness could be seen as a type of marital-distance-regulator (Byng-Hall, 1980). By focusing on Barry, father could avoid his own difficulties with drink. As father became unhappy with his colleague, mother became frustrated by her own status at work, where she felt she should be head of the department. She felt she needed to count on her own career and not on the father's. At this point, Barry was over-achieving in school and the parents became focused on his academic success and musical talents. This initially took the focus off father's lack of interest in his work as a car salesman. As Barry started to become unwell, father became his primary carer, thus avoiding his own difficulties with drink as well as the loneliness in his marriage. The parents began to focus on the issues in their children rather than in each other. I hoped that by giving meaning to some of the symptoms, the family could deal with their difficulties in more direct ways.

Re-establishing boundaries between parents and children

Barry's family was not functioning with clear, hierarchical boundaries. There was a boundary continuum with enmeshment at one end and disengagement on the other; family members often found themselves on either end but not in the middle with clear and flexible boundaries that would enable family members to carry out age-appropriate tasks. For example, at different times both mother and father appeared to be aligned with Barry, as opposed to aligned with each other. This left one spouse feeling left out and disengaged. This disengagement allowed the parents to ignore difficulties between themselves, and use the child to bring a type of stability to their relationship. Often in the session, mother would cradle Barry as if he were an infant. Because Barry could not hold his head up, it almost looked as if he was breastfeeding. I was reminded of the fathers who describe feeling left out when a new baby is born and mother is preoccupied with his care. In the same way, mother's attention to Barry left father and Barry's two older sisters and two younger brothers feeling alienated and possibly envious. It also raised the question for Barry: can I get the care that I need in health or do I have to be ill to beckon my mother to support me?

Creating a narrative of the family's experience

I think families find it helpful to periodically hear a retelling of their story based on what we are learning in the sessions. I do this by describing what I'm seeing in the family. For example, I described the way Barry might have felt overwhelmed by his feelings, the way it seemed he felt compelled to shut down rather than to try to work through the internal conflicts he might have been feeling. I wondered if the family atmosphere might not have been conducive to sharing feelings that were not "pleasant". I described Steiner's (1993) concept of "psychic retreat". The way someone might unconsciously try to reduce internal conflicts and avoid anxiety by not allowing thinking to take place. Steiner calls this an "omnipotent attack on thinking". Waddell (2002) suggests, "When psychic pain is felt to be uncontained internally and therefore unbearable, there may be a withdrawal into a closed-off state of petrified emotional isolation. The baby, or child, may retreat to a deeply withdrawn, or borderline state, unable to allow anything in" (p. 48). I wondered if perhaps Barry had taken on certain unconsciously assigned "pleasant" character traits early on in his life.

The high-achieving, conflict-avoidant, daddy's favourite was a special role within the family that helped Barry differentiate himself from his two older sisters and two young brothers. These labels might not have been realistic responses to Barry's characteristics but instead parental definitions of Barry that the parents transmitted unconsciously and then Barry took up. Zinner and Shapiro (1972) term this "defensive delineation", as it describes defensive aspects of parental personality functioning that serve to hold the child in fixed roles throughout development. It was less emotionally difficult for the parents to have an especially cheerful and pleasant, achieving son: this helped them to defend against some of their own anxieties around father's lack of interest in his work and their difficulty in facing marital and familial conflicts.

As Barry's cognitive ego capacities matured, he was particularly vulnerable to the mixed and conflicting delineations or projections he was getting from his parents. Instead of confronting his parents with the reality of who he was, Barry used protective mechanisms that were at first viewed as necessary but were later redundant. Shutting down and remaining tied to his parents was the only option that would preserve the family *status quo*, and this became his habitual way of facing life. This narrative challenged the family's belief that they lived under a "black cloud". Describing the family narrative helped the family to understand the importance of acknowledging their feelings and opened the door to looking at the inner worlds of all family members.

Containment of the parental couple

As the work progressed, one of my primary functions became containing the parental couple. This meant helping the parents to care for their children by sharing their respective concerns, supporting one another to make joint decisions, and by discovering ways of enabling their children to move forward developmentally. The parents needed help bearing the uncertainty about Barry's recovery. They felt impatient that he was not regaining his health more quickly, and they feared he would give up on life.

Hinshelwood (1999) describes containment as feeling the dread and still retaining emotional balance. It was easy to become overwhelmed with the dread that Barry could die if out of hospital. This family felt helpless and, in order to provide a containing function, it was imperative that I retain my own sense of efficacy. My goal was to tolerate the doubt and anxiety that the family was presenting, hold the feelings, and relay them back to the family in a digestible form.

But how does the therapist get a sense for what needs to be contained? The answer in one word is countertransference. Countertransference is the way the therapist's feelings serve as an indicator of the state of mind of the family. By my experiencing some of the family projections in the consulting room, these projections can be made available for understanding. These projections are unsaid and consequently remain uncompromised by Barry's non-speaking stance. Joseph (1985) describes the way in which our own feelings of countertransference help us to understand young peoples' experiences that are often beyond the use of words.

Transference is the way the child or family unconsciously views the therapist and the treatment setting through a lens of past experiences, attitudes, and feelings. Klein (1952) emphasised the re-enactment nature of transference. She viewed it as the child's way of enacting, in the "here and now", conflicts from the internal world. As I began to both highlight and demystify the family myths, I became more aware of the states of mind that were shared by various family members.

Peter Fonagy (2002) uses the term "mentalization" to describe the ability to understand oneself and others by imagining what they are thinking and feeling. In essence, mentalization is largely communication outside of language (Frith & Wolpert, 2004). It's a way of seeing ourselves from outside and others from inside. In the session, I am seeking to understand the meaning behind the family interactions and the communication behind their words. For Barry and his family, it did not seem that the collective family's mind was able to create a narrative regarding the feelings, thoughts, ideas, and aspirations of its members. Instead, feelings, worries, desires, and deeper needs were perceived as frightening or too challenging to the parents and other family members, and for this reason many family members learned to keep these experiences to themselves.

Initially, Barry's family found it difficult to focus on what was going on internally, in their own minds. Instead, they focused a great deal on practical tasks and physical problems, which consumed their attention. Fonagy describes this as a sort of mind-blindness. Family members were very drawn to stereotypical ideas of each other's thoughts and feelings as they sought to understand one another. My goal was to help the family keep their minds in mind.

Helping family members identify and own their individual feelings and anxieties

Helping the family to understand their anxiety and acknowledge a wider range of feelings, enabled them to integrate different aspects of themselves which had been previously split off and projected into other family members. Barry became the embodiment of father's unstated desire to shut down. Through my helping father to own his own feelings, Barry did not have to act them out on his behalf. Similarly, mother had a fear that any internal difficulties raised by father would lead to mental illness. Mother feared that her husband was too depressed to support himself and the family. By helping the family to understand their anxiety and acknowledge a wider range of feelings, they were able to acknowledge different parts of themselves and not resort to primitive defences of splitting and projection to manage their anxiety.

Signs of development

Barry functioning as a defence against feelings

As Barry's parents started to become aware of their patterns of relating, their communication began to change. Father started to show mother some of his vulnerability, and mother did not ask him to be different, but instead accepted what he was saying. The first time father spoke openly of his depression was the first time Barry mouthed a word in the session. As father shared that he felt his unhappiness at work was actually an unhappiness in himself, something he had never properly acknowledged, Barry looked at mother and mouthed, "I'm dying". It was as if he needed to take the focus off father, to make sure that he came between the parental couple. This pattern was repeated again in the following session as father spoke about moving from selling cars to a less demanding job as a carpenter. Upon hearing this, Barry mouthed "never going home" to mother. Barry's verbal reaction to progress in the family was a clear indication that he was making progress despite his protests to the contrary.

As treatment continued, Barry's family moved from being primarily focused on the practical and physical to showing signs of emotional attunement. They began to address issues using emotional language and thinking. Initially, they presented as persecuted and guilty, with a strong fear of being criticised by me and a fear of confrontation between themselves. As we worked together, the family became much more emotionally engaged. This engagement was evident in a number of ways including their ability to show me things besides "a perfect family": the parents responding appropriately to the children's concerns and each other's feelings, the young brothers beginning to be able to speak more openly about feeling anxious and left out by the parents' continual caregiving of Barry, and family members starting to identify their feelings instead of pushing them away. As the parental sub-system functioned more hierarchically, there was less of a need for siblings to be triangulated into the parental relationship. As family members became more capable of holding and containing feelings within their internal worlds, there was less of a need to project out the parts of themselves they found uncomfortable.

In the eleventh session, mother shared a dream she had following a session in which different family roles were explored. In that session, as father uncharacteristically began to express his opinion, mother became offended and father immediately stopped talking. As we discussed the interaction, father described feeling that mother always took things the wrong way, while mother described how she always felt criticised by father. Mother described her dream as follows:

> I am a young girl, maybe twelve or thirteen, and I'm walking along the street. It is a nice day and I feel quite happy. Suddenly, a policeman comes up and arrests me. I know I did not do anything wrong, but either I don't tell him that or he doesn't believe me. I go to prison, even though I'm not guilty.

I linked the dream to family functioning in that as mother is becoming more aware of her projections, she feels quite guilty. As we explored some of the unconscious assumptions behind mother's conscious statements such as "I'm the furthest thing from overbearing" or "There are no problems in our family", the defensive delineations seemed to be: conflict is dangerous, independent action is something to be afraid of, and acceptance in the family is conditional upon fitting into the happy family scenario.

As the boundaries in Barry's family became more flexible, family members became more capable of carrying out age-appropriate tasks. Father started to realise his conflict with his colleague in the car-selling business was actually a cover for a deeper unhappiness within himself. Mother became open to hearing about this unhappiness and did not assume it was connected with the state of their marriage. The family became less focused on external difficulties and more focused on internal thoughts, feelings, needs, and desires. Barry was able to internalise a secure attachment figure who held his feelings and gave them meaning in an empathic way. This meant that he did not need to continually cry in the absence of his parents from the unit. Barry went from only bearing weight in the presence of his parents, to allowing staff members to transfer him from his wheelchair to the sofa. When Barry was not speaking at all, I would sometimes say something like, "Tell me if I am getting this wrong, but I have noticed that you get restless and begin to cry whenever the family stops thinking about you." At times, I also would ask Barry to blink or move a finger if he shared some of the difficult feelings that another sibling had. As the family symptom of not-speaking about negative feelings was broken, Barry began to break his not-speaking stance. He went from mouthing words to whispering them. By the twelfth session, he was saying things like, "home now" and "home forever when?". As his family became more robust, so did Barry. He went from a young person who had given up to a young person with a goal: to "go home".

In one session about three months into our work together, the following interaction took place:

Father: I feel like Barry is more ready than ever to get well and go home.

Mother: Me too. It seems like something inside him is beginning to change.

Barry: As his parents speak, Barry begins to cry and shake his head vigorously, covering his ears with his hands.

Mother: I think he is hearing voices telling him not to get better.

Father: It seems as if when we talk about going home, we know it's something Barry wants, but it almost seems painful, like there is something in his mind that wants to stop his progress.

Barry stops crying and makes direct eye contact, making me wonder if he was feeling father was right.

The parents immediately move into making a hypothesis. I can imagine a few months earlier their attributing his crying and holding his ears to an ear infection or a headache. As they are able to understand Barry, so he is able to quell his sobs and show us he is really listening.

Ending phase

> We all long to share our feelings with *another* being.
>
> George Eliot (1997, p. 120)

> His heart lived in no cherished secrets of its own, but in feelings which it longed to share with all the world.
>
> George Eliot (1997, p. 120)

Role of the therapist

While we have been examining the family development throughout our work together, it may also be useful to comment on my development as a therapist during this process. The most difficult aspect of the work was being able to bear the family's unspoken, projected feelings. This was complicated by the family's virtual non-stop flow of spoken words. The pull of the family desire for concrete physical progress in Barry was often difficult to resist, and I had to stop myself at times from championing what appeared to be a flight to health and stay with the frustrating, impatient, anxiety-producing feelings.

Indicators of therapeutic progress

The ending phase of therapy is precipitated by concrete progress as well as a feeling that the family can manage with family therapy and individual therapy for Barry in an outpatient setting. As Barry's family made progress, he gradually began to access his mind, his voice, and his body, as seen in an excerpt from session twelve below:

Barry: Home forever when?
Mother: We want you home as soon as possible but not until you are well.
Barry: Now
Father: We're all really looking forward to your visit home this weekend.
Mother: I feel slightly concerned that it will be difficult to get Barry to come back to the unit.
Father: I think we have made it very clear that Barry may not come back home until he can eat and manage to walk at home. We don't know exactly what happened, but we do know that whatever it was, Barry could not speak about it and none of us could understand what he was experiencing when he retreated from life. Until he can,

well until we all can speak more about what we are feeling, I don't think he can get or stay healthy.

Barry begins to sob loudly.

Mother: Shh, Shh. She says this as she comforts Barry with her arm around him.

Therapist: I think Barry doesn't want to be quiet. He wants us to know he is impatient and unhappy. The more he can show us his feelings, the more we can help him.

Mother: Barry's got a surprise for you.

Barry is slightly grinning as he takes one of mother's hands in his hand, stands up tentatively, and walks hesitantly out of the session! This is the first time he has walked in the inpatient unit.

Here, we see the way the parents are thinking together about Barry's needs. Father makes the link between Barry's progress and the family's ability to think about him. Barry uses his voice more in this session and is quite proud that he is beginning to gain control over his physical body. At certain points, his progress appeared to be so rapid I feared I was witnessing a flight to health. I was conscious that an abrupt loss of his psychic retreat would increase his anxiety, and all members of the treatment team tried to adopt a "when you are ready" stance. Progress was noted but not highlighted so that anxiety around health could be minimised.

Soon after this session, Barry had a visit home. When the parents returned to the centre, they described all the progress he had made, including dressing himself, using cutlery, and speaking, using a wider range of words. They both felt a lot of pressure from Barry to keep him home. I suggested that the healthy part of Barry was having to remain firm under pressure from the problematic parts of himself - the voices and the fear that he could only get his needs met by remaining ill. I supported the parents to model remaining firm by acknowledging his struggle but not giving in to it.

Seven months after our initial session, Barry was given a discharge date by the multidisciplinary team. To his dismay, the date was eight weeks in advance. Once he started making progress towards talking, walking, and eating, he did not want to slow down - the opposite side of the rapid slide downwards he had taken previously. While he was desperate to leave sooner, we felt it was imperative that he and his family take the time to solidify the changes they had made. As we entered the final phases of treatment, it was interesting to think about the progress Barry had made. This progress was particularly evident in the few minutes I would spend with Barry alone after his family left each week. At first, like an infant, he would only cry to express his distress and anger. Gradually, he moved from somatising feelings, to speaking a few words like "go home now", to being able to think about his feelings. One day, Barry screamed, "No, come back" as his parents left. I sat quietly next to him, and Barry began to describe his fear that his parents would not return, that they would carry on without him and life would be easier for them. Barry had a feeling that led to a thought which he then expressed without fear of negatively impacting those around him.

In our nine months together, Barry's family changed considerably. By the ending phase of the work, there were a number of different aspects of family functioning that had improved, including: the couple working together, the family able to entertain different points of view, the children engaged in age-appropriate developmental tasks, the children turning to their parents with difficulties, the family being able to bear direct confrontations, the family taking risks in the session, and the family identifying and holding on to feelings without pushing them away. I will now illustrate each of these changes in more detail.

Couple working together and being able to entertain different points of view

Couples who work together can support each other without feeling that independent opinions are threatening. The excerpt below from session two shows father's reluctance to disagree with mother openly:

Father: We have tickets to *The Magic Flute* in Birmingham next week and I'm not sure if we should go or not. We bought the tickets before Barry was home and it would mean missing our family therapy session next week.
Mother: I feel like the routine is just getting established and it might be detrimental to Barry to disrupt things so early.
Father: You're right. We'll come here.

By session nineteen, father felt more comfortable holding his own point of view:

Mother: I think my husband should join Alcoholics Anonymous to help sort out his drinking in relation to his depression. His difficulties aren't really about work, but more about internal things and our relationship.
Father: I don't agree. I have sought help in Alcoholics Anonymous before and I did not find it that helpful. We have had almost nine months of therapy and I think I've come a long way. I want to continue thinking about things the way we've been doing here. I'm not ready to say good-bye here and then just start right away in an Alcoholics Anonymous group.

Initially, the parents would sometimes turn to one of the children to support their position. While this triangle might have stabilised the couple in the short term, in the long term it was unhealthy for both children and parents. By the ending phase, both parents were able to accept the idea that different people can hold different views and it does not mean that someone must change.

Indicators of progress

Children engaged in age-appropriate developmental tasks

Initially, Barry's sixteen-year-old sister, Lucy, very much felt that she needed to support her parents and would choose to miss school to accompany them on a journey to the inpatient centre. This made it difficult for her to establish good peer relationships, and her teachers began to complain of her difficulty in keeping up with the class. As the parents became a support for one another, Lucy was able to attend school and feel confident that her parents could manage without her. Similarly, Jaimie the oldest daughter, aged nineteen, had returned home from her travels and was finding it difficult to embark on a life of work. As we worked together, the family became less threatened by her independence and more supportive to Jaimie in her attempts to find a job and permanently live away from home. As the parents were able to support one another, so their children were able to turn their attention to age-appropriate developmental tasks.

Children turning to their parents for help with their difficulties

When children feel their parents cannot bear their difficulties, it can leave them feeling anxious and burdened with no choice but to act them out or bury them as Barry had. When the oldest daughter, Jaimie, aged nineteen, had become promiscuous, the parents felt angry and worried. As the parents became more robust, more problems could be brought to them. For example, Jaimie was able to discuss how she was frightened of her sexual identity, but wanted to have a husband and a family. She could talk with her parents now, for she did not feel that her parents would collapse under the pressure. Children need to feel they can be contained by their parents. As Barry's parents built up their capacity for mentalization, they could more easily offer a sense of containment to their children.

Family able to bear direct confrontation

As previously discussed, not speaking was Barry's family's style of communication. If someone was upset, they would often take on a non-speaking position or attempt to build a concealed coalition behind the back of the offending family member. As the family improved their communication, they became able to say directly, "That upset me"; "I don't like it when you do that"; "I disagree with you". After nearly seven months of treatment, Barry went away for weekend leave. The parents wanted to keep him at home for three nights, but the treatment team felt two nights was more appropriate. Instead of making an excuse and keeping Barry at home, the parents said directly that, while they greatly respected and were grateful for the work of the team, they did not feel they could return in the time allotted and would have to take an extra night. This would have been unheard of earlier on because so much of their aggression was externalised and projected into the external unit, leaving it feeling hostile rather than thoughtful to them. As they began to own some of their aggression, they could bear to face conflict with the unit, which was quite a distance away from their family home in Birmingham.

Family taking risks in the session

As the family felt more secure in the sessions they began to take more risks. As we looked at family interactions, family members became more and more comfortable trying out different ways of reacting and interacting within the consulting room. For example, Lucy, aged sixteen, knew how badly Barry wanted to go home permanently. While she wanted to support his desire, she was also aware of the risks he might take, for he was still so unwell. She spoke to Barry directly about her concerns, including the way Barry would sit and stare blankly with his tongue slightly protruding; the way it took him a long time to make a decision in a shop, even about simple things; the way it seemed difficult for him to interact with outsiders like shopkeepers.

Family identifying and holding on to feelings without pushing them away

It is the parents' capacity to bear and think about emotion that allows the children to elicit parental responses and receive the emotional support and understanding they require to move through to the next developmental phase. Pushing away difficult or conflictual feelings is a protection for the parents and an indication of their fragile capacity to bear intense emotion. What starts as a couple's style then becomes a family style.

If a family member became upset in the sessions, another member would often say, "Shh, shh". The message was, "keep your pain to yourself, we can't handle it". In the family therapy sessions, we practised, somewhat artificially at first, staying with the feeling, thinking about it, and trying to explain it to others. For example, when Barry's youngest brother Jonathan, aged six, started crying in the twentieth session, we sat quietly until he was able to say what was upsetting him. No one tried to tell him that he "shouldn't feel that way" or attempted to make him feel better. By listening respectfully and trying to understand, family members began to get a sense that all feelings were worth sharing. As the family internalised some of my capacity to bear and think about feelings, they too started to hold feelings, bear their weight, and think about them.

Conclusion

> You cannot acquire experience by making experiments. You cannot create experience. You must undergo it.
>
> A. Camus (1963, p. 5)

Camus was clear that we cannot create experience through making experiments, but rather must *undergo* experience. This was true for Barry's family.

Troubled aspects of Barry's family group found expression through his severe illness which included not talking, walking, or eating. As Barry became a container for the family's split-off projections, his development was severely hindered, and he became unable to maintain his thinking self, moving instead to a state of emotional isolation. Britton (1989) suggests that "curiosity spells disaster when illusion reigns supreme". In other words, initially Barry saw any attempts to explore his isolation as extremely dangerous, a disaster. His primary defence in avoiding the curiosity of family, friends, and later professionals was increasingly to move away from the external world and into an emotional cocoon protecting him from the difficulties around him. His continuous cries perhaps also represented the family's unexpressed sadness hidden under the "happy family" façade. He and his family defended against curiosity with the illusion or family script that suggested "there are no problems here".

It was as if Barry and his family had turned a blind eye to various difficulties because of their own fragility. The children did so because they did not feel they could turn to their parents. Partly because of their own lack of containing internal parents with whom they could identify, the parents turned a blind eye to their own role in influencing their son's inability to think about his feelings and develop satisfactorily. While Barry epitomised this regression to not thinking, most of the family experienced a breakdown of symbolic communication through words. Instead, their bodies began to communicate their feelings: father had migraines, mother had frequent colds, the oldest daughter became promiscuous, and the youngest siblings had nightmares, with one child regressing to bedwetting again. The oldest daughter, Jaimie, aged nineteen, did not present with any physical complaints, but she studied dance, so perhaps she was able to use her body to express her feelings.

It was as if, for Barry, the weight of his feelings became too much - too much to hold his head up, to talk, to walk, to eat. It was only as Barry's feelings were thought about by the family, and they were able to understand his non-verbal expressions of feeling, that he was able to regain the use of his mind and subsequently his body so that he could walk again. The transformation of family dynamics from expressing themselves in very primitive ways to communicating with words that provided thought around feelings was integral to Barry's recovery.

Barry's family group is characterised by a disturbance over the independent functioning of individual members. Through an examination of various excerpts from the sessions, we can infer that a number of unconscious assumptions were operating, including: 1) independent thinking and actions are threatening and should be discouraged; 2) differences between family members are attacks; and 3) independent behaviour contains a threat of separation and alienation. Initially, family members seemed to feel they must choose between two equally unsatisfactory options: the first was the loss of individuation and differentiation by suppressing their independent function; the second was anxiety and alienation through independent behaviour and separation. These distressing choices overwhelmed Barry in particular, but were stunting the development of all family members.

Through my active working relationship with the family, we were able to look at the family splits so that the underlying anxiety could be stated and understood. Family members were able to acknowledge their projections and take responsibility for them. The sense of containment that the family felt in the therapy sessions helped them to develop their own internal containing capacities. As the parents were able to contain the needy and dependent aspects of each other, the children found it easier to introject the parents' mentalizing capacities.

Through the work with Barry and his family, I have tried to show the impact of family group dynamics on the psychological development of a young person who initially did not talk, walk, or eat. I have explored the importance of shared unconscious assumptions and their impact on family group behaviour as well as subjective experience. I have also tried to illustrate the way projective identification can serve as a bridge between the family group and individual members, often leading to fixed role allocation for some or all of the family. Anxiety has been an important part of this exploration, as it is the threat of increasing parental anxiety or alienation from the parents that determines the collusion of children with parental projections. Given that projective identification occurs in all families, it is natural to wonder why in Barry's family it had such a devastating effect. I propose that the impact on a specific family member has to do with at least three things: 1) the contents of the projection; 2) the intensity of the parental defences; and 3) the parents' difficulty in integrating their vulnerable feelings and experiencing themselves as separate from their children.

As the family found their collective voice, so Barry found his mind and his own individual voice. Parents began to function much more hierarchically as parents with clear but flexible boundaries in relation to their children. Family life-cycle developmental changes began to be seen as an addition to family life as opposed to being perceived as a threat. Work with Barry and his family continued on an outpatient basis, with a different treatment team, for two years following Barry's going home. This ongoing work was essential to solidify the changes the family had begun to make. Barry was subsequently able to successfully attend university, where he studied Classics.

During Barry's last day at the centre, the tradition was to have a leaving lunch, which was attended by all staff and young people, with the designated leaver choosing the guests at his table. The dining room was arranged with six large tables accommodating six young people and two staff members. Each table was decorated with a placemat designed by each young person and usually decorated with their name and other motivational drawings or sayings. Barry asked me to sit beside him at the lunch and I readily agreed. It had been a journey for both of us and I was delighted to share in his celebration. As Barry showed me where he wanted me to sit, I saw that he had given me a placemat that said "Mum". As he saw me examining the mat, he said, "I know you're not my mum but you were kind of like a mum to me and my family". I don't know exactly to what he was referring, but I like to think it had something to do with my helping the family to learn the language of feelings and consequently to function in a more independent manner.

CHAPTER FIFTEEN

Opaque silence in groups

David Wood

"If I could tell you what it meant, there would be no point in dancing it."

—Isadora Duncan (in Bateson, 1973, p. 110)

The quote with which this chapter opens is to be found in a paper by Gregory Bateson entitled "Style, grace and information in primitive art" (Bateson, 1973), in which it is asserted that, "Art becomes, in this sense, an exercise in communicating about the species of unconsciousness" (p. 110). Bateson considers that one possible meaning of Duncan's remark was that "if the message [she were trying to communicate] were the sort of message that could be communicated in words, there would be no point in dancing it, but it is not that sort of message". Some messages cannot be communicated in words, and it is with such wordless messages, communicated through profound silence in groups that meet for the purpose of psychotherapy, with which this chapter is concerned. (I have borrowed this latter phrase from Hopper because it emphasises that, despite the group context, the individual is the focus of the therapeutic endeavour; in other words, it is not the "group" *qua* group (the group as a group) that is seeking help, but the individuals who have chosen to meet together for the purpose of getting help individually.)

Silences in group sessions take many forms. They may be thoughtful, reflective, anticipatory, embarrassed, anxious, or sullen, or many other things. Although there is not much explicit communication going on, the group still feels "together", sharing something of importance, and doing its business. As Paul Watzlawick said, "One cannot not communicate" (Watzlawick, Bavelas & Jackson, 1967, p. 48), and in these moments of silence, there is usually still a sense of something being shared, communicated by means other than speech.

These silences do not pose too much of a problem for the group therapist. It is not too difficult to infer something of their meaning from the context and they tend not to last too long. Usually, the group will do the work and think about what is happening, sometimes needing some help but often not. Here, I am more concerned with a different sort of silence; a deeper, more *opaque* silence that lasts for much longer and which seems to threaten the existence of the group as a group. (I am grateful to my colleague, Dr Jeanne Magagna, for suggesting the term "opaque", which so neatly sums up what I am trying to convey. The word "opaque" is derived from the medieval French *opacité*, which in turn stems from the Latin *opacitas*, an abstract noun derived from *opacus* meaning shady, shaded, or dark (Partridge, 2008)). These types of silences are not uncommon in work with young people who are in particularly fragile states of mind. They can feel unbearable and, without some understanding of their dynamics, it is easy to become despairing and even to conclude that these young people should not be treated in groups. However, it is the purpose of this chapter to argue that this is not the case, and that there are ways of helping a group in such a collective state of mind to move towards a more cohesive functioning that allows therapeutic transformation both within and between group members.

The observations upon which this paper is based derive from work exclusively with groups of young people who have severe eating disorders; "severe" in this case meaning that they are so ill that they need to be treated in an inpatient setting. However, the problem of opaque silence described here is not exclusive to work with young people with eating disorders but can occur in any group from time to time, and with any young people. Particularly with those who have been traumatised or who are living in contexts in which trauma has been a feature, including traumatised societies. Thus, although the clinical vignettes will be drawn from work with young people with eating disorders, there is no reason why the principles cannot and should not be applied to work with non-speaking people who do not suffer in this particular way.

A particularly challenging feature of the work with many traumatized young people is the frequent silences and inhibited communication. Such young people have been described as seeking "splendid isolation" (Willis, 1999, p. 22), with which they defend themselves from what to them is overwhelming anxiety engendered by the problem of relating to others without losing themselves. Another image is that of retreating into one's castle (Wood, 1999), drawing up the drawbridge, pulling down the portcullis, shutting and locking the dungeon door, and then throwing away the key.

> A child in individual therapy became able to tell me how even when we had metaphorically found the key and opened the locks of her "prison cell", she felt too terrified to emerge. It was like someone who had locked herself up in her castle for safety but who now refused to believe that the encircling armies had moved on and that there was no longer anyone hostile at the gate.

The deeply rooted hypersensitivity of such young people is such that the construction of an even barely adequately functioning protective ego boundary is an enormous task, which often makes them "contact-shunning" or "merger-hungry" (Kohut & Wolf, 1978, pp. 414–425).

Thus, social interaction for these people is fraught with anxiety and intensely problematic. They tend not to like being in groups, or at least not being in groups as themselves. However, despite silence continuing to be a frequently occurring phenomenon, one should not conclude that psychotherapy within the context of groups is pointless or unhelpful. To the contrary, I believe that groups offer a particularly important setting in which much psychological work can be done.

In this chapter, I will describe some of the unconscious features of opaque silence, with particular reference to the theory developed by Earl Hopper of a fourth basic assumption (Hopper, 1997). I shall then go on to show how it is possible to help the group move on from periods of opaque silence, develop a more cohesive group functioning and thus restore growth-promoting communication within the group.

Unconscious processes underlying opaque silence

It is important to begin with outlining the theory of a fourth basic assumption and the thinking implicit in it, including a brief outline of the theory of basic assumptions (Bion, 1961). Space dictates here that no more than a very superficial account can be given of these complex ideas, but as they are central to my argument, it is necessary to at least attempt to describe their essential features. The concept of basic assumptions in groups was developed by the psychoanalyst Wilfred Bion (1961), and refers to the way in which people in groups unconsciously form shared patterns of interpersonal defences to protect them from the experience of psychotic anxieties following regression in group situations. It is assumed to be a given, that, although being a member of a group can be a very satisfying and rewarding experience, it can also be a very anxiety-provoking one, particularly as a result of threats to one's identity that inevitably arise. Bion hypothesised that these basic assumptions prevent the group from working productively and that they interfere with the task of the group, although this is not always the case; for instance, a group of soldiers out on patrol may well be more effective and on task when under the sway of the basic assumption fight or flight.

Bion (1965) identified three basic assumptions: dependency, fight/flight, and pairing. In the basic assumption dependency mode, the underlying anxieties are those associated with the paranoid-schizoid position. Accompanying this is the consequent defensive idealisation of the group or group leader which leads to massive dependency from which no escape seems possible. In basic assumption flight/fight, the anxieties are again associated with the paranoid-schizoid position, but in this case defensive denigration of a person or persons outside the group leads to the group preparing for fight with, or flight from, this identified threat. In the basic assumption pairing mode, the anxieties are more those associated with the depressive position and the manic defence is that of the use of sexuality to defend against depression and despair. Bion more or less confined himself to three basic assumptions, but a number of authors (see Hopper, 1997) have observed that this does not do justice to the range of processes that occur in groups and have proposed additions.

Hopper's fourth basic assumption (incoherence: aggregation/massification) derives from his theory of the fear of annihilation (Hopper, 1991, 1995), which, as he himself states, is implicit in the work of the Independent Group of the British Psychoanalytical Society and of Group Analysis. For Hopper, the fear of annihilation is a response to profound helplessness arising from the experience of traumatic loss, abandonment, and damage. It is important to be clear that trauma in this case may relate to:

> the Chinese water torture strains of daily life, the cumulative build up of small incidents into an overpowering wave of oppression and/or catastrophic loss, abandonment and damage.
>
> (Hopper, 1997, p. 54)

Hopper (1997, p. 448) states that:

> The depth of helplessness is determined by the magnitude of event or events, the maturity of the ego, and the nature of the person's unconscious fantasy life at the time of the experience.
>
> (p. 448)

These last two are of particular importance, especially in emotionally sensitive or fragile young people, as the lack of maturity of their egos and the nature of their phantasy lives conspire together to make it difficult for them to experience anything other than helplessness. Thus, they frequently experience profound trauma in everyday life.

In early life, human infants are profoundly dependent on others for survival, a fact that has resulted in natural selection promoting the evolution of powerful psychological and behavioural systems to ensure that the infant's dependency needs are adequately met. Thus, there have evolved powerful systems for ensuring that infants signal their needs to caregiving adults, and that caregiving adults are able to "read" these signals sufficiently accurately, and respond accordingly. The attachment system (Bowlby, 1969) is one such system, and results in human infants and their carers having complex behavioural systems that maintain proximity and hence protection. As Fonagy (2002) has pointed out, the prolonged attachment of the human infant, resulting in regular, frequent, consistent, reliable, and eventually predictable interactions between infant and caregiver over time, creates the conditions necessary for the development of mind itself.

When the maintenance of these systems is threatened or compromised, particularly in early life, before the infant mind has had time to develop the necessary robustness to survive too much insult, or to develop a sense of agency, the (partial) collapse of these systems threatens the fragile development of the self, resulting in a sense of annihilation or falling apart, or dissolution, or profound helplessness. It is, of course, only possible to infer what the experience of these states might be like for the human infant, from the impressions that older children, adolescents, and adults (including ourselves) give at times when they have felt themselves to be falling apart or profoundly helpless.

Coltart has coined the term "grenvy" to refer to a primal emotion of greedy possessive desire (Berke, 1989, p. 26), that can be imagined to be a component of the state of mind of an infant in a profound state of dependency. When this dependency fails, from there follows the experience of profound helplessness, a splitting of "grenvy" into, on the one hand, greedy desire, and, on the other, envious hatred, resulting in both greedy desire and malign envy being directed towards objects who are perceived as able but unwilling to help.

> Objects of failed dependency are subjected to annihilating attacks... and, in turn, they are imagined to retaliate... The secondary fear of annihilation is then likely to develop.
>
> (Hopper, 1997, p. 449)

These combined primary and secondary fears of annihilation are expressed as intrapsychic fission and fragmentation and become associated with typical anxieties such as fears of disintegration, or dissolution, or falling apart. These are followed by a compensatory introjective fusion and confusion with the lost and abandoning object, which is associated with anxieties such as fear of suffocation, of swallowing or being swallowed, being crushed, trapped, or petrified. At this time another compensatory swing back to fission and fragmentation is likely. There then ensues a non-dialectical oscillation in which there is incessant psychic activity, but no change and no development, which becomes encapsulated within the psyche and which produces two autistic forms of self-protection: "crustacean" and "amoeboid" in Tustin's terminology (Tustin, 1981, 1986), or "contact-shunning" and "merger-hungry" (Kohut & Wolf, 1978). When in groups, young people under the sway of these unconscious processes, will tend to oscillate between avoidance of contact, on the one hand, or merger with the group (thereby losing any sense of themselves as individuals), on the other. Both these positions are likely to result in silence: in the former, communication is avoided as it is dangerous; and in the latter, it is avoided as it is "unnecessary".

As stated above, these patterns are considered to arise as a result of traumatic experience, the primary feature of which is the experience of extreme helplessness. As well as the more usually recognised catastrophic types of trauma, trauma can also arise as the result of low levels of helplessness, which are maintained over a prolonged time. In this case it is not the severity of the trauma but the accumulation of repeated experiences of helplessness which may be traumatogenic.

It is also crucial to be aware that the degree of helplessness depends not only on the intensity of the event, but also on the sensitivity of the person involved in it. Some young people have the misfortune to be born sensitive. Recent developments in neurobiology and genetics have clearly demonstrated that certain genotypes, in combination with certain kinds of intrauterine experience, lead some people to be predisposed to experiencing as overwhelming and traumatising what to others might be normal and manageable degrees of frustration. From this point of view, those individuals who develop extreme sensitivity to experiencing helplessness are extremely vulnerable to developing particular forms of defence associated with these types. In particular, the crustacean characteristic of desiring a "hard, bony shell" with no soft or fleshy areas can be seen as protecting from the fear of an amoeboid merger with an object (usually maternal) who is felt to be wanting to engulf them or swallow them up.

As an example, bulimic young people demonstrate this non-dialectical oscillation particularly clearly and concretely, by oscillating between a state of aching emptiness, loneliness, and despair, which stimulates uncontrollable and escalating "greedy" desire culminating in a binge, which is only terminated by the physical impossibility of cramming anything more inside. Usually within seconds or minutes, the sense of pleasurable fullness becomes the object of an envious attack from within, and turns into a sense of being filled up with, and being taken over by, overwhelming feelings of badness, disgust, and fear of a loss of any sense of self. The sense of badness can then only be dealt with by physically cleaning out the badness through vomiting and/or purging. Of course, this is then followed by the recurrence of the emptiness and so on. (Although the above examples are drawn from experience of people with eating disorders, these intrapsychic processes are not exclusive to them; their symptoms exemplify them in particularly concrete ways and therefore have a particular heuristic usefulness.)

These sensitive young people are therefore prone to adopt these patterns of defence when they fell threatened, and, as they feel threatened much of the time, these patterns become very deeply entrenched. When a number of these people come together in a group, processes of unconscious communication and resonance conspire to create patterns of group defence that utilise similar mechanisms.

The concept of the group matrix

Foulkes (1964, 1975) used the term "group matrix" to refer to the field of interaction within which the individuals in a group communicate; the person is seen as a "nodal" point within this field. The field of interaction not only links the individuals but "passes through" them so that communication is not only "interpersonal" but "transpersonal". The word "matrix" conveys the sense of a network, but also the sense of something maternal out of which the individual emerges. Thus the individuals within a matrix both create it and are created by it. Foulkes's concept of the "foundation" matrix refers to all that is communicated within the matrix in which we are born and reared, and which becomes "part of us". As Hopper (2003) puts it: "The foundation matrix meant that people and groups are rooted within species, societies, cultures and systems of communications" (p. 128). Therefore, as persons, we can no more separate ourselves from the society and culture within which we have grown, than we can separate ourselves from our bodies. For many today, particularly females, this is a particularly painful fact. They are caught between having a body that has found it difficult to develop adequate regulatory systems (secondary to hypersensitivity), and a society that has virtually stopped valuing restraint or regulation in the matter of desire. This fact contributes to daily life becoming suffused with the experience of helplessness.

The rationale for conducting psychotherapy in groups

Speech and language emerge within a social context. A group cannot be a group without communication, and a person cannot become a person without communication. There is a lot of communication without language being the medium used to relate to another person. Although we are almost certainly born with innate capacities to develop language, we cannot do so without interacting with others, without hearing them speak, without "being with" them. When the development of "personhood" goes awry, then it is likely that being in a group for the purpose of psychotherapy will have the potential to address some of the problems even if at the same time it is experienced as being overwhelming and daunting. However, in order to make this a therapeutic experience, there is a need to vary technique in working with the group.

As Willis (1999) has pointed out, in group therapy, the fundamental factor associated with change is the interaction with others in the group-as-a-whole, which Foulkes (1964, p. 82 and 129) referred to as "ego training in action". It is the richness of perspectives and the possibility of a greater freedom of interaction in groups which results in repeated, corrective, emotionally charged experiences, which in turn foster maturation.

Coherence and incoherence

It is necessary to view the "group" level of interaction as representing a different level of organisation and structure than an individual or dyadic interaction. The group has properties that are "more than" the sum of its constituent parts and these properties emerge from the constitution of the group as a group; they are not properties of the individual members.

In order for a group to be a group, it must have a certain level of organisation that defines it as a group rather than a number of individuals who happen to be standing or sitting more or less in the same place. How group-like the group is depends upon a number of factors including the extent to which it is "cohesive". Hopper (1997) reminds us that cohesion differs from adhesion in that when persons, particles or unities bond together cohesively they do so in such a way that they do not lose their individual identity, and when the group dissolves they do not suffer damage to their individual boundaries. In contrast, when constituents of a group are bound together adhesively then they lose their individual identities, and thus when the group is dissolved they are severely if not fatally damaged. "A cohesive bonding implies that the resultant body is only temporarily unified. An adhesive bonding implies that the resulting body has become a new entity" (Hopper, 1997, p. 197).

The manifestation of encapsulated traumatic experience in groups: the basic assumption of incohesion: aggregation/massification

Of particular significance is Hopper's proposal of a fourth basic assumption of incohesion: aggregation/massification. Hopper considers that:

> When people have been traumatized, have experienced the fear of annihilation, and subsequently, have encapsulated intrapsychic oscillations between fission and fragmentation and fusion and confusion, then, on the basis of various kinds of externalization and internalization, especially projective and introjective identification, their groups are likely to evince processes of incohesion. In the first instance this is characterized by aggregation in response to fission and fragmentation and then by massification in response to fusion and confusion and in turns by oscillations between massification and aggregation.
>
> (Hopper, 1997, p. 14)

One manifestation of incohesion is profound opaque silence. In basic assumption incohesion, the massification pole describes the shared unconscious phantasy that there is no differentiation in the group, that the individuals have merged into oneness, and that therefore, verbal communication is unnecessary. Moreover, the very fact that verbal communication implies that there would be a difference, and therefore differentiation (if there was no difference, there would be no need for verbal communication), means that it is fiercely resisted. Verbal communication itself becomes the signifier of difference, and difference means separation, and separation means aloneness, and aloneness means abandonment and therefore annihilation. When the basic assumption massification is present, verbal communication as the signifier of difference must itself be annihilated.

At the aggregation pole of basic assumption incohesion, each group member has retreated into his/her own space and become isolated from the group. Aggregation implies a collection of constituents with little or no interaction between them. Verbal communication is resisted because communicating verbally will threaten the aggregated state and risk the loss of any sense of self. In this state of mind, verbal communication becomes the signifier of merger and, for this reason, has to be annihilated.

The group's opaque silence referred to here has a very particular feel, and is often extremely painful to experience. It may be so intense as to be difficult to find words for it; nothing quite conveys its primordial, inchoate nature. Perhaps the nearest one can get to it is a sense of intense rejection coupled with profound helplessness or paralysis. There is a sense of being in the presence of people who are completely unwilling or unable to even recognise that you exist, and that one feels there is absolutely nothing that can be done about it. Even direct questions are met with a total lack of any observable response. Here is a vignette drawn from a group of eleven- to sixteen-year-old young people illustrating opaque silence:

> Fairly soon after the beginning of a group session, the atmosphere began to feel very tense. Four members of the group were clearly very withdrawn. Two sat on their chairs with knees drawn up under their chins, long hair over their faces, two others curled up on the sofa so that no facial expression could be seen. Some of the other members bravely tried to start a conversation, but somehow the silence was such that even to speak at all felt extremely dangerous, as if one was breaking some sort of taboo. The conductor tried to share some thoughts about what might be going on, but found himself beginning to feel full of rage which made him think that he had better be very careful about what he said in case he was unable to control his emotion. He felt in danger of losing his temper with this silence, and he found it harder and harder to think of anything to say at all. In the calmest, gentlest manner that he could muster, he addressed a number of direct questions to one or two of the silent ones. There was no flicker of acknowledgment that he had even been heard, let alone that any response might be forthcoming. He felt as if he did not exist for these young people, that he had been annihilated from their universe.

It should be emphasised that silence can occur in groups in which any of the Bionic basic assumptions are currently operating, and of course can occur in groups that are on task and working well together. But these are not the silences that are the topic of this chapter. It is argued here that opaque silence is a property of groups under the sway of Hopper's (1997, 2003b) fourth basic assumption, and it may be a feature of either or both of the poles of massification and aggregation.

Therapeutic factors promoting transformation of opaque silence

Setting

Opaque silence is a manifestation of the operation of basic assumption in cohesion: aggregation or massification in a group. This basic assumption is a defence against very primitive anxieties associated with the fear of annihilation. Therapeutic work is required to address the source of those anxieties. Primitive anxieties associated with the fear of annihilation arise from the experience of extreme helplessness. Helplessness is engendered when an individual perceives himself/herself to be under extreme threat and feels that there is no source of help, either from internal or external resources. The principal psychobiological system involved in the generation of these appraisals is that of the attachment system (Bowlby, 1969); a biological system that has evolved to ensure as far as is possible the survival of vulnerable infants by maintaining proximity to protective adults. Thus, the first parameter that has to be addressed is that of the security and safety of the group, by ensuring that the basic and familiar rules of stability and predictability of the boundaries of the group in time and space are maintained. In particular, the room needs to have been prepared properly and should be consistent in its furnishings, with little (or preferably no) sign of previous use, the chairs being fit for purpose (i.e., comfortable without being too casual); the conductor needs to arrive on time, and in a proper state of mind (i.e., not rushed or distracted by other events); and notice of absences needs to be given well in advance.

If the group is being conducted by co-therapists (I have increasingly come to value this way of working with these particular young people), the conductors need to reserve time together before and after the group session to think about their experiences. They need to have developed sufficient confidence and trust in each other to be able to be very direct and honest about their countertransference during the session, especially when this involves difficult feelings about each other.

However, in thus addressing the need for structure promoting security it is also important not to do so in a way that becomes excessively rigid, bureaucratised, and inflexible; in other words, care has to be taken not to stifle freedom and creativity.

Context

Any group is always part of another group; in other words, groups are always brought together as part of open systems and attention needs to be paid to the context in which any group meets, be it an outpatient or an inpatient setting. In relation to groups that take place in inpatient settings, one needs to consider what is happening in the wider milieu of the institution, particularly in relation to events that may activate attachment systems. Questions to be considered are: have there been any significant staff changes or absences?; have new patients arrived or others left the institution?; has the timetable changed (e.g., school holidays in a young person's setting)? Consideration needs to be paid to how the group is relating to the whole larger institution, to what is being projected into or out of the group; is it holding any split-off transferences on behalf of the whole, what is the group wanting to rid itself of into the wider community? In relation to opaque silence, thought should be given to whether the group is holding something particularly toxic on behalf of the community.

It is not uncommon in the setting in which these observations have been made, and in which the community divides into two small groups which run in parallel, to find that, when one group has been immersed in opaque silence, the other has been particularly active and talkative. It is always important, but particularly in these situations, that all the conductors of both groups meet together after the session, and think together about how the themes in each group might reflect processes occurring in the wider community. It is even important to consider what may be happening at a yet wider level, that of the social context in which any group may be existing. Have there been any particularly anxiety evoking events, such as recessions, wars or disasters? At an even more deeply embedded level one needs to consider the time of year, particularly the onset of winter which still carries with it, at a deeply unconscious level, the primordial fear of the ever darkening days and the anxiety as to whether spring will indeed return.

The conductors' and eventually the members' therapeutic stance that promotes development

The experience of opaque silence invariably signals that members of the group are experiencing intense and overwhelming painful affect related to very primitive anxieties, but it is likely that they are not aware of this. Indeed, the very reason that the group is so profoundly silent is in part because these painful affects are so overwhelming and threatening that being aware of them is out of the question. In particular, what is often being projected is the experience of being annihilated, and it is important that the conductors of the group are able to accept these projections without fear. Bearing the brunt of this mental pain, particularly the experience of being annihilated, is not easy and requires considerable emotional maturity and robustness on the part of the therapists. It is vital, in the face of this, to hold on to the belief and hope that by bearing it, gradually the patient will become able to bear it too. "Bearing it" here means being prepared to feel it, in all its raw and painful intensity, to experience it but not to act on it, or turn away from it, to be able to face thinking about it, not necessarily immediately (which may be impossible), but as soon as it becomes possible.

Eventually, words may be found for it, but not too quickly, as putting it into words too soon can be felt by the young person as an attempt by the therapist to push the feelings back into them when they are not yet ready to accept them. To these young people, "plunging" interpretations, in which the therapist plunges into the depths before allowing the young person to become familiar with the surface, feel like intrusive attempts at taking over their minds, and this nearly always results in increased withdrawal. The projection of feelings of annihilation into the group conductors can also arouse anger. When this occurs in their private thinking, the conductors need to examine their own historical and unconscious personal responses to the experience of rejection and feeling annihilated in order that their projections into the group members are elaborated upon and understood.

The group conductors may need to make their interpretations silently to themselves, sometimes for some considerable time, before the group will be ready to hear them. What the act of silent interpretation does is to allow the therapists to reach some sophisticated understanding of what is going on that then allows them to respond, not necessarily verbally, in an understanding rather than a defensive way. Silent interpretation changes the therapists' state of mind, which then, in turn, alters the subtle, barely perceptible (perhaps only unconsciously perceptible) responses that the therapists give to the group which, in turn, influences the experience the group is having. Later on, when the mood feels right, co-therapists may discuss their experiences between themselves in front of the group, demonstrating the capacity to think about feelings with curiosity, to wonder why they might have felt that way, or experienced it in that way, demonstrating a "mentalizing" (Allen, 2003; Bateman & Fonagy, 2004; Fonagy, 2002; Skarderud, 2007) approach.

Here is a description of one of the weekly therapy group sessions that illustrates the therapists' *silent reflections*, which are subsequently reformulated into non-intrusive comments for the group members.

A brief vignette

> The two conductors enter the group room and sit down. The other members of the young people's group are already present. As soon as the conductors enter there is a sense that communication has been shut down, in that before the group "started" there seemed to have been some interaction, which now suddenly ceased. All heads, but those of the conductors, are down, eyes looking at the floor making it impossible to make eye contact ("I" contact?). After a few minutes the conductors are beginning to feel mildly irritated, having an "Oh no not this again" sort of feeling, with the anticipation that they are going to have to work far harder at facilitating than they would like (in the sense that having to work hard at facilitation makes it more difficult to reflect on what is happening). After a while, one conductor says (to the group as a whole): "It seems that is it is difficult to start this afternoon, it feels like everyone seems to be in their own world". There is absolutely no response of any discernible kind. This lack of response feels hostile and it would have been easy to have said something along the lines of, "It feels as if the group is angry this afternoon". However experience has shown that this sort of remark inevitably makes things worse. The silence continued. It seemed that there were nine individuals in the room, each in their own world, if not universe, with no possibility of linking between them. The group seemed to be an aggregate rather than a group.
>
> The conductors openly discuss between them why the group might feel this way today, but they are not able to pick up any particular clues as to why. At one point the male conductor (DW) asks a direct question but there is no discernible response (this leaves him feeling ignored and rather hurt; he wonders to himself if this was retaliation for being away last week but this seemed too far from the group's conscious experience to interpret).
>
> The conductors comment on this complete lack of response but there is little, if any, interest in their comment. Then Wendy says, somewhat angrily, "People don't always have to talk, that's what is wrong with this place, no one leaves you alone for a moment, you can never have a moment to yourself to think". DW questions this: "Is it really true? What about evenings, etc?" Wendy responds, "Staff always come and ask you how you are." DW suggests (as gently as he could, hoping to convey curiosity) that, in that situation, she might say "I don't feel like talking at present, I need some time on my own".

Wendy then becomes very disparaging of the clinic. DW (probably feeling defensive and getting caught up in a symmetrical position) challenges her and says that it seems that whatever he says, she will disagree with, on principle, as she is in that space where she is not prepared to let anything help.

Annie says that she does not want to talk because she might cry. DW asks, "Does it matter if she cries; might she not get support for her unhappiness?" There is again no response from the group. DW points this out. Wendy is again indignant and says that Annie knows that she cares because they have talked about it, just the two of them, outside the group. DW says, "But it would be difficult for Annie to know that anyone cared at present, here, now."

CL comments that she is worried that some people who are nearing moving on from inpatient treatment seem unable or unwilling to speak to one another, which they need to be able to do if they are going to manage when they have less support available. There is no response. CL comments that Maria is looking very withdrawn and wonders what might be the matter.

Maria whispers an inaudible response. CL and DW say they cannot hear. Eventually it becomes clear that she has said that, "Something has happened but I don't want to talk about it". DW says that it might help to talk about it. Maria replies that she has already discussed it with a nurse and does not want to talk further. CL comments that it looks far from resolved. DW tries again and is then challenged by Wendy who takes him to task for "pushing". She says, "What are we meant to do? Staff congratulate people in the morning meeting for having said that they do not want to talk, and people apologise for pushing people, and yet DW is still doing it." DW states his view that it might help Maria. Wendy repeats and elaborates upon her pejorative remarks. DW tries to make clear where he is "coming from", that, "It might help, not that you have to, or that I will be upset or cross if you don't talk" and he goes on in this vein.

There is some talk about trust and privacy. Annie talks more about what she misses from home, "her mum"; specifically comfort, support, care, etc from parents. "I just want to be with them". DW raises the question of whether they might think about how not to get into a position where it is "either/or"; at least get some comfort rather than none.

The group seemed in a "livelier" place by the end of the session but three members had said nothing at all and one said very little and that was mainly, "I don't know".

As stated above, it is impossible to discuss any group without consideration of its context. This group was meeting once a week on Tuesday afternoons for one hour as part of an intensive inpatient programme for the treatment of young people with eating disorders. The size of the group varies between five and nine members depending on how many young people are resident at the clinic. There is another group of similar size that meets at the same time in a room next door. The average age in the group is about fifteen. Clearly, as part of a residential programme, all members of this group are members of a larger group, "the community of staff and young people", in which they meet each other throughout the rest of the week. The group is conducted by two therapists, one of whom (DW) is the senior Consultant Psychiatrist to the Clinic and also the Clinical Director (and also one of relatively few males working in the institution). The other (CL) is the Clinical Nurse Leader (the second most senior nurse in the organisation), and one who has responsibility for managing the nursing team. Thus their "parental" roles as father and mother of the institution are very prominent. In particular, DW's significance is worthy of further discussion. It is an often observed feature of families with an anorexic member that the daughter-mother relationship is particularly intense and the daughter-father relationship relatively weak. It is also of note that anorexia nervosa would appear to be more prevalent in societies (i.e., Western societies) in which fathers are often, in reality, relatively absent and in which men in general appear to be undergoing a crisis in identity.

Of further significance is that this session occurred during a period of significant upheaval in the organisation of the clinic. A number of relatively senior staff had recently left, and either had been replaced with relatively inexperienced staff, or some posts were temporarily vacant, leaving the team somewhat "thin". There had also been a greater than usual turnover in the young people's group with a number of young people leaving and new ones joining. In other words, the matrix of the group as well as that of the whole organisation felt less secure, consistent, and predictable than usual.

The first impression of the group was that of an aggregate of individuals; no eye ("I") contact, no "we-ness", each person isolated and encapsulated and afraid to make contact. There was the impression that this had developed rather suddenly as soon as the staff entered the room. There was a sense of disappointment at having to have to work harder at facilitating than hoped, perhaps in the sense that a mother trying to feed a reluctant infant may feel frustrated that she has to work hard at getting the infant to feed and therefore is less able to relax and enjoy her reverie and profound sense of connection to her infant. From his countertransference early in the session, DW felt ignored, excluded, left out, and it was very painful as if he was being shunned, or even "annihilated". He linked this in his mind to his absence the previous week. The significance of his absence may have been increased by the fact that the previous week had included a bank holiday (the Monday), meaning that fewer senior staff were around in the early part of the week, DW had worked on the Tuesday but had been absent on leave Wednesday, Thursday, and Friday. (It should go without saying that his absence had been announced several weeks before this, so was expected.) By coming in on the Tuesday, he had perhaps inadvertently communicated that he could look after the group, but his absence on the following 3 days could have been interpreted as his choosing not to do so. Thus, the absence of DW on holiday assumes particular significance. His absence could be expected to evoke experiences of failed dependency that would be likely to arouse particularly intense anxieties.

However, previous experience suggested that interpreting this sort of thing too early often evoked a response such as, "You think you are so important but you are not, it doesn't bother me that you have been away", and leads to increased defensiveness and less capacity to get in touch with the pain of loss and abandonment. He therefore kept this thought to himself. In particular, although the group felt very hostile, to respond with a comment such as, "I think you are all angry with me for being away last week" would almost certainly have been heard as, "How dare you be angry with me, you ungrateful children". In any case, it is very likely that the hostility was too far from consciousness for any of them to have been in touch with it. The conductors focused more on containment and support than on interpretation. They gently invited the group to wonder why it might be hard to talk today, although this was met with no response at first, and then with a rather cross "leave us alone" type of comment that suggested that trying to draw them out too soon was being experienced as an assault. A retaliatory accusation was made that, "No one leaves you alone for a moment; you can never have a moment to yourself", suggesting that the idea of making contact risked losing your self (i.e., moving from fragmentation to fusion), and that the oscillation at that moment was towards aggregation. DW responded with a suggestion that implied it was not necessary to have either fragmentation or fusion. His remark came in the form of, "It might be possible to be oneself in company" through stating "I don't feel like talking at the moment". This met with a defensive disparagement, suggesting that she or the group were not yet ready to move out of the defensive isolation. This left DW feeling alone and rejected, and there was almost certainly more defensiveness in his response than was helpful. However, this did seem to allow another young person, Annie, to share her fear of falling apart, "I might cry". DW gently questioned the belief that this would be a disaster by inquiring as gently as possible, "Does it matter if you cry? Might you not get some support from the group if you were able to communicate your distress?" The group responded by enacting Annie's fear, as if to say to the conductors, "Don't you know anything? Of course we can't say that we need something - stupid!", and not responding to her in any way. Wendy took up her role of group elder sibling (she has a valency for this role as she is an elder sibling whose parents have been very preoccupied with their own difficulties, and have not been able to give sufficient attention to their children for significant parts of their lives) by implying that a dyadic relationship with just one other is all that is required and is certainly more useful than the group which is useless and therefore not needed. Wendy suggests that she is able to offer Annie all she needs. DW tries to bring it back to the here and now in the group and think about what is needed now.

The attention turns to Maria who is communicating non-verbally that she is very upset by demonstrating the depth of her withdrawal from the group by drawing her knees up, almost curling up into a ball like a hedgehog. When asked a question she whispers an inaudible response. Maria is a member of the group who is often very articulate and certainly does not lack a voice when she wants one. She then states clearly that she does not want to talk, she needs nothing from the group as she has "already talked about it". When DW tries gently to encourage her, Wendy again steps in to "defend" her from this phallic "pushing" father. She is unable to make a distinction between the encouragement of more open communication and the intrusive penetration of a defensive barrier. For her and the group, at that moment, giving up the defensive isolation and fragmentation risks the loss of self inherent infusion and merger; there is no concept of personhood available.

Annie begins to talk about missing home and the comfort of her mum; she just wants to be with them. For her, there is little or no concept of an internal sustaining maternal object; she needs to be physically with her mum or she feels completely alone and abandoned. Here the oscillatory process swings back towards the pole of fusion and merger with an idealised mother who will provide everything that is needed.

The next week's group was very different, with some quite lively conversation throughout.

> The session began with a few minutes silence. Wendy began by saying "can't we meet outside". She went on to question why we have the group; it does not feel that it is a good use of

> time etc. Maria joined in a bit, then began to think about how it would be easier if DW and CL were not present. DW/CL gently questioned why this might be, and an idea was put forward that we are a bit like teachers or parents. Maria began a sentence, referring to DW, by using his first name, but then quickly changed it back to the more formal surname. DW picked this up and was curious about what it was about his role in particular that inhibited people or made them feel that they could not talk freely. There was some discussion about how it seemed difficult to think of using his first name even though first names are used for everyone else (possibly connected with a difficulty in keeping him in role if a first name were to be used because of the wish to be close to him). Wendy introduced the idea of how strange language was when you stepped back from it and just listened to the sound of the word; it seemed odd. They explored what teenagers talked about together that they did not talk about in front of teachers or parents. Wendy talked about how her brother talks to her about girls; asking her for advice as to how can he "get" a particular girl that he fancies, "and he is only 12!"

The group now began to feel more interested and interesting. It had moved from basic assumption incohesion: aggregation/massification to basic assumption pairing. Other members seemed much more involved even though they were not saying much; their silence was more to do with their lack of confidence than a defensive aggregation. The principle theme was connected with questions about what it was possible to talk about in front of the "grown ups" and what wasn't, with an explicit theme of adolescent sexuality and a wish to get rid of the parents in order to have some fun! In other words, they were using the excitement of talking about sex as a defence against the pain of acknowledging their loneliness and anxieties about growing up and leaving homes that for a variety of reasons had not been able to provide them with what they had both needed and wanted in order to enable them to feel more equipped to face growing up. The feel of the group was very different; it was a cohesive group, not an aggregation of individuals.

In subsequent meetings, these themes continued, and the group was able to continue to talk together about their worries about growing up and the overwhelming fear of abandonment that this induced. There was a wish that they could return to 'things as they were before', to the Garden of Eden, and their unawareness of their aloneness and the parental intercourse.

Implications for technique

The idea advanced here is that profound, opaque silence in groups is a manifestation of the operation of a fourth basic assumption, incoherence: aggregation/massification (in particular the aggregation pole) as proposed by Hopper (1997, 2003b), and that this is likely to occur when members of the group are in touch with anxieties associated with the fear of annihilation. The fear of annihilation is associated with the experience of extreme helplessness and is in turn associated with the experience of trauma, whether it is of the catastrophic or cumulative strain type. It is also proposed that some people are particularly prone to this anxiety due to their exquisite sensitivity to change, which leaves them very vulnerable to the experience of trauma and the subsequent development of particular patterns of defence associated with the traumatogenic process. It follows then that what is required from the group conductors is particular attention to the factors which provoke these anxieties, while finding ways of working with both the factors and the resultant anxieties which continue in the here and now.

Particular attention needs to be paid to the "attachment" context of the group. That is, to the regularity, predictability and reliability of the context, and all factors that promote secure attachment. It is suggested that when groups are evidencing the need to use the defences associated with the fear of annihilation, that is, basic assumption incohesion: aggregation/massification, the conductors need to pay special attention to containment. In our experience, interpretations, when used at all, need to be focused on the experience of profound helplessness. It is rarely helpful to focus on the hostility as this just provokes further retreat. Often, the conductors need to make relatively few interpretations as such, but what is important is to convey their understanding of these deep fears and anxieties through their tone of voice, facial expression and other containing non-verbal forms of communication.

It is also important to remember that, even when individual group members are silent over prolonged periods of time (months or even years), it does not mean that they are not learning from their experience of others or the group as a whole grappling with these difficulties. As long as the group as a whole is doing some work, all members of the group will be learning something, even if it is not easily apparent. During the pupa stage in the life cycle of a butterfly, there is no visible evidence, viewed form the outside, of the active reorganisation of the internal physical structure of the caterpillar as metamorphoses. Similarly, there can be no evidence of the internal change taking place in some profoundly mute young people, until, one day, like the butterfly emerging from the pupa, they will begin to speak and subsequently make clear that they have heard and understood everything.

Opaque silence is very difficult to experience and bear, as it evokes very primitive anxieties of abandonment. It is therefore not surprising that therapists may easily (and defensively) conclude that patients who are very silent in groups should not be treated in groups, or groups in which there is a lot of silence should not be continued, or more "active" techniques need to be introduced in order to fill the silence.

It is the contention of this chapter that this is not the case; that groups can provide a very therapeutic space in which these issues can be addressed, provided that the therapist is prepared to tolerate feeling terrible now and then, and is prepared to work with the group at a pace that its members can manage. Then, just as inevitably as, after the winter solstice the days begin to lengthen again, and light again begins to counteract the darkness, the silence can become less opaque as the group once again finds its capacity to think and talk together.

PART IV

CREATIVE ACTIVITIES FOR NON-SPEAKING CHILDREN

CHAPTER SIXTEEN

The creative group experience

Tara Pepper Goldsmith and Naomi Ben Simon

In this chapter, we will explore the unspoken communications between therapists and the young people in an inpatient group that we run on a hospital psychiatric ward specialising in work with children. One of the tasks of such a unit is to help each child build up a capacity to think more about her emotional life and thereby remove some of the impediments to development. We established a creative group on the ward to help the children begin to represent their state of mind through artwork, and then to think and talk about their feelings. We will describe how we have drawn on the Tavistock Model of Infant Observation to understand what the children are communicating, through body movement and facial expressions, and by exploring our experience of the transference and countertransference.

The psychiatric unit takes children with very entrenched eating disorders and somatic disorders, including a pervasive retreat from life. In this chapter, we will use the feminine prefix to refer to children of both sexes. A child pervasively retreating from life may lie immobile, mute, and withdrawn from the world for weeks or months, communicating a silent terror of treatment, with the nurses keeping her alive with naso-gastric feeds. An anorexic child may also refuse all food and drink, and require feeding through a naso-gastric tube, sometimes actively sabotaging a feed by pulling out the tube, by vomiting, or physically attacking the nurses giving the feed. She may exercise constantly, moving her legs in rapid, repetitive cycles, doing "star jumps" and skipping. At bedtime, she may attempt to sleep standing up, or condition herself to wake early or throughout the night, interrupting sleep to exercise when no-one is there to challenge this. When she does speak, it is often to express a wish to be thin or to die.

Our aim over time is to help young people replace their symptoms with an ability to mentalize, that is, to develop a mind that can mediate their experience of the world through communicating to oneself and others (Fonagy, Gergely, Jurist & Target, 2004). Bion described how a mother receives her infant's powerful, unprocessed emotional states, and by mulling them over herself, is able to return them to her in a form that is more manageable (Bion, 1962). By using her mother's mind in this way, the infant introjects the mother's capacity for containing and thinking about her feelings. This is the nature of the help that the children with whom we work need, and which we try to offer. In this way, we hope that they may gradually be able to replace symptoms with symbols. We hope that harsh and punishing internal objects may to some degree be mitigated by the internalisation of more helpful ones, and that these changes may be acknowledged by our patients. The process of thinking about emotional experience has barely begun for most of the children with whom we work. When a child has not developed the capacity for mentalization in the context of a good enough infantile experience, she is left very vulnerable to any difficult experience, lacking the resources to think through everyday experiences as well as traumatic ones (Fonagy, Gergely, Jurist & Target, 2004). A difficult or traumatic experience, such as illness in the family, or bullying at school, unhappy events that many encounter, can then, for these more vulnerable children, feel like an overwhelming and powerful attack on the self, and necessitate a retreat to primitive forms of protection against anxiety.

Symbol formation

To examine how participation in a creative group helped ameliorate the life-threatening symptoms and deadly states of mind of the inpatient children with whom we worked, we will explore briefly how a capacity for symbol formation develops in the context of a healthy parent-infant relationship. We will then discuss how it can be derailed. In normal development, a baby will, during the first year of life in particular, have experienced the transformation of his bodily sensations and expressions of distress, crying, body gestures, and psychosomatic responses, into meaningful communications by a thoughtful parent (Bion, 1962; McDougall, 1989). With repeated experience of this process, the infant develops an understanding that he too has a space inside for containing and thinking thoughts. As the good object is more securely established within the ego, the fear of bad objects, and anxieties around the loss or inaccessibility of good objects, can be displaced onto the external world, and symbolic representation of these anxieties becomes possible (Segal, 1957). This allows difficult emotions to be communicated and thought about.

This process may be seen in the following extract from the observation of a thirteen-week-old baby girl, Lucinda:

> Before leaving the room to help her toddler get ready to go to the park, mother lay Lucinda underneath the baby gym. This had two arches over her, with toys hanging from them. Lucinda grasped a soft snail that was hanging down above her, clutching its two raised horns. Lucinda fingers the horns, then starts pulling the snail towards her open mouth, using both hands, straining with the effort. She then lets go of the snail, and waves her arms, making a low, grunting noise, then grabs it again, pulling the raised horns towards her. Mum comes back in and kneels down to watch. Lucinda does not turn to her. She is holding the snail,

> pulling it towards her, letting it go. Her eyes are fixed on the toy. Suddenly Lucinda lets go of the snail, which snaps away from her. She starts to sob. Mum picks her up and holds her close. Lucinda calms quickly.

It seemed that initially Lucinda wished to use the snail to plug herself up in her mother's absence, perhaps using it in the form of a symbolic equation, to deny the absence of the breast (Segal, 1957). However, in her play, as the snail snapped back, and she pulled it forward, there seemed to be an element of more genuine symbol formation, as Lucinda experienced the anxiety of the loss and her wish to re-create the object. It seemed that in mother's presence, the sense of loss Lucinda had experienced and played with moments before became concrete and overwhelming. She projected this outwards in her sobs, and her mother responded with close contact that helped the baby feel her painful state of mind had been understood and contained.

Once another person has provided this containing function, in healthy development, later in therapy, or within a group and ward such as ours, and the idea of a container has been introjected, there is a growing interest in and engagement with the world. This corresponds to the shift identified by child development researchers that occurs around the end of the first year, from a powerful dyadic relationship between parent and baby, to a state of "secondary intersubjectivity", in which the infant becomes increasingly aware that there can be a sharing of objects and events and communication about them can occur (Trevarthen, 1978). This common interest in another object, and the idea that it might have meaning both for oneself and for another, makes possible new forms of thought and communication (Hobson, 2002). The ability to create symbols enables us to conjure up absent realities and imagined worlds, "fix objects and events as experienced, and then… think about them" (Hobson, 2002). Symbolising enables us to explore different attitudes and approaches, to move away from entrenched ways of being and relating, particularly important when established modes are destructive (Pepper Goldsmith, 2009). It is a lively, vital link between internal experience and external realities, suffusing the latter with personal meaning, ensuring the former is submitted to reality-testing (M. Klein, 1930). Philosopher Mary Warnock suggests that if we are successfully imagining something, then, this is what we are doing: 'either by means of physical or non-physical analogues we are calling up the sense or significance of something which is not present to us in fact.' Thus the absent object is conjured up, present in affect. (Warnock, 1976, p.171).

But the route to the development of symbol formation is paved with the acceptance of sharp realities. As Edna O'Shaughnessy points out, initially, it will be difficult for the infant to hold on to the good aspects of the absent object. It may be perceived not as a good object absent, but as a bad object present. Its harshness forces reality on the child, and breaks the hold of phantasies, which protect him from the realisation of his vulnerability and dependence (O'Shaughnessy, 1964, p.34). There must be an increasing awareness of the difference between internal and external worlds. Omnipotent identifications must lessen. Objects can then be recognised as having their own qualities, and standing for some other object, with quite different properties.

Defences

These unpalatable realities take a good deal of ego strength to negotiate. Faced with them, the child can choose, as Bion (1962) wrote, "between procedures designed to evade frustration and those designed to modify it" (p. 29). If a parent, for one reason or another, has not been able to help the child take in such painful experiences, modifying them so that they are meaningful and can be used to aid development, the infant "reintrojects, not a fear of dying made tolerable, but a nameless dread" (Bion, 1962, p. 116). If this occurs repeatedly, an internal object is formed that destroys meaning and leaves the subject in a bizarre, meaningless world (Bion, 1962). Then, the existence of the object and awareness of separation are attacked, as they are a painful reminder that "the source of life and goodness lies outside" (Segal, 1983, p. 270) and that the child is vulnerable and dependent on an object that lies beyond its control (Rosenfeld, 1964). The very apparatus of the mind which is becoming aware of this situation, felt to be intolerable, may come under attack. The ability to perceive and think about need and dependence, and the capacity to think itself, may also be dismantled (Bion, 1962). These confused, and confusing, states of mind were often projected into us as we worked, and I will discuss the way in which they made participation in a creative group extremely difficult.

Deficits

These defences exist alongside, and sometimes develop from, deficits in a capacity for mentalization and symbol formation. Recent child development research has confirmed the connection, first postulated by Bowlby, between disruptions in early attachment relationships and later tendencies to cope with stressful situations in ways that are maladaptive (Bowlby, 1969). While it is not possible to speculate about the nature of the early relationships experienced by the children on our ward, we know that many had experienced different kinds of trauma, including parental illness, bullying at school, or abuse. Incidents of trauma involve a range of experiences in which, rather than helping the infant or child modulate her emotional states, a caregiver induces levels of stimulation or arousal that are extremely high in cases of abuse, or very low in instances of neglect (Schore, 2002b). Along with this, the caregiver is unable to help the child process these states, responding to her in a way that is frightening or detached (Schore, 2002b). A terminally ill parent for instance may be so preoccupied with her mortality that she may be less available to help a child with her own heightened anxieties about death.

Describing neglect, Tronick and Weinberg explain that:

> when infants are not in homeostatic balance or are emotionally dysregulated (e.g. they are distressed), they are at the mercy of these states. Until these states are brought under control, infants must devote all their regulatory resources to reorganising them. While infants are doing that, they can do nothing else.
>
> (1997, p. 56)

In the absence of help with modulating and thinking through stressful experiences, the physical response becomes entrenched. In later life, such a child may move very swiftly from feeling mildly anxious to profoundly threatened or terrorised, or she may swiftly regress into a state dissociated from external reality (Perry, Pollard, Blakely, Baker & Vigilante, 1995). Once this trait is established, it can be difficult to help a child to hold in mind and think through painful emotions. It is important to acknowledge that this combination of defence and deficit can make treatment and further personality development difficult.

Establishing the group

To foster communication between staff and children, the unit's multidisciplinary team felt it would be helpful to develop a creative group. If the children were not able to put words to their states of mind they could begin to express their feelings through art. Members of the team agreed to set aside a specific time once a week during which the group could work undisturbed on the ward. It was agreed that the group would be staffed by Naomi, a nurse therapist, along with a nurse from the ward. Later, Tara, a psychotherapy student joined the group. Our aim was to give children the opportunity to begin to think about and communicate very powerful emotions first in their art and then in words. This reflected the aims of the ward as a whole. We followed a therapeutic milieu approach, in which children are offered "supportive containment" within a mutually cooperative multidisciplinary team, including nurses, therapists, physiotherapists, dieticians, and social workers (Flynn, in Lanyado & Horne, 1999, p. 168). The aim of nursing in this context was to explore the children's capacities across a strict daily routine, using ordinary human reactions or responses (Flynn, in Lanyado & Horne, 1999).

We saw often on the ward how, in the absence of words, strong feelings would be expressed by projective identification. This is a process in which feelings that were too unpleasant or painful for a child to acknowledge were simply cut off and evacuated; projected into a convenient staff member, such as one of the nurses who work so closely with the children (M. Klein, 1946). The nurse might then find herself representing or acting out this split off part of the patient's experience, feeling the child's experience of being enraged, denigrated, humiliated, or useless.

We wished to help the young people take a first step towards acknowledging these unbearable states of mind through the creation of artworks, which might help bring painful emotions into the realm of the symbolic (Case, 2005). Moreover, by being aware of the feelings aroused in us by children's projective identifications, we considered that we could gently, in a very gradual way, begin to reunite the child with these painful, split-off parts of their experience. With this in mind, there were certain factors that we considered to be integral to the successful working of the group. It was vital to have in place a strong, containing environment so that these powerful feelings could be first firmly held, then thought about and discussed. Elmhirst (1988) has discussed the particular importance of ensuring regular, punctual sessions at an established time and setting when, as she writes "working in the white-heat of the infantile transference" (Elmhirst, 1988, p. 7). Establishing the continuity of staff was paramount, so that the children would always know who would be there. A therapist is the recipient, in the transference, of powerful anxieties related to early experience. For this containing relationship to develop, it was important that the group be run by the same staff members each week (Daws & Boston, 1981). We had to make a strong case to the ward manager for assigning one nurse to work consistently with the group. In the end, this ideal situation did not prove to be possible, as there would always be at least one week a month when our designated nurse would work night shifts. So we agreed to have two rotating staff members. Staff made time before each session to think about the group and any changes that might have occurred during the week. We also set aside time afterwards to think together and process what had happened in the group.

Once it had been decided to hold the group on the ward, the continuity of this setting was also important. The group took place in part of the large common area, which was also used for meals and some meetings and other groups. There was a large table, surrounded by chairs. Nearby were cupboards and drawers with art materials, and also a piano and shelves of board games that the children use at other times. The space was closed off with curtains from a corridor and a second part of the room, which contained a TV, DVDs, and sofas. We were not given a choice of rooms; we simply had to make the best of the space we were offered despite some drawbacks.

It was a practical challenge on a somewhat run-down psychiatric ward to create a space that felt sufficiently secure. There were physical obstacles, which could not initially be overcome, such as curtains that were missing, leaving part of the room exposed, so that the space felt very large and uncontained. In addition, we needed support staff to be aware that the group was happening, as cleaners and administrative staff regularly came into the area to ask questions or to do their work. It was helpful to discuss the nature of the group with everyone involved with the ward, so that interruptions could be avoided if at all possible. As the space which we were offered for the group was not only used for therapy, the transference became complicated. In a neutral environment, the child can freely project painful feelings and anxieties to the therapist, opening these up for thought (Daws & Boston, 1981). In this case, the room already held some different, strong associations for each of the children. Some had difficult experiences around this table at mealtimes. Others had more positive associations, of family visits or playing games together during free time. This complication was heightened by the fact that the group took place immediately after lunch. We often came in to the tail end of a conflict over eating, or to a table still covered in bits of food; a concrete reminder of the difficulties of thinking about the mess inside.

The creative group was set up as part of the weekly programme in which all the children participated as part of their treatment. It was not an option, but an integral part of the schedule of meetings, therapeutic groups, and individual sessions designed by the unit to facilitate communication among the children. Each child had weekly individual work, usually with a child psychotherapist or clinical psychologist, regular meetings with a nurse keyworker, and a weekly family therapy session. The ward was run by both mental health and paediatric nurses, along therapeutic community lines, with a strictly timetabled weekly routine. Children attended morning community meetings three times a week, during which it was hoped that they could discuss any issues which arose on the ward or on visits home. They attended school, organised social activities such as going to the cinema or park, ate meals together, and helped with shopping, cooking, and keeping the unit tidy.

The realities of work on a hospital ward posed additional difficulties for working together as a group. The group's membership fluctuated as new patients arrived and others went home. Children stayed in hospital for anything from a short, six-week admission, to a long-term stay of over a year. Leaving hospital and returning home happened gradually over an extended period, so that the child would know the exact date of her departure, perhaps a month in advance, and could begin preparations for returning home. Thus, a child who was on the ward at other times might miss this group to spend a day at their home school. This made it challenging to hold on to a sense of the continuity of the group. However, these comings and goings were routinely discussed among the members.

The children came from a range of ethnic backgrounds, and were drawn from across the country. They ranged in age from nine to nearly sixteen years old, and there were usually between four and six children in the group. Most had been referred to our unit for specialist treatment after spending several weeks or months in hospitals closer to their homes, with little or no improvement in their condition. They might have experienced intrusive physical tests and medical interventions over several years before doctors began to explore the possibility of psychiatric treatment. Many defied conventional diagnoses, or had the symptoms of several, such as eating difficulties along with severe muscle pain that had no organic explanation. Their silence might convey a powerful feeling of hopelessness; a powerful unconscious assumption that they could not be helped. Almost all the children had strikingly different ways of relating, making communication within the group difficult at times.

Using themes

We discussed, and at times tried to run, an open-ended group in which the children used the materials supplied for the group as they liked (the only stipulations being that they could not use them to hurt others or damage the room). There is a powerful case to be made for this type of non-directive group. The introduction of a theme may feel like an unwanted intrusion, akin to medical interventions or the naso-gastric tube feeds that are used to nourish very anorexic children on the ward. It is important that the therapists explore among themselves how far the theme is helpful for the group, and to what extent it might be used to assuage the therapist's own need to have a structure and to feel confident in holding the strong emotions that might be expressed (McNeilly, 2006). Offering a theme may adversely affect the dynamics of the group, as the therapist takes on the role of the good, providing mother. The children in turn may feel placed in a position of dependency on the therapist which can, along the lines of Bion's description of the "dependent group", limit the development of interrelationships among the children (Bion, 1961; McNeilly, 2006, p. 32).

At times, we found we had a group who were able to feel contained by the strong structure we provided and work in a self-directed way. An idea suggested by one member might be taken up and form a running motif in the work of the others; each exploring it differently. At one stage, we had a group of five girls and one boy. They had been on the ward together for many months, and four of them were moving toward health and returning home. In the first session after a Christmas break, Miranda, aged twelve, the first child about to return home, painted a deadly-looking skull and crossbones, which she said she had learned to do from Lydia, a very anorexic patient who had recently returned to a unit nearer home although still very ill. Miranda finished this piece of work, then took another piece of paper and painted a heart with a jagged line through it, as if it were broken. She filled it in with hollow eyes that echoes the skull, and a frosty white border that cut the heart off from the rest of the page.

Over the next two weeks, other group members were able to take up and explore these strong images of death and life, and death-within-life in different ways. Hearts might start off red and vibrant, and become spoiled and poo-coloured. Joanna was a twelve-year-old girl who had been admitted in a state of *pervasive retreat from life* and had made great strides towards recovery, including spending time at home. She asked Miranda to paint her a skull and crossbones, then surrounded it with hearts and wrote: "PAARTY!!" in big letters. We wondered about acknowledging a feeling that some deadly thoughts still plagued her, even as she began to return to normal life. In the third session after the break, one of the newer admissions, Jean, aged ten, continued the heart theme by creating heart-shaped badges for each of the children, to signal their membership of the group. In this group, Miranda returned to her initial image and painted a heart filled with a richly coloured, ornate abstract design, suggesting to us an internal world that was coming to life in the context of group relationships, a step forward from the ghoulish heart cut off from lively contact with others by its frosty barrier.

At other times we found it helpful to offer the group a brief suggestion of a theme. This was particularly useful when there were a number of new or very ill children on the ward. Such a group, left completely undirected, might be overwhelmed by the powerful projections of profoundly ill children, some of whom were being kept alive against their will by nasogastric feeding, to which they objected, and constant supervision. As therapists we might face a tremendous attack throughout the hour on what we had to offer, on our capacity to continue thinking and engaging with the children, and on the whole idea of a "creative" group. Within the firm boundaries of the group setting, the gentle introduction of a theme could awaken in the children a deeper awareness of their thoughts and feelings about issues they had in common: sharing space, whether with siblings or other patients, for instance, ideas about growing up, or being apart from their families.

Before the group, the co-therapists met and discussed a possible idea for that week's session. At the start of the group Naomi, as co-leader, introduced the theme. She spoke gently, as if offering an invitation, and used as few words as possible, to leave the idea open to interpretation. The therapists might then elaborate and discuss the theme a little among themselves, opening up the idea to the children. The suggestion was that we welcomed the children's help in developing the theme but also that there was no requirement to participate. If we had a group with members who struggled to remain seated, we would generally move around the group as little as possible. However, often Tara and the nurse who was working with the group, would sit with the children, arranging themselves next to those who might need extra support, while Naomi would stand. Placing herself a little outside the group in this way helped reinforce the feeling that she was there to observe and contain the group, but was without expectation that the children would work or behave in a certain way. We had two brief guidelines in forming themes. Usually, the idea came from the children's own concerns or experience, or from an idea or issue raised in a previous creative group. When we suggested a theme, we tried to include the idea of opposites, in order to stimulate thinking about different possibilities. For instance, near the time of a young person's returning home to live, we might suggest thinking about, "saying goodbye and saying hello". If one week we sensed a preoccupation with the difficulties of sharing the materials or the attention of staff, with one or other child dominating the group, or pouring out vast rivers of paint, we might try to explore the idea of, "too little, too much".

When there were new children on the ward anxiety was often high. Then, we used simple exercises to encourage the group to begin working together. We might suggest that they write or paint their name and decorate it in a way that said something about them. We hoped this might encourage them to begin to explore their internal worlds and communicate these within the group. Occasionally, we felt we had a group with a broader cultural frame of reference, which could try something more ambitious. Then, we might suggest illustrating their favourite fairy story, and telling the group about it. A theme beginning with a round of speaking or suggestions often worked well. Even very resistant children were excited and interested in the idea of "opposites". They took turns to suggest pairs of contradictory concepts ("dark and light", "life and death", "calm and anger"). They then illustrated these, and began thinking about extremes of emotion that they might experience, and the possibility of a middle ground between these.

Groups with more time available to them might find that after a small settling in exercise, the children are more able to work on their own ideas. If the children are not able to begin thinking, or indeed, if they are actively avoiding thinking about something that might be painful, such as a departure, a small suggestion such as this may help them begin to make use of the materials and the time, which in our case was limited to just one hour. A good resource for further themes, which covers working with eating disorders on an inpatient unit, is *Art Therapy for Groups: A Handbook of Themes and Exercises* by Marian Liebmann. In the Appendix, we have also suggested some themes for groups.

At the end of each group, we set aside ten minutes for group members to share and think about each other's work. Many found this period extremely difficult. Some would try and continue painting until the end of the hour, filling more paper with paint in order to avoid thinking. Others refused to show their work at all, or discovered that they needed to go to the toilet very urgently and could not wait. We gently encouraged them to pause and at least remain seated so that those who were able could gather and share some thoughts with each other. We also felt it was important for the children to experience the end of the group together.

Beginnings

Despite their different symptoms, all the children in our group had great difficulty putting their thoughts and feelings into words. They did not verbalise their anxiety or distress, but showed it in non-verbal ways and through their symptoms. We aimed, then, to help them begin to express themselves through the medium of art, using colour, plasticine, and different kinds of paper, paint, pastels, pencils, or pens. As the children handled and used these very concrete, tactile materials, we gradually observed developments in their capacity for symbolic thought. Powerful internal feelings and conflicts became more visible when represented in their clay work and paintings (Case, 2005). As these slowly came to be shared and thought about within the group, the children made moves, small ones, towards leaving behind their extreme isolation, even beginning friendships with others in the group.

Very primitive states of mind could be absorbed and held within the artwork and the group setting over time. These intense feelings could be reflected on very slowly when there was a sense that the child was ready to digest the meaning contained in her artwork (Killick, 1993).

With a very ill child we would let her be, and observe, for several sessions. It might take weeks for a child to move from doing nothing at all, sitting with eyes shut and body slumped in a wheelchair, to looking, then touching some clay, or tearing at some paper. She might gradually signal an interest in one material or another, simply by looking at it for a prolonged period of time. Observing this, we might offer her the plasticine or the paper she had been looking at, to hold and feel. She might then notice the presence of another mind, considering her needs and wishes, with whom she could begin to communicate.

It often took several months before a severely ill child was able to participate in the group in any way at all. During this period, we observed closely the way she used bodily movements to communicate states of mind. After several weeks of sitting motionless in his wheelchair, with his eyes shut, Oliver, a fourteen-year-old boy *pervasively retreating* from life, began to lean more and more to the left, until it looked like he might fall from his chair onto the floor. We noticed this and reflected aloud on the idea that he might be protesting about being in the group, trying to take himself out of it by keeping his eyes shut and forcing his body away from the group.

Each part of the body might communicate a different state of mind. Lydia, a severely anorexic twelve-year-old, would often extend her legs out stiffly under the table, moving them rapidly up and down. This might signal an attack on the group, and an allegiance to an internal "gang" state of mind (Rosenfeld, 1971). But on top of the table, her hands might be drawing quick, sharp lines on the paper. Her eyes would dart from one child's page to another's, taking in their work and ideas. Thus, parts of her were able to participate in the group work, even though the constant, repetitive movement of her legs helped her avoid thinking and using her creativity.

When a new child entered the group, she might hover at its edges, joining in at times, unable to participate at others. She might communicate her difficulty in participating by acting out physically, standing away from the table, or going back and forth. On one occasion, we planned a session on the theme of "we are" to try and encourage the group to begin to work together. At this point, the children were either avoiding the group altogether by standing away from the table, or drawing the staff into very powerful dyadic relationships. It was difficult to think about the existence of a group at all. The exercise involved tracing around the hand of a partner, and decorating it. The children then glued the cut-out hands onto a large sheet of paper. We considered that this might inspire the children to begin to think about the other group members and reflect on what it was like to be together. There were four members of the group present in this session, ranging in age from twelve to fourteen.

Although she had been in the group for nearly a year, Lydia was often unable to participate in the work. We experienced her as cold and aloof, isolated from the rest of the children. In this session, she chose to stand in the corner of the room, near a long counter, looking away from the group. Her chin jutted upwards defiantly, and her dry lips were pressed firmly together, letting nothing in. She moved slowly from one foot to the other, staring at the bare wall with blank eyes. As the session progressed, she glanced over furtively, eyeing from behind her hair the colourful materials and the other children working together. Her jogging on the spot became more frenetic as the session went on. The other children's creativity and efforts to work together may have evoked increasingly intense anxiety and envy. She kept moving her legs, concentrating on the constant, physical repetition, to help her avoid thinking about these painful feelings.

When the group had finished and the table was tidied up, Tara, one of the co-leaders, observed Lydia still standing on her own by the counter. She was tracing around the edge of a coin, using it to draw a number of circles that came together to make a flower. In plain pencil on white paper, it was a stark contrast to the richly illustrated and colourful hands the other children had created. It highlighted an important point about the nature of Lydia's relationships at this time. Just as she had determinedly held herself aloof from the group, drawing around an inanimate object signalled that she did not wish to think about anyone else too deeply, nor have another person "get under her skin" by tracing her hand. Moreover, by doing her work outside the group's time and setting, she was effectively attacking the group itself.

Lydia's isolation illustrates many of the difficulties of establishing a group with this type of young person. To enter a relationship with another person might evoke feelings of dependence which were, for Lydia, unbearable and unthinkable at this time (Rosenfeld, 1964). Money, symbolised by the coin around which Lydia chose to draw, enabled her to cling to the notion of her omnipotent status without the need to encounter her own sense of responsibility, her own vulnerability, or concern for another person. During the session described above, we observed Lydia's stance and movements. We reflected on these aloud to encourage the others to keep her in mind, and bring her within the life of the group, asking, "I wonder how everyone feels about Lydia, standing by herself over there?", and, "Can anyone think of something that might help Lydia join us at the table?" These anxieties were powerful and her desire to sabotage the group often, as in this case, proved destructive to our attempts to think and work with her. The possibility of coming together to think seemed too painful for her to bear (Rosenfeld, 1964). For a long time, Lydia projected quite a deadly state of mind, into us and the rest of the group. As we attempted to talk about what might be going on with the children, our thoughts were cut off, we would struggle to continue thinking and observing the children as we came under this deadening attack. We often felt confused, wondering, "What on earth is the point of all this?" At other times, we found ourselves feeling very anxious that the group might fall apart.

At the beginning of working with such very ill children, we relied a great deal on our awareness of the countertransference: the feelings evoked within us by the group. During the session, we might be aware of bearing intense confusion and deep anxieties. We might feel hopeless, as if the effort was pointless; upset and anxious about the mess created by the group, or angry or frustrated as our few, carefully chosen words met with blank, uncomprehending stares. Throughout the session we kept an observant eye on the development of these feelings within ourselves, noting carefully how they might be linked to a particular state of mind that the child was projecting. After the group, we discussed these countertransference feelings along ourselves and tried to make sense of them. By doing this, we were beginning the process of communicating with the child; and in turn by keeping his or her mental state in mind, demonstrating that these feelings could be given words. All of the children with whom we worked had a very intense wish for an all-consuming dyadic relationship with the group's therapists. We often felt drawn to talk with or think exclusively about one child in the group. It was a constant challenge to keep the entirety of the group process in mind.

Developing communication within the group

Isabel

In order to develop communication within the group, we paid close attention to their non-verbal interaction. Isabel, aged twelve, who was *pervasively retreating from life*, spent her first months on the ward hunched over in a wheelchair, without moving or speaking. Her hair covered her face, and saliva and urine dribbled from her. The group leaders observed her, and reflected on how withdrawn she seemed. After a while, co-therapist Naomi began to ask if she wanted to touch something, indicating the materials on the table. For many weeks, she refused. One week, Naomi placed some pink, orange, and green coloured tissue paper in front of her and, after looking at it for a while, she took the orange tissue paper and began to tear it. She then ripped up the rest of the paper, taking more and more, until it had all been shredded. She sat back, looking exhausted, the pile of torn paper in front of her. Tearing tissue paper was the beginning of Isabel's participation in the group. It became her lifeline to the rest of the group. Its softness, pliability, and transparency seemed to appeal to her. As she tore it, it became a container for her anger. The other children watched, and seemed to be thinking about what she had done. One by one, they reached for the torn paper and considered it, looking at it, and getting a feel for it themselves. One child began to experiment with making tissue-paper flowers from the shredded bits, and gradually the others joined in, creating something quite beautiful out of the fragmented, angry mess Isabel had dumped on the table. We came to see the tissue paper as serving the function of a placenta for Isabel. It held her toxic, destructive feelings. It also offered her the possibility of containment and nourishment from the rest of the group, who explored the torn shreds and returned them to her transformed (Bion, 1962).

This session showed us how Isabel had an embryonic notion of a mind that might help her contain her strong feelings and think about them (Bion, 1962). In the sessions that followed, she continued this theme, tearing and cutting tissue, getting rid of her anger. After a number of sessions, perhaps recalling the way the group had used the shredded tissue paper, she began to stick it in colourful patterns onto a sheet of paper. In subsequent groups, she chose to work with other tactile materials, moulding plasticine and playdough. Her progress was not straightforward. In the first session after the Christmas break, she regressed:

> Isabel was pale, with a sad face. She started spitting again and she was looking down. She refused to touch the paint or paper, but as the session went on she started to look at them. At one stage she raised her hand, as though she wanted to start, but she did not.

In the next session, the theme was "a fantasy island in the sea". Again, Isabel was pale, looking down, and did not respond to the group leaders' welcome.

> Andy, a fellow young person, sat with Isabel. She didn't show any interest to start with but slowly, with an agonised face, she started to look over at what he was doing. She stopped spitting and looked tense, but looked and nodded as she gradually became involved in what Andy was doing.

The following week, Isabel was sitting up straight and was not spitting. As Naomi, one of the group leaders, came into the room, Isabel looked up, looked startled for a moment, then smiled.

> During the session, Isabel's face was shining with excitement and laughter. She was moulding the playdough into different animals. From time to time, she looked straight at Naomi, nodded her head and made a sound, to indicate that she wanted another colour of playdough.

During the following week, Isabel started crawling around the ward, moving her lips and trying to whisper, although she was not speaking audibly. One step forward in the group created anxiety in her, and she was ill during the next session, and spent it sleeping on a sofa, away from the group. Her head was covered by a blanket, and the group expressed their concern for her. The next week, she was waiting expectantly in the room. The theme was "under and above".

> One by one they started. Briony began talking to Isabel, suggesting what Isabel could do. Isabel asked Briony to guess what she was going to do, then requested tissue paper. From that moment, Isabel was busy. She took a piece of paper, cut out a circle, then took some tissue paper and stuck it on, making eyes and a smiling mouth. Then she stuck silver stripes on the figure. When she was finished, she showed it to everybody, looking very pleased and proud of herself. This was a huge step forward for her.

Isabel continued with her own theme of cutting and tearing tissue paper, but her work had begun to take on more of a symbolic feel (Segal, 1957). There was a sense that she could begin to tolerate her emotional experience rather than closing down her mind and her body. When a new child, Jenny, joined the group a few months later, Isabel chose to sit next to her, and very gently and with sensitivity helped her begin to look at the materials. In one session, the theme was "day and night". Jenny found it difficult to begin, but Isabel's warm encouragement helped her.

> Jenny chose to paint the dark night. All her flowers and trees were dead. Isabel painted a bright sun in the middle of the page. She painted some colourful flowers, but empathising with Jenny, she also painted a tree with a few autumn leaves falling down, close to Jenny's dead tree. As she worked, Isabel seemed serious and grown-up. When she looked over at Jenny, her gaze was warm and maternal.

It seemed that by this stage, fifteen months into her admission, Isabel had internalised a helpful, caring object through her participation in the group. She became one of the most popular children on the ward, talking and laughing confidently and listening to others. At times Isabel still seemed to retreat from the world, but she was more resilient than before as shown, nineteen months later, by her capacity to integrate into mainstream school.

Making interpretations

It was a constant challenge to develop the therapeutic nature of the group. Although we frequently reflected on Lydia's behaviour, for instance, and encouraged her to show her work to the group, she was rarely able to do so. Any talk or interpretation was anathema to her, and to most of the children. Thoughts or reflections offered by the staff would be belittled or fiercely rejected. On one occasion, feeling intruded upon, Lydia demanded furiously, "Can't I keep something private, for myself?", leaving us feeling violently pushed away. Observing the strength of her feeling, we interpreted it as a countertransference, communicating to us the force with which she herself had felt attacked by our words. In general, we tried to address the children's states of mind less directly, addressing our thoughts to the group as a whole, in the hope that each child might be able to take something in.

This group often retreated from our comments. The children might be able to access painful experiences momentarily, but this was often fleeting and such difficult feelings were sometimes rapidly expelled. Occasionally, we offered interpretations to the children. However, it was our experience that these must be very well-digested, "chewed-over" interventions if they were not to be experienced as violently intrusive, and increase the child's already profound anxiety (Steiner, 1993). In the case of Isabel, Lydia, and other patients suffering from anorexia nervosa or *pervasively retreating from life,* it seemed more important to bear consistently within ourselves what was so unbearable for the child: the profound anxiety or "nameless dread" (Bion, 1962) against which their symptoms of not speaking, not eating, and not walking were so powerful a defence.

This approach enabled most of the children to begin gradually to open up to the group. We encouraged this process by consistently trying to extend a comment made by one group member to the others, inviting them to share thoughts and experiences. They began by sharing materials, requesting pencils or scissors, passing them back and forth between each other as a way of being in the group. Gradually, they shared ideas and commented on each others' work. One week, Melissa, a twelve-year-old girl with severe obsessive compulsive disorder, had drawn dark shadows in charcoal and covered it with gold glitter. We had reflected on the extremes of darkness and light in her picture. She had gone on to paint a well-rooted, leafy tree surrounded by blue sky, which the group felt represented something more grounded, an idea of growth and development. Having kept in mind the previous drawing and the discussion surrounding it, the next week Lydia used the paints for the first time in the group, painting blue waves. These echoed Melissa's sky of the previous week. The group experience had enabled Lydia to experiment with an idea of something more hopeful.

Lydia increasingly made sure that her work was seen by the therapists, initially holding it up backwards in front of us, so that the light would shine behind the paper revealing the image on the other side. Then, she began to leave it openly on the table during the session so we could look at it. If we spoke about it, she would retreat rapidly, hiding the paper or throwing it away. It seemed enough that she knew we had seen her work and were holding it in mind. Initially, she was preoccupied with drawing figures that looked like the sketches of couture designers: stick-thin girls drenched in stylish clothes. Over several months, Lydia put one or two pieces of work in her folder rather than in the recycling bins. Each week, she would make a tiny addition to one of these, before returning them to the folder and starting on something else. We spoke to the group about our feeling that some pieces of work represented something perfect and beautiful; while others were unsatisfactory, ugly, and were thrown away. Lydia did not speak, but she listened with interest as the others discussed having a "perfectionist streak" and not liking their own work very much.

Gradually, Lydia's work began to capture more of the terrifying objects that peopled her internal world. In one session, for instance, she drew in pencil on plain paper a very thin, unclothed figure in a small cubicle reminiscent of a changing room in a clothes shop. Around the girl, she sketched thin, black figures, prodding at the girl with outstretched spikes that looked like little devils attacking her. In a later group, she drew a large shark with very prominent, sharp teeth. Near the shark's mouth were three small fish, one of which had a speech bubble, saying, "We've got to get out of here!" Lydia may have been developing a perspective on the deadly object within which she felt trapped. Here, she was able to represent this and think about it. She seemed to express a wish to escape the biting teeth that snapped at her, representing, perhaps, very entrenched, destructive parts of the self (M. Klein, 1958).

In one group session, four children were present, all of whom Lydia knew very well. We chose not to have a theme in this instance, as the group were all very familiar with each other and seemed to be working well. There was a lot of banter back and forth over the materials, and the children, including Lydia, passed pens and a rubber across the table, sharing them and perhaps feeling that this was a way they could all come together. In this session, Lydia drew a three-dimensional picture of a house with a door and, inside, a cosy sofa and a cabinet with drawers. We wondered whether, in the safe confines of the group, she was beginning to have an experience of herself as person with a space inside for thinking and containing thoughts (Bion, 1962).

Progress was never linear, and a thoughtful, working group might be followed by one in which the children seemed to move backwards, spurning all attempts at communication with words. As they settled in to the group and began to participate, they might start to draw more on other defences, such as sarcasm, singing loudly, laughing, or denigrating what the group was doing. Even as she started making her work more visible to the rest of the group, and standing at the table, rather than some way away, Lydia might say that a theme was "boring" or tell us, disparagingly, that we "sound like therapists". Moreover, one effect of a very ill child joining the group, as happened at regular intervals, was that the others might revert back to earlier ways of interacting, showing how difficult it was for them to continue to participate.

When Oliver, a Polish immigrant boy aged fourteen, pervasively retreating from life, first joined the group, his verbal communications were limited to muttering, "yes", "no", and "ow". He sat immobile, physically cut off from the rest of the group by his immense wheelchair, a deep, black cocoon covered in wires and buttons. At this stage, Oliver's eyes were always closed and he held his head tilted upwards at an uncomfortable angle that ensured he was facing away from the group. In Oliver's second session with the group, four children were present, working on a group project called "A Garden Centre".

> Oliver is sitting in his chair, eyes closed, hands in his lap, lank hair covering his face. He begins to say, "Ow, ow". "Are you in pain, Oliver?", asks Lydia. "Does your head hurt?" asks Lydia. Oliver murmurs, "Nuuuhh". His head is bent down so that his chin almost touches his chest. "Does your stomach hurt?" Oliver persists, saying, "Nuuhhh ...". "Is it a physical pain?" Lydia asks. He seems to say, "Yuuh". We wonder what it might be, and Tara asks if he could give us more of an idea of how we can help. Tara suggests that it might be difficult to be part of a group that seems to be doing something interesting together, and yet not to take part. Oliver begins to say, "Ow" again. Tara asks if he would like to hold some plasticine, and he says, "Nuh" again. He seems to retreat entirely from us at this point, his eyes close firmly.

During this session, despite having participated and worked well together the week before, none of the children seemed able to think about the topic or the materials. We had encouraged them to consider all the different elements of a garden centre; plants, animals, sacks of fertiliser - whatever struck their fancy. Sophie, aged twelve, had talked a lot about what she would do, wondering about creating a shop full of pots and trinkets. In the end, she simply made a criss-cross pattern of flat, black strips of paper that looked like a trellis, saying she didn't feel like creating a shop after all. It seemed Sophie had backed away from the idea of a shop, which might have contained some rich, interesting objects, and held on to the safety of this simple, repetitive framework. A sense of flatness, and desperate boredom, was something that the staff on the ward often noticed in the countertransference when working with Oliver at this stage of his admission. It seemed that this numbness had been projected into the other children in the group as well.

As we began to get to know the children, this kind of countertransference information could also be used within the multidisciplinary team at the hospital to help teachers, social workers, and nurses understand how the children affected other people, and help them grasp, and perhaps mitigate, some of the difficulties they might encounter in everyday relationships. In the session above, co-therapist Tara considered that at times she had been overwhelmed by Oliver's anxiety, resorting to asking repeated questions and trying to help fix and assuage his painful feelings, rather than thinking about them. In fact, we realised during discussions within the multidisciplinary team that this way of interacting with Oliver followed a similar pattern to that noticed in his family therapy. His family seemed to have difficulty being aware of his painful feelings. The parents felt the need to make everything better for him by ensuring his physical comfort.

Oliver began to build an increasingly warm and trusting relationship with the therapists and the other children in the group. Lydia, in particular, seemed to develop her own capacities for relating to her silent peer, thinking about what Oliver might be experiencing, and wondering how to help him. Her questions, in the session described above, and at other times, seemed in turn to foster Oliver's ability to be with her and with the group. He became increasingly able to express himself, and began to state more clearly what he wanted. He started by making simple choices about what to cut out and which colour pen to use (at this point, he was still far from being able to hold the pen himself). In the session described below, Oliver was cutting out pictures from magazines to make collages:

> Naomi asks Oliver what he would like to look at. She mishears what he says, "Buuhhh", thinking he has said, "Birds." She says they can look through and find pictures of birds. Oliver tips back his head, and although his eyes are still closed he starts to laugh. He repeats what he has said, it is, "Bikes" His laughter is deep and genuine and his shoulders are shaking. Naomi laughs too and they begin to look through the magazine about bikes. Oliver is very definite that he wants her to cut out the picture of a motorcyclist on the front cover.

Oliver's laughter in this session was a world away from the profound depression he had communicated just weeks earlier. Following this, Oliver gradually seemed more alive and at home with the other children. He started to open his eyes, looking around, dazed and blinking, as if waking from a long sleep. He began to try to communicate with the other children, laughing at their jokes, and participating in a group discussion about whether or not they liked being part of a group, saying that he had enjoyed sleepovers at home. He also began to talk in the group and to nurses on the ward about feeling that his work was rubbish and that everything that came out of his mind was useless nonsense.

Towards the end of the year, two sessions before we would take a break for the summer, we used the materials as a theme, putting lots of coloured tissue and crepe paper on the table, along with glue and newspaper. We briefly showed the children how they could model a doll out of newspaper, with a ball of paper for the head. Some children chose to cut up and stick the paper. Tara, the group's co-leader asked Oliver what he would like to do, and he looked at a ball of paper we had used to show the group how they could make a doll's head. He asked her to cover it in blue tissue paper, and studied it again. He said that the doll looked like a woman in a wedding dress. Then, he moved away from this thought and decided it was a superhero, first called "Paper Boy", then, "Tree Boy". Tree Boy could move across continents by flying underground through the mud, which then settled back into place as though he had never been there. Oliver wondered where Tree Boy might live, thinking about America, then Mars, then decided this was too unoriginal, and settling on Saturn. He talked about this superhero in sentences, albeit in a voice so low Tara had to lean over him to catch his words. This was such a startling contrast to Oliver's arrival as a nearly mute boy, *pervasively retreating from life* with his eyes shut and his face tilted away from us. At the beginning of this session, Oliver had picked up the ball of paper the art therapist had made, and considered how to use it. He seemed to acknowledge a wish to forge a creative and thoughtful link, represented by the woman in the wedding dress he described. Yet he needed to move away quickly from this idea and perhaps the feelings of vulnerability and dependence it engendered within him (Rosenfeld, 1964). "Paper Boy" was too close to the original material, "Tree Boy" perhaps one step further removed. It seemed that the wish for a connection then took a very concrete form in his mind. He could not continue holding onto and working with the materials symbolically. Moving away from the experience of a connection, Oliver became a superhero, omnipotent and far removed from the anxieties stirred up by everyday experiences of desire and separation, and the relationships he needed to sustain life. He struggled to grasp and spell the name of the city he had in mind; then moved away from these feelings of frustration to settle on a distant planet. Describing the mud through which he flew, Oliver seemed to be articulating an experience of trying to stir up others with these muddled feelings in which he was trapped. Yet he found that they settled back again as if he had never been there, leaving these emotions unacknowledged and unmentalized, in the realm of Bion's beta elements (Bion, 1962). As he spoke, we had the sense of a frightening, disorientating experience that might lead one to question one's own existence.

Over the summer break, Oliver started to hold a cup himself to drink, raising it slowly and shakily at first, then more confidently. In the first session after the break, he picked up a pencil for the first time and began to draw.

> He points at one figure, and says this is a monster on a plank. Below him is a second monster, with very sharp teeth, resting in some deep water. Oliver says he has written, "Help me!" coming out of the first monster's mouth. Underneath the monster he has written his own name.

However, when, at the end of the session, Oliver shared his work with the rest of the group, he changed the story. This time, he said, the monster on top was stamping on the monster on the bottom. The sign that said "Help me!" was actually the monster's foot, stamping down on the biting monster below. It seemed that he had altered his story to communicate something hopeful to the rest of the group: that the monster illness could be stamped on. He seemed to agree with this idea, then let his head droop, his eyes closing slightly as if he was exhausted.

We recalled the seemingly endless weeks of watching Oliver sit nearly motionless in his chair, with his head bowed and his eyes closed, and the deep anxiety and frustration with which we were filled at the time. We considered that the time we had spent holding his then "nameless dread", which perhaps had not been well contained before. This allowed him, after six months, not only to make the breakthrough of holding a pencil, but also to communicate to the rest of the group a message of hope and recovery.

Endings: developing symbolic thought

Oliver's last session came about suddenly. He had successfully attended school one day a week, and it was decided that this would be extended to two, meaning that he would miss the group for the last weeks of his admission. For some months, he had been walking unaided, eating well, and chatting, albeit often in a low, hesitant voice, with the other children. He came to his last session early, and got down to work straight away. He spent the first few minutes looking through the work he had done in previous sessions, and we reflected on how far he had come.

He then took a pencil, and a large sheet of paper. He seemed to have confidence that he could fill it. He drew a giant sketch of a man on a motorbike, leaning sideways as if turning a corner at great speed. His pencil strokes were bold and dark, full of potency and movement, and the group commented on how different this was from his more hesitant, smaller drawings of previous weeks. He then turned the paper over. He drew a much smaller figure of a boy, holding a skateboard. He then drew something in the boy's other hand. Unsure of what it was, we commented that it looked like the knife he had drawn a couple of weeks ago. Oliver turned it into a plank of wood with a nail in it. We asked whether it was to hurt someone or to build something, and he said he didn't know. He drew another, shadowy figure behind the first. The group wondered about this figure: was he friendly? Oliver drew a speech bubble saying "Hello!" coming out of the shadow's mouth, and another saying "Shit!" coming out of the skateboarder's mouth.

This prompted a group discussion about the difficulties faced by those leaving the ward. Would the world outside be a scary place? Would they need to be armed with strong defences? Would people be welcoming and friendly, or hostile, and how can one tell? How could they hold on to feelings of friendship and an idea of health and potency nurtured on the ward? Can these feelings of potency be creative and aggressive at the same time? This group seemed to have developed some capacity to bear the anxiety that might have been raised in considering these difficult transitions. Oliver had represented his feelings of nervousness and defensiveness, as well as a sense of his own potency and a wish to move forward. No longer overwhelming, dreadful, and unnamed, these feelings were opened up for thought and discussion.

Conclusion

We have shown how establishing a creative group on an inpatient psychiatric unit including children pervasively retreating from life, not talking, walking, and eating; those with eating disorders; somatising disorders; and other diagnoses, enabled non-speaking children to make significant advances in their ability to think symbolically and creatively. This in turn aided their recovery from illness. At the beginning, the non-speaking child is communicating in other ways, using the body and symptoms. As she develops her ability to represent her internal state in art and, gradually, with words, these symptoms were less needed as protections against anxiety.

In working with the children on our ward, we encountered a complex interaction between deficit, defence, temperament, and life experience. Deficits in mentalization made it difficult for children to process painful emotions. A fragile ego, without the resources to integrate distressing experiences, or overwhelmed by traumatic ones, needs to evacuate these using powerful defences of splitting and projection in order to survive (Bion, 1962). Disowned, these states of mind are no longer available for integration and development, weakening the ego further and increasing its reliance on defensive processes that make further development difficult. One aspect or another may predominate in a particular child, but the whole picture must be kept in mind (Alvarez, 2006).

Working with very ill children, it was particularly important to ensure that the group had a strong containing structure (Elmhirst, 1988). We negotiated a regular time and space, and consistent group leaders. In addition, we arranged to have time before and after the group to think about the work, and had weekly supervision. This gave us the space to explore what had been communicated non-verbally in the transference and countertransference, and to consider how these thoughts might, over time, be reflected back gently to the children in the group. We have suggested that this valuable information could usefully be fed back to the multidisciplinary team, enhancing others' work with the children on the unit. We have drawn deeply on the Tavistock's Model of Infant Observation. We have shown how we used this attention to unspoken communication through the body, facial expressions, projected states of mind, and the countertransference to develop our understanding of the children in the group. We deployed the same technique to help us understand how the children used movement and their bodies as a communication. We have shown how different parts of the body might be simultaneously communicating different states of mind; how a wish to work with the group might co-exist with an equally strong desire to run away from it or attack it. When a child did not speak, we regarded everything that she did in the group as a communication, from her choice of crayon colour and the force with which she put the crayon to the paper, to whether or not she was able to sit at the table. In an infant observation, we observe how the baby communicates his inner state through the way he uses his body: fists tightly clenched or legs kicking. In the absence of a mother's holding arms or containing mind, an infant will turn to repetitive activity, moving his legs backwards and forwards, for instance, to avoid a feeling that he is falling apart, dissolving into nothingness (Bick, 1964). In normal development, the baby experiences his mother's thoughtful processing of his different cries and body language, and begins to take in the idea that he can communicate with another. As he introjects mother's containing capacities, he begins to develop his own ability to think and tolerate psychic pain in the interest of development. Mindless actions and somatisation in response to intense affective states are decreased.

Often with the profoundly ill children on our ward, the process of recovery begins with work on these very infantile feelings. We considered that many of the non-speaking children with whom we work might have suffered a catastrophic series of failures of this kind of communication and containment in infancy, of primitive anxieties left for one reason or another too often uncontained and unmodulated by an empathetic caregiver. If this has not happened sufficiently in a child's early life, he might have to continue to rely to a great degree on very primitive processes, expelling or somatising painful feelings.

At the beginning, the non-speaking child will use the therapists and other members of the group as containers for these unprocessed emotional states. It is the role of the therapists to begin to help him to think about them. The team members must also spend time understanding the unsymbolised physical and mental states that have been projected into them.

We have discussed ways of gently offering insight and interpretation to the group. A mother who cannot receive her baby's communications, due to her own depression, preoccupation, or illness, is internalised as a hostile and cruel internal object. If she has also used the baby as a container for her own anxieties, his mind will have developed, from its earliest moments, as a vehicle for evacuating experience rather than for thinking thoughts (Mitrani, 1995). These were some of the harsh internal objects that we as co-therapists might meet in the transference. They made it difficult for the children to begin to imagine that we could offer benign, possibly helpful, ideas, which did not need to be expelled. We participated in a wider multidisciplinary team, whose dedicated work enabled the recovery of these profoundly ill children who did not speak. Their capacity to express their feelings through symbols, in drawings, artwork, and words, increased. Along with this, each non-speaking child developed her capacity to bear and think about the everyday difficulties and the ordinary pain of life. "Much will be gained", wrote Freud, "if we succeed in transforming... hysterical misery into common unhappiness" (*SE* 2, p. 305). For the children with whom we work, this meant a return to life and common pleasures too: talking, eating, walking, becoming closer to and more trusting of family members, making friends, and going to school.

Appendix

Themes that have been used for the creative group

Below are some self-portraits which have been drawn by children when they were withdrawn and not speaking

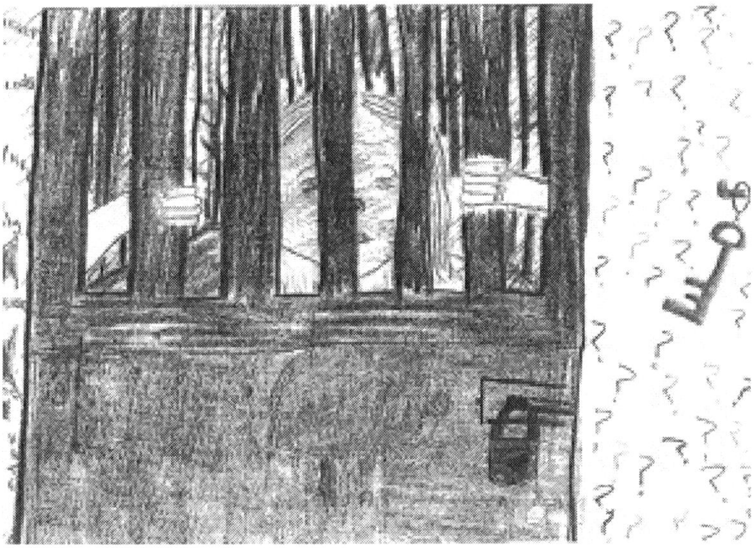

Figure 16.1 A child feeling imprisoned.

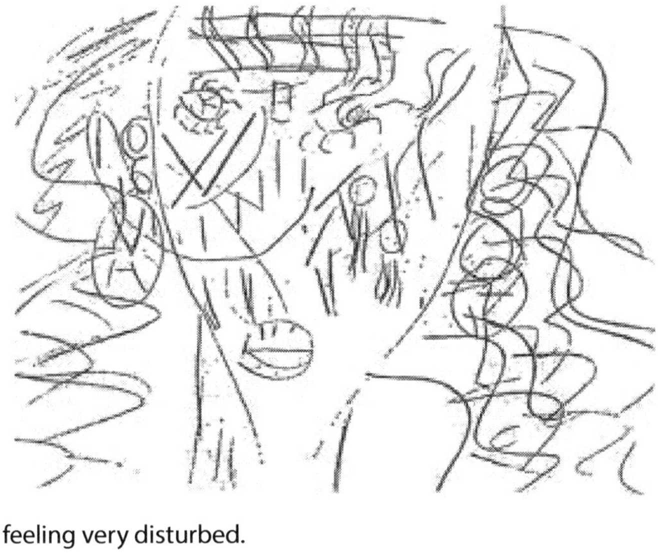

Figure 16.2 A child feeling very disturbed.

Introductory themes

Below are some introductory themes for groups in which several new non-speaking children are beginning to get to know each other and work together.

- Decorating folders: (which are then used to hold the child's work for the duration of her time in the group). These can be added to and altered throughout a child's time in the group.
- Self-portraits: These can be created using a variety of materials, including clay and paint. A child can explore how she sees herself. More established groups can add, how the child thinks others see her, how she would like to be seen.
- Names: write and illustrate your name.
- "We are a group": the children trace around each others' hands and illustrate the drawings. The hands can then all be pasted onto a larger piece of card and paper, representing the group coming together.
- Patterns: this can be a useful exercise when it seems difficult to begin. The child can choose a simple shape and repeat it in different ways, varying the size, colour, and overlap, and using different materials. It can be as simple or as ambitious as she wants.
- Materials: one kind of material could be put out for the children to explore. One week it might be tissue paper, which can be torn, cut, pasted and used in different ways to make sculptures and designs. Another week, paints could be put out with a variety of rollers and brushes so that the children can experiment with colour and texture.

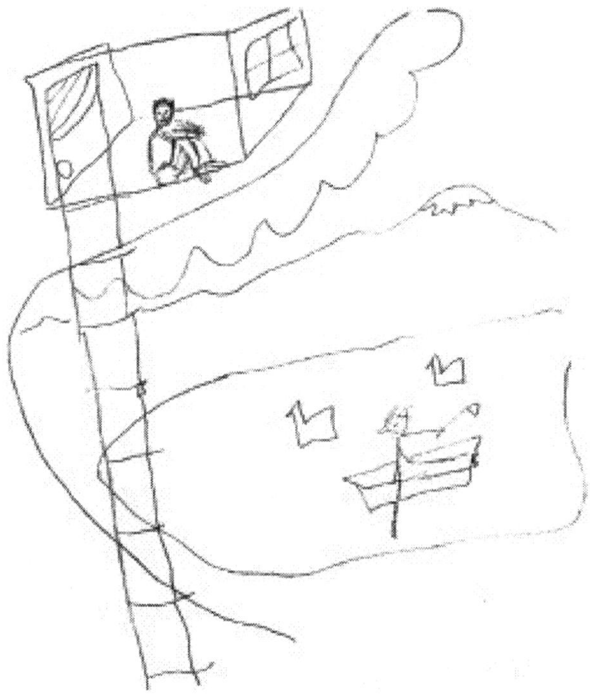

Figure 16.3 Boy feeling isolated from life.

- Variation on the Squiggle (Winnicott, 1958): the therapist draws a "squiggle" on a large sheet of paper and passes it to the child next to her. The child adds to the "squiggle" and passes it on. Each child develops the drawing, and it could go round the group several times. There is time for discussion afterwards about what has come out of this group effort.

More ambitious themes

These can be used for groups who have been working together for awhile. They are left deliberately open so that the children can place their own interpretation on the ideas.

- 'Being in and being out': the children can explore the idea of being in and out of the group, the family, or anywhere.

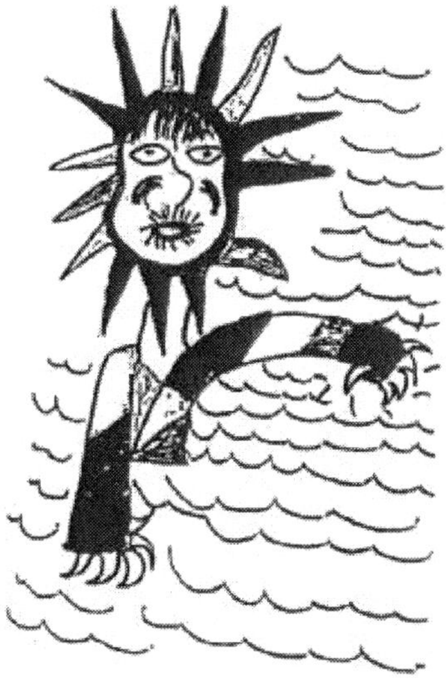

Figure 16.4 Nightmare of a terrifying lion drawn by a physically abused girl.

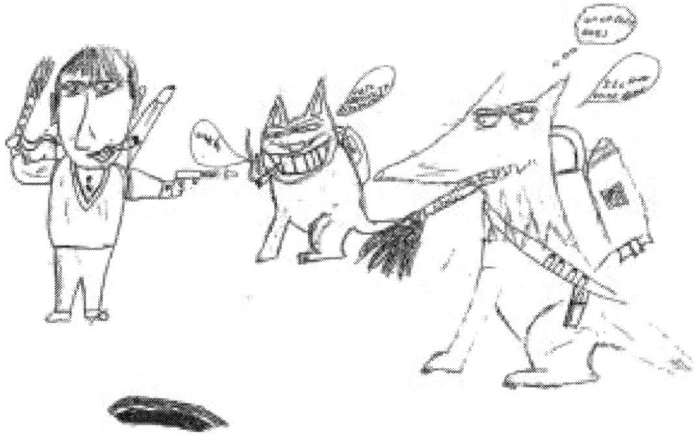

Figure 16.5 Fury with others.

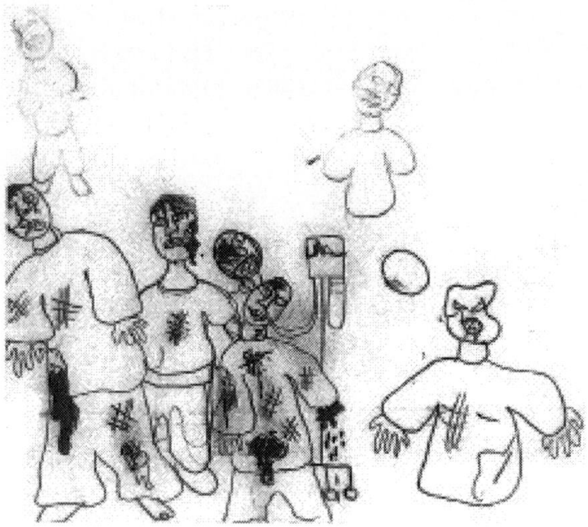

Figure 16.6 Persecutory ghost-like damaged figures: terror after being aggressive.

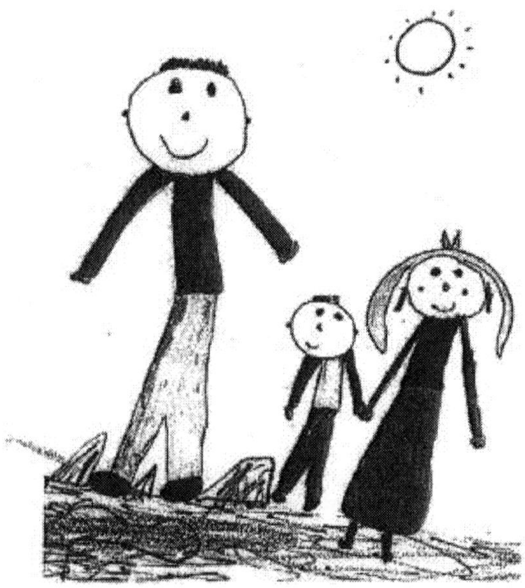

Figure 16.7 Idealised biological family of a physically abused, adopted boy.

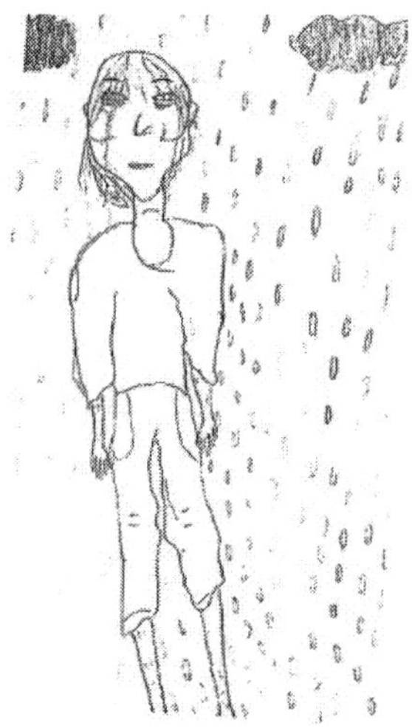

Figure 16.8 The sad girl.

- Seasons: "Now we are coming toward spring/summer/autumn/winter". As the year turns, the children can think about what each season means to them.
- "Opposites": the children take turns suggesting pairs of opposites, and someone writes them down. After they have gone round the group several times, the pairs can be read out, and each child can choose one set of opposites to illustrate.
- "Dreams and nightmares"

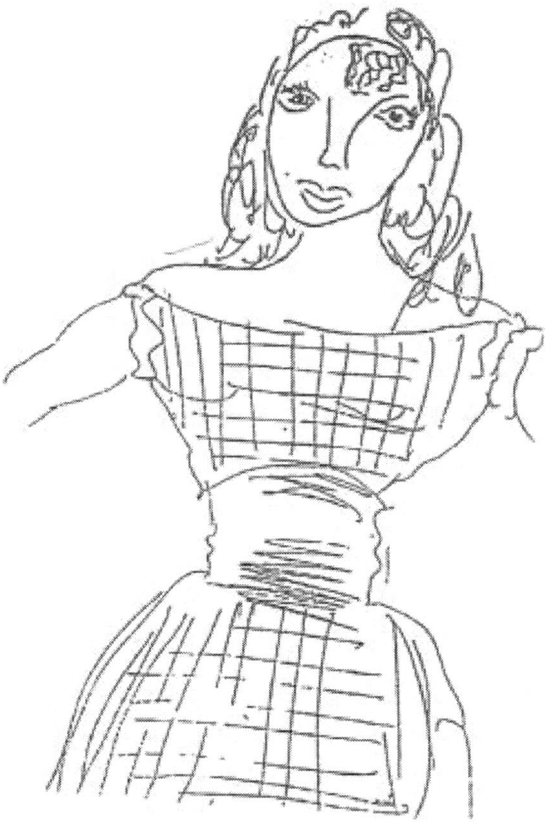

Figure 16.9 Drawn by previously mute, anorectic girl as she is becoming physically and mentally healthy.

- "Superheroes and villains"
- "Lies and truth—who is lying?"
- "Lost and found"
- "Leaving someone, or someplace" or "Saying goodbye": these are useful during the last sessions of a departing group member.

CHAPTER SEVENTEEN

Roar and rumpus: engaging non-speaking children through stories and songs

Charlotte Wormald and Natalie Le Clézio, with contribution by Ankur Sharma

Stories are central to every culture, to every family, and to each individual. Any understanding of who, where, and why we are, exists as a unique narrative thread that tells "our story". The power of the story partly comes from its nature as a two-fold, interconnected system: our story is how we understand ourselves and how we connect with others, while to connect with others is to share our story and to listen to others' stories. The listener makes space and time for the teller, and the teller offers a story for the listener. Listening to another's story, we identify similarities and can feel validated, understood, and even appreciated. We can see reflections of ourselves in these stories and use them to guide and develop our individual selves. In sharing a story, we can experience empathy and sympathy. Crucially, stories can inspire an understanding of a different perspective. The importance of differences reveals another fundamental role of stories: connecting the unknown with the known.

The sharing, building, and shaping of narratives underpins almost all therapeutic processes. The non-speaking child's story is being expressed through symptoms and illness, and so it comes to exist in a lonely and painful internal twilight, remaining untold and feeling "untellable". This chapter describes how the creative and thoughtful use of stories, poems, and songs can help the child to rediscover or develop his voice so that his story can be heard and understood.

We will trace the developmental challenges a non-speaking child might experience along his psychological journey, suggesting narrative forms that could be used to work on themes that are relevant to that particular stage. Each stage will work on a particular theme, but most themes and tasks can be interchanged with different stories.

Throughout this chapter, Jake, a ten-year-old Polish child, will be featured to exemplify our work with a child who is not speaking. His parents are over in the UK whilst his father undertakes a two-year business administration Master's Degree. Jake was admitted to the inpatient eating disorders unit six months after his arrival in the UK. This chapter will focus on the work being undertaken by his keyworkers, who are a therapeutic care worker and a nurse, assigned to Jake for the length of his stay. Their role is to manage his care plan and work with Jake alongside the members of the multidisciplinary team assigned to his care. However, the underlying principles, sharing a space, connecting and engaging with a non-speaking child through story books, poems, and music, can be taken up by any practitioner or parent. In the case of Jake, picture books seemed to be the most appropriate narrative tool with which to engage him; however, where appropriate, songs and poems have also been incorporated and explored as alternative examples of narrative, which might be more suitable for an older child.

A third narrative

Stories, poems and song lyrics can be used to reach out to and connect with a young person who has become isolated and disconnected. They can be used as tentative bridges between reality and fantasy connecting the known and the unknown and offering a containing space for thinking about that which has become intolerable. Narratives have beginnings, middles and ends, boundaries that give shape and structure to the experiences they describe. To a non-speaking young child, feeling chaotic and out of control, these narratives offer a safe, mutual space, a place from which to step back and reflect. Through them they can experience sharing words in a controlled and creative way even if at first their role is simply as the listener. Later the stories can be used to shed light on a situation and, eventually, to think about a problem in a different way. In time, the narratives might evoke a greater capacity to share the story of one's internal world of relationships with parents, siblings and significant others.

The reading of stories together is particularly suited to working with a younger child but might also be appropriate as a shared activity for an older child who has regressed psychologically, and for whom this type of nurturing activity can be a comfort. Often however for the older child reading has become a solitary activity and for him a connection can be made more readily through the oldest and most primal shared narratives: music and its close relative, poetry.

Music in particular is a salient tool of popular culture. It brings groups of young people together and helps them find both group and personal identities (Laiho, 2004; North & Hargreaves, 1999). A smash hit on MTV will be heard, downloaded, talked about, danced to and shared by young people worldwide. More importantly, music seems to be something that young people in distress still might seek out and maintain a connection to: via the radio, television, MP3 player or via each other. Music and poetry are narrative tools that are designed to be shared and experienced collectively. They are very emotive, and not only through their words, but also through their melody, mood, timbre and rhythm.

Stories, poems and song lyrics can be used to introduce communication and thinking about emotions into the non-speaking child's world in an indirect, non-threatening way. They function as a third narrative; an "in-between" story that is not about the young person or the person they are with, therefore offering a freedom to explore and imagine without fear of intrusion or giving away of the self. The most useful tools for this task can be any kind of human story that can be shared: picture books, poetry, music, paintings, old newspapers, in fact, even a particular ensemble of clothing, if one is to really engage the imagination.

Silence as communication

> On admission Jake was very distressed. He curled up in a ball and tucked himself into a tiny space between the sofa and the wall. His head was lowered and his face was covered with his hands. He made no noise, but his body seemed to shake with his crying. The other members of the group, including young people of different ages, tried to comfort him and offered him tissues and a glass of water. He did not respond to them and remained disconnected and very withdrawn from the group for several days. In meetings and at the table, he covered his face with his hands, and his head was lowered into his chest while his body was hunched.
>
> Later in the week, Jake is expected to attend the morning meeting at which the whole community is present. He has spent a long time in the toilet and his keyworker has had to knock on the door to remind him that the meeting is about to start. As he makes no response, the worker voices the dilemma that it is hard to know if Jake is okay or if he needs help, but lets him know he is there for him. Jake eventually comes out, and as they approach the meeting room he sees that everyone is seated in a large circle and they are waiting for him. He freezes outside the door. His not-speaking makes it difficult for him to explain his late attendance to the group. It also prevents him from describing how he might feel when he sees the whole room of staff and young people waiting for him. Collectively, these experiences combine with the feelings and thoughts that caused him to hesitate initially, pushing him further into his non-speaking retreat from others.

A non-speaking child, new to a group of young people and staff, particularly those in an inpatient unit, could be experiencing terror, fear, and mistrust. Like Jake, as well as trying to bear the separation from his family, he may be feeling that he is imprisoned in the inpatient setting and surrounded by strangers who are potential threats. His non-speaking may be accompanied at times by a profound and complete withdrawal. This physical manifestation of a child retreating into a disconnected, foetal space can make those working with him feel helpless, overwhelmed, and anxious as they feel unable to reach or comfort the child for whom they are meant to be caring. The child's not-speaking and *pervasive retreat from life* can feel very powerful, making the members of staff feel deskilled, and they may feel less self-confident and even less effective. The child's utter rejection of words and friendly approaches that would usually be accepted and even welcomed can leave staff feeling lost, confused, and frustrated.

A key point to keep in one's mind is that the non-speaking of the child does not need to silence others' words! The child's not-speaking can feel like it wipes out the thoughts and words of those around them, and staff can feel controlled and stuck for things to say because they don't know what to say that will make a difference. The second key point, however, is that staff, in their anxiety, should not try to "absolutely fill" the silence created through the child's not-speaking.

The child's not-speaking does not need to control the thoughts, feelings, and words of those around the child, for he is still *communicating without words*! It is helpful to remember that vocal silence is always accompanied by potent non-verbal communication, and the absence of speaking leaves more potential space for observing and understanding all non-verbal communication.

At first, Jake insisted on sitting on the floor, curled up and hunched over with his back keeping him safely hidden from his keyworkers. Often, he would stand with his back towards them, or with his face covered and his arms crossed around his body. This may have been his way of communicating that he could not trust his keyworkers enough to sit alongside them. It may have felt easier for him to put barriers up, until he is sure of communications about what he is feeling towards them. If the child is not covering his face, the direction of his gaze and level of physical activity can also be used to inform a sense of communication. The staff's experience in the moment with the child, their countertransference, is essential in understanding the non-speaking child's emotional experience. His keyworkers ensured that they coupled use of their countertransference experiences with verbal communications, as they maintained the belief that sharing their understanding of the present moment in empathic words would enable Jake to begin to lend words and meaning to his feelings, and that this would eventually result in Jake's own spoken words.

In this very first phase, when the child is completely in retreat from the external world through not speaking, not eating, and perhaps not walking, the temptation is to try to "pull the child out" of that state rather than first providing understanding of where the child is in that *present moment* (Stern, 2004). It is particularly difficult to do that when a child is not speaking, but perhaps this poem addresses the non-speaking child's retreat from the world:

"A Sudden Darkness"

I have lost my way.
My mind is numb.
In my gut I feel
a fearful twist
that strangles me
today.

Whence does such darkness
of my once bright spirit
come?
I cannot think.
My numbed mind
does not have the power
to find.

What load has fallen
upon my spirit?
Crushed, bruised and dim.

It tries to move
But the self stays perplexed,
Like the pinned butterfly,
Unmoving.

Seervai (2003, p. 14)

Later, instead of questioning Jake, his keyworkers would "wonder out-loud together" in his presence. They would think understanding thoughts alongside Jake and then voice them to each other. To acknowledge Jake's uncomfortable position on the floor, one said, "We would like you to come and sit on the sofa because it would be more comfortable for you and the floor is very hard", while the other might say, "Maybe it feels too difficult just now for Jake to respond to us or sit on the sofa". The keyworkers thought out loud together for Jake and about Jake. They tried to be empathic in thinking about his anxieties, voicing the idea that he may feel mistrustful or unsafe and how new and even threatening everything may seem. They then aimed to offer nurture in thinking what could be comfortable for Jake or what might help him to feel safe and supported. They strived to achieve a balance between this way of thinking out loud and giving Jake space to just "be" so that they not only acknowledged the possibilities, but that they also gave Jake space to feel them.

A place for mindfulness

Adopting the mindfulness model when working with a non-speaking child can be a rewarding and helpful framework for everyone involved. The concept, based on the work of Jon Kabat-Zinn (1990) incorporates several principles:

1. Listening with full attention and focus to the person who is communicating. If the communication is silent, this can include a focus and attention on non-verbal interactions.
2. Being and staying in the present moment.
3. Being emotionally aware, which is simply to be aware of the emotions that are being elicited within oneself in that present moment.
4. Being non-judgemental of who and what is happening in that present moment, and being non-judgmental of the emotions and thoughts of anyone in that moment, including one's own.
5. Being self-regulated, which involves being able to "stand back" and think about the emotion instead of automatically reacting to it. This principle focuses on being objective about experienced emotions, which might give one time to stop, think, and choose how to respond to them.
6. Feeling compassion, which involves being compassionate to oneself for feeling whatever one is feeling, and also being compassionate and empathic with the child.

For the purpose of this chapter, mindfulness can be used in four ways. First, the keyworkers could adopt a mindful approach in relation to each other and the non-speaking child. Second, they can apply the mindfulness principles to the text or poem they are reading. This especially invokes the compassion and emotional awareness principles. Third, through the reading, responding and interpreting the texts offered in this chapter, the concepts of mindfulness can be identified and named when they are found in the narrative. They can be located in characters, in narratives and in the poems and lyrics. Lastly, if the concepts of mindfulness are adopted by the keyworkers and modeled through the stories, songs, and poems, they can eventually be encouraged and developed in the non-speaking child himself.

The narrative session

Given what we have described about the complex nature of the communication between a non-speaking child and keyworkers as well as the high level of distress and fear the child may be experiencing it is essential to provide an appropriate and containing context within which to introduce the idea of working with narratives. This narrative time should adhere to the principles of the therapeutic milieu, using clear boundaries to keep the child safe, structured and supported during the session. With this in mind the keyworkers drew up a timetable for Jake to keep, so he knew exactly when to expect his key sessions.

The child's family should also be involved where appropriate, as should the rest of the team. Jake's keyworkers thought with his family about what stories, poems or music he liked when he was younger before he became ill. They fed back to the multidisciplinary team any development or outcomes arising from the narrative sessions, and often ideas for new key work would come from case discussions where it would be decided that certain themes could be approached most appropriately with his keyworkers. Regular supervision was an essential part of the process. During the supervisory process, keyworkers were encouraged to create their own narratives of their experience of the child and imagined narratives of what the child might be feeling, giving words through writing about their experiences so as not to feel so compelled to "get information" from the non-speaking child. Writing also enables workers to bear the pain of what they understand about the child. Writing for the clinician involves searching deeply into one's own countertransference and seeking to identify with the whole being of the non-speaking child as much as possible. Here is an example of such a writing exercise involving identifying with the regressed, non-speaking child *pervasively retreating from life*:

> As I walked home along the wintry path, I felt a pain in my ear. It became more and more intense until it drowned my dreamy thoughts about my boyfriend Samuel. The pain resulted in my screaming out so loudly at night that my parents brought me to a paediatrician who immediately placed me in a paediatric ward. The nurses gave me one painkiller after another, to no avail. A series of brain scans ensued. It was scary as can be!! But they revealed nothing of interest to the doctors. "Nothing is wrong with you", said Dr Mann. But the pain was there regardless. "Maybe mastoiditis is brewing", he said, "but there is nothing visible at the moment".
>
> Dr Mann decided to keep me in hospital for several nights because the pain simply didn't subside. My parents weren't allowed to stay overnight because since I was twelve, the person

in charge of hospital beds felt my family had low priority. There were babies on my ward and they needed their parents! But I did too! I had never spent a night away from my parents, my older sister, Sarah, and my best friend, Bobby, my Alsatian dog.

I fought the doctors and nurses, experiencing them as prison wardens. How dare they make me spend a night alone without my parents! It was cruel, and I screamed hysterically, shouting, begging, crying, "Please don't leave me here! Please! Please! You are torturing me!"

I yelled loudly as never before at the nurses and the doctors. I know my mother doesn't like nurses and doctors either, she stays away from them. But, my parents did as they were told and left the hospital that night. I spent one month of long, scary nights with babies crying and dying, appendicitis victims moaning as their anaesthetic wore off, and children going through the corridors with other undiagnosed problems. They terrified me with the strange yellowness of their skins, their lack of hair or bandages covering various parts of their bodies. Worst were the young people lying rather comatose on their bed moaning.

Gradually, I left my body and began to look down on myself talking to my parents. The doctors' voices became dimmer and dimmer as they argued about what to do with me. My head continued to ache. The pain spread to my whole head until gradually there was just a deadly numbness, no sensation of hot or cold, pain or pleasure. No sound. There was no mouth to receive food, no eyes to see light or darkness. I'm in Sylvia Plath's "Bell Jar". I had a dream that a man had plucked my brain out and put it in a vase. Was I alive? Or was I dead? I was in some black chamber in which nothing existed. Perhaps I also ceased to exist. This went on for days until I awakened in another unit. One day, I heard my mother's voice and then it floated away. I moaned and moaned, but I could not hear her voice again. After another time when she came and then left, I began scratching my face and punching my eyes. Then my silent scream froze inside, "Don't go! Don't go!" But my parents couldn't hear, they didn't speak to my mute corpse-like body. They betrayed me. They left me there in that inpatient unit.

I lay there with some liquid arriving in my stomach giving me a horrid stomach pain. I spoke to no one, moved no limbs, but the pain was excruciating. One day, a doctor performed surgery on what I later learned was an abdominal obstruction.

Days became months as I lay there, gradually peering at disappearing bodies of nurses in jeans and T-shirts, a young deaf boy in a wheelchair and two skeletal young girls who futilely tried to talk to me. I could see again and hear sounds, but I couldn't make out what the sounds of people's voices meant. Words were unintelligible, but I could hear loud or soft, friendly or irritated, in the tone of voice spoken to me. I had no words, there were no words for me to speak to this cold, uncaring world into which my parents had abandoned me. Lost was my memory for words, but along with it went pictures; pictures of my bedroom, of my dog, of my sister. There was only one place, these pale green walls of my hospital prison. The teacher tried to read to me, showing me pictures in the book. When occasionally I covertly looked at the page, it was filled with hieroglyphics. In what country was I living? What were these pictures in the book? There was no alphabet in my head, no pictures.

Then my mother came one day, and I heard her say, "This is your dog." She was pointing to some animal photo. I didn't know what "dog" meant. I didn't know who this strange girl was that she called, "your sister". Did I have a sister? I only "knew" my mother.

I was dead-alive with no anchoring point in being alive. There was nothing, no one but my mother who came and went. As she went, I began punching my eyes, then scratching my face and moaning. They put mittens on my hands and restrained them when she was departing. There was just this pale green room with faces appearing and disappearing.

Then finally a little man appeared on my hand. He spoke to me. He seemed to say, "You have been killed", and later, "I am your friend". He would stay there with me, in my hand. When the room was empty, I turned to him and he said, "I have been sent by God. I will rescue you. Don't listen to them. They are enemies. They wish to hurt you." At times I looked with fascination as he stood on my hand pointing to the nurses as my enemies. But then he grew taller and taller until soon in the dark nights he was filling the ceiling. His long legs descended to the floor. I became frightened of him. His face turned into that of a menacing monster. He was no longer a friend. I was terrified to be left alone in the dark with him. I was alone and terrified in the world.

(Magagna, 2009)

Writing such a story about the pieced-together non-speaking child's experience helps the clinician to get to grips with the sensation of pervasively regressing to not-knowing, losing words, losing memory. It is a terrifying experience, but also very painful. It is important for the clinician to tell stories to herself about encounters with the child so she doesn't "cover over the brunt of the pain" of the child's experience (Magagna, 2009).

Stage 1: Engaging a non-speaking child

Initially Jake refused to participate in any of his key sessions. His keyworkers acknowledged that this was his choice at the moment, whilst remaining clear that these key sessions and activities were an important part of the programme and that there was an expectation that Jake attended the sessions. They let him know that they planned to bring stories, songs and poems to the sessions to share with him and he could participate or not as he wished. His keyworkers held in mind an idea that he may use gestures to signal how he felt in the sessions and that he may later feel able to write things down as steps towards more direct communication.

In the early sessions, Jake refused to look at them and did not appear to respond to their suggestions or thoughts. The keyworkers felt Jake's fear and terror and this also felt uncomfortable for them; however, over time, the sessions became a refuge for both Jake and his keyworkers. It was a dedicated time when they could get used to being together and could engage in a shared activity of looking at pictures and listening to stories.

Initially, direct communication using the word "you" was not part of the sessions, for this way of speaking created the risk of intimidating Jake. Instead, there was a creation of a third space, where everyone could feel safe. The keyworkers took it in turns to bring a picture book, poem, or piece of music and would briefly say why it had been chosen before reading or playing the music while the others listened. At the end of the session, the workers would spend a little time talking out loud about what they had heard and how the session went. The sessions seemed to help Jake, as they gave him time out from focussing on his symptoms of

> retreat from talking, walking, and eating. Listening to music meant that he was still attending to the structure of the unit. Gradually, he began to connect with his keyworkers in this non-confrontational space with the focus on sharing a regular time, place, and thinking together. His keyworkers remained mindful and patient and Jake was allowed to go at his own pace in getting to know them and trusting them.

The point of narratives at this stage was not to fill the space where no words were present. Instead, they are offered as a creative and dynamic process of establishing a rapport and engaging with, shaping and thinking about emotional experiences. For example, if music is being used, keyworkers might explain the purpose of the session as "listening together to see what we hear in the music". They might start with a fairly calm piece of music, perhaps even a piece without words. After the song is over, keyworkers could reflect on what they might have imagined in the music: the sounds of the sea, a journey, perhaps. They could then reflect on what the song was about: summarise what might have "happened" in the song in terms of lyrics and melody, rhythm, and mood.

After this initial stage of reflecting on the song or story, keyworkers could try to take a step back from the actual narrative and name some of the main themes. This should be done in a generalised and accessible way such as, "It might be about the main boy going off and having a bit of an adventure and then coming home and feeling pleased to be back". It's important for the keyworkers to say "it might be" about something rather than "it is" about something, so that they model the ability to see the same story or song from several different perspectives.

Next, the keyworkers could talk about where the same theme has come up in other narratives. These could be from recent popular films, on TV or other books, songs or poems. This is for two reasons. First, it validates these themes as being significant and universal: it sends a message to the listener that these things happen to other people. Second, this is important as it connects "one" to others and illustrates the shared experiences. This not only challenges their feelings of being isolated, but also enforces the immediately present shared experience of the story listener and story-teller. This can then be a contained context where the feelings of the people in the stories, poems, or songs are suggested by the keyworkers, and they think together about what it might feel like to own them. There can also be a helpful focus on the courage of the characters in the stories or songs, how they expressed themselves, resolved conflict, developed emotional integration or shifted from a stuck position.

It is always very important to leave a space for the young person to enter the spoken communication at any point should he feel able. In the meantime, when ready, the young person can be encouraged to keep a private diary of thoughts, or perhaps to write, draw, or make a collage or model with plasticine in response to the sessions. Even if this space for non-verbal activities is not taken up for a good long while, perhaps many months, it is important that creative material is available, thus allowing for the possibility of creative expression of feelings.

Stage 2: The terrified and imprisoned child

Recalling the distress, fear, anger and withdrawal of Jake when we first met him, an appropriate story to use at this stage is *I'm Really Ever So Not Well* by Lauren Child (2008). This book is part of the popular Charlie and Lola series and documents the experience of Lola getting ill. To cheer her up, Lola's big brother brings her a tray of her favourite pink milk and some biscuits but Lola says, "My pink milk tastes green. And the biscuits are too prickly to swallow. I don't feel like eating or drinking anything" (p. 4). After this, she says, "I remember when everything tasted yummy" (p. 5). This memory is pictured with a huge glass of pink milk with a straw looping across the page, upon which some cartoon birds are singing. Lola is cut off in a red frame on the side of the page, small in comparison to the glass and looking sad. This frame is repeated when Lola says, "My nose hurts, and nothing smells" (p. 7) after Charlie has bought her some flowers. This time she is in a black frame, which is cut off from a bright pink page full of different flowers. The pink page represents the memory, "I remember when I used to be able to do smelling" (p. 7). When Charlie tries to sing her a song, she says "I can't do singing, Charlie... my throat hurts and my voice is all quiet" (p. 9).

Later on, she asks Charlie, "Why do I feel so really, really not well?" (p. 14), and Charlie says it's because of the "germs". Lola looks into her mouth in the mirror and what she sees is represented by a double-page spread of "thousands and hundreds of germs... 1... 2... 54 billion... a trillion" (pp. 16–17). The page is completely black apart from neon, spiky, nasty-looking germs with sharp, crooked teeth and evil-looking eyes. Lola is floating around amongst them and some are bigger than her. However, Charlie finally gets her to cheer up by playing games with her and playing make-believe where they go cloud-hopping to catch butterflies. The next day, Charlie is ill in bed and Lola is going to look after him.

Often, when a non-speaking child has progressed along his psychological journey and moved out of the phase where he is silent, he has reflected that his silence was extremely frightening and lonely but that he was even more afraid of getting well as he believed he would be moving to an overwhelming unknown. Like Lola, he can feel lost and bewildered in the changed landscape that is illness, where he feels he cannot be reached and he holds no hope in the possibility of being well. One way of engaging with this stage of terror could be to gently revisit specific events when "things used to be nice" before illness. This gives structure and boundaries to the narrative and experience of illness and also suggests the possibility of a self that exists, or at least has existed, outside life with illness or trauma.

For an older child, a poem that seems to deal with these issues particularly well is "I know why the caged bird sings" by Maya Angelou (1969), which can be found in its entirety on the internet. This poem contrasts the "songs" and experiences of the caged bird and the free bird. Most poignantly, the poem describes how trapped and angry the caged bird feels, and how desolate and yet silenced he feels as he watches his silent shadow. The cage seems to echo this position of feeling stuck in silence, it is a tightly boundaried, yet very painful, space. The poem describes how the caged bird is able to observe the experiences of the free bird that is able to fly unencumbered through the whole of the sky. Importantly, the poem emphasises the fear with which the caged bird observes this life of freedom.

Even though the caged bird feels like he cannot move at all, he is still able to sing. In fact, the caged bird's song has great power and is heard from afar. The power of the caged bird's song could be thought to parallel the communicative power of silence.

The poem uses very vivid imagery to conjure up an appreciation of how it might feel to live without a cage and of how it might feel to fly freely through different spaces. Although the caged bird expresses fear of the unknown, he still longs to experience these new and unknown things. Moreover, the caged bird is still able to sing despite his constraints and the fear and anger he feels. Ultimately, the poem tells of the caged bird singing a song of freedom. That he is still able to do so from both the pain and safety of his cage suggests great hope and imagination.

The poem talks of what it might be like to feel caged around people who seem to be "free". Yet, it also opens up space to think about what the caged bird can see from his or her cage; the experiences of freedom he or she might have had in the past. These ideas and feelings resonate with the experiences of a non-speaking child, new to a unit, feeling very alone and afraid; frightened to leave the boundaries of not-speaking, opposed to those things that threaten it and yet, also feeling trapped and imprisoned within the silence.

Both the story and the poem offer voice and structure to the experience of these feelings, thus implying that there was a time before and that there might be a time after these feelings: Lola's illness ends and she can now care for Charlie. The caged bird is able to imagine the life of a free bird and is able to sing of freedom. This dual function of naming such powerful feelings and also thinking about a time when they were/might not be so powerful can be applied in a host of different ways with the non-speaking child. In the case of the story, the book is made from collages; so one way of working with these ideas is to revisit things that the child used to enjoy by making collages. Similarly, the poem is a collage of evocatively described images and thus could be built on through collages of words or images chosen by the child.

For example, in Jake's session, one of his keyworkers simply read the book out loud and when they had finished, the other pointed to the pictures he thought were particularly good and interesting. Both the keyworkers and Jake were able to spend the first session just being in the room together, sharing a story.

Later when his parents came to visit him that weekend, his keyworkers used the opportunity to continue the work they had done in the initial story session. The keyworkers asked Jake's parents what Jake used to like doing with his friends and his big brother, who had recently gone to university, thus trying to build a picture of a time before his non-speaking and pervasive retreat from life. Jake's parents had recently separated, but they were coming to visit him together. Each parent thought about past activities and wrote down hobbies, colours, places and animals that Jake used to enjoy. In the next two sessions, the keyworkers brought old magazines, scissors, card, and glue. They began working on a couple of simple collages made up from the things Jake's family had said he liked before he got ill. Jake was given these collages to keep as a reminder of the sessions in which he was better known and nurtured by the workers, and was supported in participating in activities which were important to him.

Stage 3: The curious child

> Jake's keyworkers thought it was important to think with the larger community about Jake's not-speaking, but communicating without words. For this reason they raised the general topic within a holiday programme which they were running for all the young people. They

> set a task where everybody was divided into groups and given a form of communication. One group was given "acting", another was given pens and paper, another was given hand and body movements, and the last group were given dolls. Each group had to come up with a way of showing "not-speaking" without saying it or writing it down. The acting group showed someone who was trying to shout and get another's attention while being silenced and restrained by two bodyguards. The drawing group drew pictures of faces with eyes that were crying, but left a blank space where the mouth should be. Another drawing showed a thin horizontal line for a mouth. The dolls group positioned the dolls all close but with their backs to each other and the hand and body movements group wrapped their hands and arms around their head to block everything out.
>
> Jake refused to join his group, which was the drawing group. He sat hunched in the corner with his face covered by his hands, but occasionally looked up to peek through his fingers. When they had finished, the group talked together about how creative everyone had been and how strong the representations of not-speaking were, despite the fact that no-one was allowed to say the word "silence". The keyworkers suggested that it showed that not-speaking in itself is communicating something, because in each group people looked sad or angry and others looked scared or lonely. The group agreed that not-speaking itself is a way of communicating and that if you can't use words, there are other ways of expressing how you feel. Jake's direction of gaze suggested that he was listening to the other members of the group talk.
>
> Later that day, when one of the young people asked for the water to be passed down the table at tea, he pushed it along with one of his hands, while keeping his face covered with the other one. It seemed that through their creative expression of understanding, the young people had shown Jake the possibility that the group outside of himself may not be as threatening as he had feared. This allowed him the possibility of being willing to tentatively join them.

The Tiger Who Came to Tea by Judith Kerr (1999) is a much-loved children's picture book that can be used both to broach themes, which are salient to the non-speaking child's tentative curiosity, and to help build his confidence in the face of the unknown. In the book, Sophie's tea with her mother is interrupted by a large but polite tiger that explains that he is very hungry and asks if he can have tea with them. He is so large that Sophie has to stand on her chair to feed him, but he manages to sit properly on the chair at the table. However, when offered cakes, he eats them all and the story goes on to describe how he eats and drinks with a seeming insatiable appetite. The more he eats, the bigger he gets. With each page he is growing in size and Sophie and her mum are shrinking in proportion. On the next page, he is down on all fours for the first time in the book and looking "around the kitchen to see what he can find". The picture is quite ambivalent because, although Sophie has her arms around his neck and is cuddling him, his gaze is averted and his body has taken on a tense yet dynamic pose, making the reader slightly unsure what he is going to do next.

This four-page feeding frenzy ends with his drinking all "Daddy's Beer and all the water in the tap". After this, he leaves, and Sophie's mum then stands in the middle of her kitchen, which is in chaos, looking distressed. The kitchen that was tidy, clean, and previously full of food has now been destroyed, with food and implements all over the floor, and cupboards and drawers hanging bare. Sophie cannot have a bath because there is no water.

At this crisis point in the book, "Daddy came home". Sophie's dad has a hero's arrival; he has a firm, wide stance and lifts off his hat as if to say, "I'm here!" In proportion to dad, Sophie and her mum are very small. Sophie's mum looks upset, but Sophie seems to be smiling to herself. Dad rescues them all by taking them out for dinner, and the story ends with a resolution as the next day Sophie and her mum go shopping to replenish the food supply, including a large tin of tiger food in case the tiger should come again.

Through the sharing of this story, the keyworkers were able to explore the experience of unexpected and chaotic events. The tiger is wild and demanding and represents the chaos both external and internal that the child may fear or have lived through in his reality. It offers an opportunity to look at how order and safety can be restored through trusting relationships and a secure environment and suggests that we can not only survive chaos but that it can be a learning experience that can help us feel more prepared for the future.

In terms of music for the slightly older child, a suitable song to use could be "Human" by The Killers (2008). The song sounds like someone running or looking for something. It questions whether the singer is still human, or merely a "dancer". The words ask for the singer to check if he is still vital and alive and explores how he can let others know this. As such, the song touches on themes of being different: human or dancer, of uncertainty about one's identity, and of the difficulties in connecting with one another and letting each other know of how we are feeling - the state of our own vitality. Nonetheless, the song demonstrates a curiosity and a desire to make new connections, and to try new things while tolerating uncertain outcomes. The song suggests that even though one might be nervous when confronting unknowns, one might acknowledge this fear but try out new things anyway. The song also suggests letting go of fears or ways of interacting that may have kept one stuck in unhealthy relationships or ways of being. Also, the lyrics bid adieu to ways of being that have kept the singer in dark places.

The song seems to be inviting the listeners to "dance" with it while searching through uncertainty. While there is no clear resolution of the uncertainty and an element of fear attached to it, there is a spirit of adventure in the music: a sense that trying new things, making new connections and asking new questions might be liberating. There is a sense of adventure and anticipation inherent in the beat and melody of the music. There is also an implication that one can initially join others in ways other than speaking.

Connected to the theme of curiosity, is one of safety and trust. The child has moved out of the terrified and invaded stage and is starting to wonder if it would be possible and safe to connect to others. As well as being curious about those around him, the non-speaking child may be curious about whether he feels safe enough to think about himself. Can he think alone? How does it feel to be in an inpatient unit away from his family? Both the story and the song raise these issues in a variety of ways. Thinking about these tentative gestures of thought, Jake's keyworkers, decided to think about safety and danger in a broad and indirect way. They decided to compose a newspaper article together, as the story of an escaped tiger is quite sensational and newsworthy. The narrative was constructed as something possibly dangerous and scary that worked out all right in the end. Using the medium of a newspaper article offered Jake a different format for the creative expression of all the feelings involved in the frightening and chaotic story while keeping the session structured, thereby meaning he had the experience of mastery over the situation and its outcome.

The song could have been worked with in a similar way. Keyworkers could use a variety of media and narratives to explore how someone who has always been a human might use other qualities of the self (such as "dancer" or "drawer" or "musician") to navigate a variety of situations. For example, keyworkers could draw a cartoon together with the child (much in the spirit of superhero cartoons), showing how the "human/dancer" uses his or her extraordinary quality to achieve a difficult and perhaps dangerous task. The nature of the task could be related to current news stories, or to something relevant to the unit, or to activities that the child used to enjoy. Like the creation of a newspaper article, this activity also provides a structured experience of trying something new and scary, with a positive outcome, and also incorporates the idea of using a contained space to explore different ways of communicating or different ways of viewing the self. Drawing cartoon stories or newspaper stories can be facilitated through keyworkers using the book *Picture This: The Near-Sighted Monkey Book* (Barry, 2010), which is replete with illustrated ideas for collage and cartoon stories.

However, the beauty of music, in contrast to drawing, is that by its very nature, the media for consolidating and building on the shared musical experience need not be limited to using drawing materials or newspapers and words. Dancing and movement, drawing, playing other instruments, humming, whistling, diary reflections, creative writing - all these can follow from the inspiration of a movement and/or musical experience and become invitations to the non-speaking young person to participate. As such, keyworkers could be quite creative as to follow-up activities, while bearing in mind the importance of structure and containment during that activity.

Stage 4: The split child

Jake began to experiment with communication by pointing to things he wanted or needed. He also would point to direct the gaze of another child in the unit, if he was looking for something. (Pointing is one of the first ways a young baby begins language communication, for in pointing he is saying "look here", and thus Jake can be seen to be evolving from his cocoon in which he does not use language.) The other children in the unit seemed to feel encouraged by this and in return, they started thinking more about ways of being "alongside Jake".

When his parents left after a visit, or a phone call with his parents ended, Jake became very distressed. He would appear very stuck often refusing to leave the area in which he had been talking with them. When staff tried to help Jake express what was wrong, a few of the other children replied saying, "I think Jake might be feeling really homesick" or "I think he is really missing his mum because he spent all day with her and now he won't see her until next week". When staff asked Jake if this was right, he nodded his head.

When Jake "spoke" to one of his parents on the phone, although he was not-speaking and just listening to a parent musing aloud in conversations with him, he would refuse to end the

> phone conversation. Even if his parents hung up, he held onto the telephone, despite the fact that another young person had a telephone call booked into the slot immediately after him. Other children started to say that they felt angry or frustrated with him, because they thought he knew that they had a phone call and this allowed them less time to make their call. Jake's not-speaking and not showing facial expressions in response to their complaints seemed to involve his not apologising to them or not acknowledging their distress and the anger they felt. The staff felt that in this way Jake might be projecting his own distress and anger at the ending of his parents' telephone conversation. The tentative connections and friendships he had made would be set back by these episodes. At times Jake's forming of links with other young people was further interrupted by Jake's rejection of his new friends' efforts to be friendly to him in the evenings after his parents had left.
>
> As Jake settled into the centre and began making some warmer contact with young people, he began to appear quite split, showing friendliness in the unit and coldness to one or the other of his parents. Sitting with him in a key session, his keyworkers wondered aloud whether it felt like part of him was in the centre and then part of him was still at home. As Jake was becoming ill his parents separated, so they wondered whether the split between the home and the centre reflected the split Jake was feeling between his parents, and the further fragmentation he may have experienced when his older brother left to attend university.

It is known that children in this position have expressed that they feel like part of them is at home, while part of them is at the centre, and they get filled with feelings of guilt and loyalty to each place. They can feel very stuck and can get angry and frustrated while they try to acknowledge and manage these feelings of being split between loyalties to the staff and loyalties to separated parents. It is particularly difficult to keep loyalties to both parents if they are still in serious conflict with one another despite being separated. The child can feel trapped in a "go-between" position rather than firmly connected to either parent.

Missing Rabbit by Roni Schotter (2002) is a good book to use with a younger child who is in this position of having separated parents and/or two places to live. In *Missing Rabbit*, Kara has a dilemma. Her parents have split up and she divides her time between her mum and dad's house; however, when she leaves her dad's house, her toy Rabbit asks her, "Where do I live?" She doesn't know the answer. Rabbit tells her that he wants to stay at dad's house, so she leaves him behind. When she gets to her mum's house, though, she misses her dad and she misses her rabbit. They call dad and he brings Rabbit back to mum's house. The same thing happens when Kara moves from mum's house to see dad. Rabbit is confused about where he lives and whether or not he wants to stay behind. But Kara misses him too much, so decides that Rabbit will stay with her wherever she goes, otherwise there will be "too much missing". Then Rabbit asks Kara, "where do you live?", and Kara doesn't know. She tells her parents that Rabbit wants to know where she lives. Her parents respond by saying that sometimes she lives with mum and sometimes she lives with dad, but wherever she is, they are always thinking of her and they still love her.

The strengths of the character can be named as toleration of uncertainty and bravery. Kara has a dilemma and she tries to do something about it. When her plan doesn't work, she asks her parents for help. Their answer is not clear-cut, but they model the idea that things can both change yet be safe and consistent.

A way of working with this theme is to focus on the core or central dislikes and likes of the child. This can be done using a collage, placemat, or mobile. Keyworkers can ask parents and siblings about these things, and then spend time with the child making the mobile and giving it to him to keep. This can then be used to think about the key and more stable elements of the child's life with each of the parents, whether they are together or separated. Some elements are that the parents and child can all think of one another, get in touch with one another and love one another whether they are separated or together. To address the pain and possible freedom of separation, the song "Little Bird" by Annie Lennox (1992) is suitable either as a poem, using only lyrics, or as a way of thinking while listening to her singing. The song is about separation but also about having the strength to "fly away" and let burdens go. It can allow the listener space to acknowledge the difficulty of separation and the pain, but also the freedom it engenders to have a separate space in which to find oneself and be oneself.

Stage 5: Anger and hostility

> As Jake progressed he started engaging in more non-verbal friendly overtures with some of the young people and his parents. He would also whisper the occasional word to his parents and write down messages to his friends in the centre. At this time, his parents noticed that there were scratches and wheals on his legs. When asked about this, Jake refused to respond and started crying. At the same time he started showing strong feelings of anger towards his keyworkers and was erratic in his non-verbal overtures towards them. He would slam doors and run away from keyworkers when they were talking to him about things about which he felt too emotional to consider. Sometimes, he would walk into areas of the clinic that he knew were out of bounds. At times he would engage responsively with his keyworkers and at times he would not respond to what they were saying. He ripped up his work at school and threw away gifts and cards that people had sent him.

One of the recurring feelings and experiences of working with a non-speaking child can be intense and acute projections of very powerful anger. At times a child's not-speaking is done with expressions clearly showing the child is feeling furious with those around them (but there is more vitality in aggression than in persecutory retreat from terrors of life). A child's fury can be shown through aggressive physical resistance to care or engagement. A possible way to understand this is to use the concept of "identifying with the aggressor". A child who has experienced traumatic events out of his control can shift out of the position of being a victim, helpless and experiencing pain, when he feels a tiny bit stronger. Instead, he may identify with the aggressor who causes his pain, and inflict the hurt, rejection, and sense of inadequacy onto someone else. We will look at a good illustration of this later in the chapter. Jake's keyworkers thought about Jake's aggression and what it evoked in them in their supervision and work discussion seminars in the centre. They also felt it was necessary to do some work with Jake thinking about his anger as well as thinking about his sense of being rejected and the responses he had to feeling abandoned or having limits placed upon him, which at times also felt like a rejection of him and his wishes.

The non-speaking child may be in a double-bind of wanting a connection and love but feeling furious and destructive towards those same people, such as his family or therapist for leaving him and causing him pain. His lack of control over his parents or therapist to make them do exactly what he wants may cause intense anger and he might feel furious that they cannot make things better quickly. He may also experience feelings of rejection, guilt, and shame as his anger creates damage to his internal parents, keyworkers and therapist, leaving them "bad inside himself". He may be experiencing this in the present moment, but it may also be tapping into stored pain and responses from very early infantile feelings of abandonment and/ or non-attunement by primary caregivers. Anger connected with a fear of abandonment is a common theme in children's story books due to the inevitable developmental anxiety concerned with growing up and separating from one's parents.

A very useful picture book for thinking about the angry non-speaking child and his identification with the aggressor is David McKee's *Not Now, Bernard* (2005). The book begins with Bernard cheerily walking up behind his dad and saying, "Hello, Dad" (p. 1), which causes dad to bang a hammer into his fingernail, turn green, and say, "Not now, Bernard" (p. 2). This all happens without his turning around to look at Bernard. This pattern is repeated straight after with mum; Bernard's greeting of, "Hello, Mum" (p. 3), is met with, "Not now, Bernard" (p. 4), and mum's face changes from neutral to a look of exasperation. Although the house is colourful, it distinctly lacks any evidence that a child might live there, making it appear unfriendly and even hostile. Bernard then tells his mum that there is a monster in the garden and it's going to eat him. Again, the response is, "Not now, Bernard" (p. 6), and the exchange becomes destructive as Bernard's mum spills her water. So far, the reader can see that not only do Bernard's parents ignore him, but also he has a negative impact on their lives, causing them to break things and hurt themselves. This raises the theme of subjective appraisal, which is crucial for the book. How Bernard's parents treat him morphs into a representation of his self-esteem. This creates inner conflict and confusion within Bernard. On the one hand, he is being ignored and rejected by his parents from whom he dearly wants attention; on the other hand, he is a destructive, horrible person who makes bad things happen and exasperates his parents so that they are at the end of their tether with him. What has he done that is so bad that they ignore him yet also means he has a terrible effect on them?

The next page sees Bernard going out into the garden, approaching the monster and saying, "Hello, Monster" (p. 8), then, "The Monster ate Bernard up, every bit" (p. 9). The scenery and landscape suddenly changes from a blue sky with a green tree and grass to a pink sky, an exotic pink and yellow spiky tree, and a yellow ground. The monster is suddenly sitting on top of some rocks licking his lips and brandishing Bernard's shoe. The sudden harsh terrain reflects the wild and dangerous nature of the monster.

Having consumed Bernard, the monster goes into the house and the text describes the next event, "'ROAR", went the monster behind Bernard's mother" (p. 11). The pattern is repeated, as without turning around, Bernard's mother says "Not now, Bernard" (p. 12) and spills her paint. Then the monster tries biting dad, but still he gets the same response, and dad doesn't even realise that he has been bitten by a monster instead of Bernard. This interaction is especially interesting as Bernard's father flails about in pain after the bite but still doesn't look at the monster.

Bernard's dinner is left for him in front of the television, and so in the next few pages the reader sees the monster misbehaving in a very monster-like way while engaging in Bernard's solitary routine. Eating the dinner involves standing on top of the table and tipping the whole plate into his mouth. Watching TV is done by climbing up the wall and standing on top of it. Then the monster becomes more like Bernard, sitting on top of his shelves with his legs crossed while he seems to be quietly enjoying a comic. But then, instead of playing with one of Bernard's toys, he breaks it. Mum's response is to say, "Go to bed, I've taken up your milk" (p. 21), and monster climbs the stairs dragging a teddy behind him. In this picture, he is proportioned like a child as the stairs loom above him. The last page sees the monster tucked up in Bernard's bed with a cup of hot milk and a teddy bear while mum is turning out the light. Again, as in every page, her eyes are averted away from the reader and from the monster. Looking shocked, surprised, and even upset, the monster looks straight at the reader and says, "But I'm a monster" (p. 23). The inevitable response comes in the last words of the book, "Not now, Bernard" (p. 24).

Bernard was scared of being eaten by the monster, but because his parents didn't care, he turned into the monster. Therefore the identification with the aggressor is played out, as Bernard merges with the monster. Second, this could also connect to a child's fear that if his parents' caring eyes are not on him, something very bad will happen. Third, a child could feel horror and get scared about the overwhelming nature of his own angry feelings towards the parents he feels "don't care". He becomes consumed with anger; then the child may see himself as a monster. Working on the theme of anger, the child can draw a picture to describe an angry monster. The picture can use words and non-verbal icons, such as colours, shapes, and even thunder and lightening. He can explore the things the monster might do when he is angry and then think about why he might be angry. On the other side, the keyworkers can think about a letter that Bernard/monster might write to tell his parents why he is angry. What words would he use? How would he explain it? For further exploration of why there are monsters, and ways of exploring this subject through collages and writing, are found in *What It Is: Do You Wish You Could Write?* (Barry, 2009, pp. 58–61).

Much music deals with the emotion of anger: anger at betrayal, being left behind or abandoned, anger with others or with oneself, anger at political regimes, a lover, or one's peers. One of the most poignant songs that speaks of anger is "Crucify" by Tori Amos (1992). It is especially powerful because it covers anger from so many different perspectives: anger derived from fear of being inadequate among others, anger at others for not accepting oneself, anger at oneself that comes from a sense of guilt for having got oneself into, and choosing to stay in, a state of despair and difficulty, acting out on one's anger by hurting those around one, and finally, suggesting that acting out one's anger is also a communication and sometimes can be a plea for help.

This spectrum of thoughts and feelings echoes the confusion which a non-speaking young person be may experiencing and may reflect the internalisation of the feelings of shame, rejection, and guilt that underlie the acting out of anger and the use of anger to disrupt relationships. For example, "Crucify" begins by speaking of anger born of fear of being rejected by others if the singer reveals her true nature and anger to them: Amos sings of feeling as though everyone in the room is accusing her of something and the anger she feels as a result of this. Often, a non-speaking child will later report having had a similar fear saying he was too scared of how his parents would react to express his anger for fear of the consequences. He therefore became impotent in relation to expressing himself directly. The fear, not letting the anger out, and not speaking all give rise to more feelings of anger, both with others and oneself for being "put" in situations where the young person becomes the focus of disturbing, uncomfortable discussions about his not-speaking. These are situations that not-speaking is designed both to avoid and yet, contradictorily, into which the young person and his family, peers, keyworkers, and therapists are forced.

The song "Crucify" also speaks of anger with others for not accepting "the monster", the victim, and the vulnerable part of oneself. Amos uses the very powerful verb "crucify" to speak of how this experience feels for her. The song also suggests that the writer feels abandoned in her pain and her "monster" state. It tells of how she seems to wander alone with her difficulties, desperately searching for some solace. The song tells how the singer is searching for a rescuer in the world around her, and not finding one. This is not unlike the angry and hostile non-speaking child who both seeks connection with others and yet disrupts it through anger and not-speaking. He seeks "a saviour" and yet might believe that the "saviour(s)" are rejecting him for not being good enough, or he might feel that the "saviours" are failing in their task. This can give rise to immense frustration, anger, and destructive, rejecting impulses as the child fights against owning his own emotional needs and fights against those he sees as causing him pain.

However, the song "Crucify" also speaks of the singer's difficulties in embracing and integrating those shadow parts of the self and describes how she punishes herself; her daily self-crucifixion for her feelings of anger, fear, abandonment, despair, vulnerability, and impotence, as they feel unacceptable to her. The non-speaking child who then begins to speak again will frequently talk about this self-punishment, even self-harm, which is used when overwhelming uncomfortable feelings and situations come to the fore. Thus, the idea of "crucify" can be thought about in many ways that are applicable to the angry non-speaking child; as an act of aggression towards the self, as an act of punishing others by asking them to witness this self-punishment, as an act "done to" a victim by an aggressor, or as the physical enactment of mental and emotional pain which is too difficult to bear alone.

These are all vital themes in the unpicking of the angry projections of the non-speaking child and can be addressed in a number of ways after a shared listening to the song. These themes can also be raised in more subtle ways. For example, the song is sung in a plaintive, angry, and desperate tone. The melody is haunting, pained and angry. The singer is "alone". Keyworkers might have a joint discussion in front of the young person regarding the mood of the music, or the idea that the singer is alone behind the microphone as she sings the lyrics and what that might feel like. Does she sing in order to be heard? Keyworkers could also discuss the roles that the different elements of the music play and the contradictions between them. For example, the drums add to the anger, the guitar to a sense of desperation and aggression and so on. Musical instruments could be brought to the follow-up session and the different elements or characters of the young person's anger could be "played" out on these instruments. This music could act as a prompt, like the story of Bernard and the monster, which would enable working towards thinking about how the non-speaking child could begin to symbolise his anger in a wide variety of ways.This could include drawing graffiti on large sheets of paper, writing letters, stories, or songs. At this point, group or individual drawing and thinking about feelings in key work sessions can be facilitated by using Margot Sunderland's drawing and writing workbook, *Drawing On Your Emotions* (1997).

Stage 6: Exploring loss

> Eventually, both Jake and his parents began to build a close therapeutic alliance with his keyworkers. Jake's parents brought up the loss of Jake's maternal grandmother, which had happened around the time of the onset of his illness. They stated that it was a very difficult period particularly as Jake's dad was working and his mum had to go back to Poland for the funeral. Jake did not attend the funeral and became angry and distressed when his parents mentioned his grandmother to his keyworkers. Alongside this, the keyworkers had been trying to explore Jake's relationship with his older brother. Jake had not replied to any of the letters that Jake's brother had written him and on a few occasions had refused to talk to him on the phone. Jake's parents referred to this older brother as "really strong", "capable", and "unaffected" by their marital conflict and subsequent split.

With his therapist, Jake's keyworkers identified that they should do some work on loss and bereavement. They were concerned not only by Jake's reaction to his grandmother's death but also to his sense of grief when his older sibling left home and went to America to study.

A good book to use when thinking about loss is John Burningham's book *Granpa* (1984). The text and pictures are both dynamic and fluid. They lend insight into Granpa's memories and experiences and his relationship with his grandchild. These drawings are a cross between nostalgic memories and imagined adventures. This contrast serves to emphasise the pairing of Granpa and his granddaughter, reflecting both his past life and the life he now shares with her.

His voice is represented in normal text while hers is written in italics, underneath his. Each person is talking from his/her own perspective on the current scene in which they are occupied. This emphasises both the grandfather and grandaughter's individuality and their connection to each other through shared experience. Each page is a snapshot into different activities that they do together, gardening, playing with dolls and the text offers snippets of their conversation.

About a third of the way into the book, there is nothing on the double-page spread apart from the little girl standing in the far left corner, and Granpa standing on the far right. Both have their backs to each other after the little girl has said something not nice to her grandpa, and the text reads, "That was not a nice thing to say to Granpa". The body language is a very striking representation of conflict between the two and feels very uncomfortable. This page could be referred to when thinking about conflict. What is Granpa thinking? What is the little girl thinking? The teller could ask the listener when he experienced something like that and what happened? How did he or could he have made it better?

The next two pages are in full colour, depicting a garden tea party. The little girl is serving imaginary ice-cream made of soil and Granpa comments, "This is lovely chocolate ice-cream", to which his granddaughter replies, "It's not chocolate, its strawberry" (pp. 12–13). The representation of Granpa indulging in the make-believe game offers a reassuring resolution of the previous conflict. This sends an important message suggesting that it is OK to have disagreements and that the person in the adult role can manage the conflict. Often, a child who has experienced trauma and who has assumed an inappropriate parental role with his caregivers, reports feeling unable to risk any conflict with that caregiver because he thinks they are too fragile or will be too upset. This conflict resolution between Granpa and the little girl could be used to model a safe experience of resolving distressing emotional conflicts.

The sense of connection and collaboration is emphasised later in the book when Granpa says, "When I was a boy we used to roll our wooden hoops down the street after school" (p. 18), and the girl responds, "Were you a baby as well, Granpa?" (p. 18). This is an interesting interaction that could be used to help think about the roles people take up in their family. The keyworker and child could think together about what roles mean, what it means to be a child, son or daughter and how these roles relate and change over time. The story could also use be used to think about the child's own parents or grandparents. Pretending to take up different roles in the story may help the child think about taking up different roles in life.

The structure of the book seems to pass through the seasons, with summer on the beach and then a vivid depiction of autumn, through to winter, when the girl says, "You nearly slipped then, Granpa" (p. 21). Granpa looks thinner and more frail, and the girl is depicted as taller and bigger in comparison to her Granpa. The next page is Granpa tucked up in the armchair, the same place that he was at the beginning of the book. This time he is not holding his arms out for his granddaughter. He "can't come out to play today" (p. 23), and the colours are pale and the palette is limited to a variety of dull greens. There is an implication of illness and the pencil drawings on the opposite page have changed from memories to medicine and a hot-water bottle.

The last two pages have no words and instead depict a faint pencil drawing of the little girl perched on a chair on one page looking across the opposite page at Granpa's empty armchair. There are no traces of Granpa and the reader does not know for how long he has been gone. The silence is almost overwhelming, as the absent text seems to hang in the picture. To think about loss and bereavement, the keyworkers made an "all about me" sheet about the little girl in the book. They drew a picture of her and wrote down the things she liked, and then wrote down the feelings she may have experienced, which included all the diverse emotions associated with grief. Jake's keyworkers did an "all about me" about Jake's brother and asked Jake to fill in things about his brother's personality, likes and dislikes. Although he remained silent, Jake agreed to write a few words down. Then they used this to think about the role that Jake's brother used to take, possibly protecting him and looking after him and that he may have served a parental role. They then did an "all about me" about Jake's grandmother who died and, with the help of Jake's mum, wrote down things that she used to like. They used the *Granpa* story to think about how precious memories and shared experiences can be, and how we can hold onto the good things about a relationship even if that person has gone away.

Part of grief comes when an "old way" or ideal must be surrendered and when loss must be accepted. In order to move on from grief, there must be compassion and empathy, and hopefully the forgiveness of the self and others. Brian Patten's poem "And Nothing Is Ever As You Want It To Be" (2007), could be a useful poem to use in this stage. It is about love, but it is more about the difficulties in loving, allowing it in, and the dilemmas of not knowing and of loving freely.

Stage 7: Exploring the inner mind

> At the table, Jake suddenly stopped eating his lunch. He would lift his fork up to his mouth to eat and then suddenly stop and appear unable to eat the food. He sat hunched over the table covering his face with his hands. The other young people at the table appeared concerned and asked him if anything was wrong. He did not answer them and did not appear to acknowledge them. Then his keyworkers asked if something was wrong and they got the same response. Every time someone engaged with him, Jake seemed to withdraw more and became more hunched and blocked himself off even more from the rest of the table. Jake had recently been communicating with the young people by nodding and shaking his head and by appearing to be actively listening. His keyworkers voiced that it seemed like Jake was going back a bit, maybe because he felt unsafe and had to retreat to the safety of withdrawal.
>
> As this conversation unfolded, Jake became more and more distressed and started crying. The sound of him crying increased and other young people around the table stopped eating. Several of them became distressed and one young person spoke crossly saying, "He's making it really hard for everyone else". At this point, Jake got up and ran out of the room. Staff followed him and supported him to come back. When he returned Jake sat at the table appearing very hurt by the boy's crossness and he needed extra time to try to finish his lunch. It was discovered later in a therapy session that Jake often felt unable to ignore 'something inside him' telling him not to eat for eating was wrong. The voice threatened him saying something bad would happen if he did so.

It is known that a non-eating child who is also not-speaking, yet beginning to explore thoughts and feeling may experience hearing voices. These voices are inside his head and this can be a frightening experience for him. He might not choose to or be able to tell anybody, but this is a very useful time to think about the differences between reality and fantasy. Work can be done at this stage on differentiating external fantasy from inner phantasies and feelings. One book to use, is *Come away from the water, Shirley'* also by John Burningham (1992). This is a beautifully illustrated picture book that contains humour and irony, but its main function is to clearly illustrate the difference between reality and fantasy. On one hand it could be used to encourage a child to think about stories and use his imagination. It also shows how fantasy can be incorporated safely and contained within the limits of reality and the everyday.

The story follows a family trip to the beach. Throughout the book there is the same tension between the didactic text presented on each of the left pages which are adjoining the right pages having vivid, colourful pictorial representations. This tension represents the difference between "reality" on the left side of the book and Shirley's fantasy life on the right side of the book. Shirley's parents remain on the left-side pages throughout the book and the drawings use pale almost translucent colour with large, blank empty spaces. In contrast, Shirley's pages are illustrated in deep, full colour.

At the beginning of the text, the parents are facing the storyteller and listener on the left page and on the right page Shirley is standing with her back to them. They see what she is seeing, which could connect both of them to her and this implies that they are both going to share her adventure. By simultaneously accessing reality and the fantasy, represented through the left and right pages, the storyteller and listener literally and metaphorically become the bridge between reality and fantasy. This connection is also emphasised by the meta-fictive text in the book, which uses humour and irony to connect the reality of the left pages to the fantasy of the pages on the right. Initially, Shirley's parents' banal and didactic comments communicate to the reader that the corresponding pictures of Shirley's actions are happening in her imagination, however, irony is introduced when her parents say, "Why don't you go and play with those children?" (p. 4), while in Shirley's picture, a pirate ship looms. Again, her parents make a comment, "Don't stroke that dog, Shirley, you don't know where he's been" (p. 8). Simultaneously, on the right side, the dog is attempting to rescue Shirley from being made to walk the plank. This use of irony could be a useful way to bring a sense of fun and humour to the session. At the same time, the fact that Shirley's parents are nearby, but not involved, could be representative of a child's need to feel safe and contained in order to be able to go off and have these adventures. This is in line with John Bowlby's (1969) work on attachment and secure base behaviours.

In order to work further on the theme of the splitting between reality and fantasy, the keyworkers can write a letter from Shirley's parents to a friend or grandparent. This can be a postcard, detailing what actually happened on that day on the beach, not including Shirley's adventure. The next can be a letter and pictures pretending to be from Shirley, revealing all her adventures, which could be written in the style of an old pirate adventure story. From this, keyworkers can tentatively explore the difference between what is internal and what is external. What happened outside in the world and what happened inside Shirley's mind? How did Shirley put what was in her mind outside into the real world? Then they could think about the things that people put from their mind, onto the external world. Thoughts, beliefs, and expectations can all be offered as examples by the keyworkers, to model this distinction between reality and fantasy.

Stage 8: The cocoon stage, "'trapped"' in the safety of the unit

> It became apparent that Jake was experiencing regular headaches. After a consultation with a doctor, he was referred to an optician, who said he needed to wear glasses. Jake struggled against his parents taking him to the optician's to decide on which glasses he needed. Being also opposed to putting his glasses on, he would hide himself away from the rest of the group, in a crouched, hunched position and cover his face with his hands. During these encounters with both the outside world and the glasses, he would cry, recoil from any support, and appear to very strongly resist any of the staff's attempts to help him. On one occasion, he got so cross that he stamped on the glasses. They were replaced, and he was given a sanction. He then wore them, but covered his face with his hands and took them off whenever he could.

> Jake's resistance to wearing glasses seemed to be linked to a resistance to learning at school. He had been in the centre for quite a while and appeared settled and comfortable with the routine. When his core team started talking about future plans and going back to school, Jake became very upset. His keyworkers wondered whether he felt threatened by the idea of leaving the unit. They decided to do some work thinking about hope and positive change. They wanted to think about how the unit could be a different kind of place for Jake. This could be a space for him to think about change, development, and hope instead of a place in which he could remain cocooned as an ill child. As the keyworkers experienced Jake beginning to develop more of a sense of himself, they tried to help him develop some faith in his inner resources and hope for something better in his life.

A good book to use for a young child in this stage of development is Eric Carle's (1969) *The Very Hungry Caterpillar*. This is a classic picture book about hope and growth. It can be used to work on the idea of the hard work involved in taking on and processing change, and the security in being stuck and not making changes. At the beginning of the story, there is nothing but a "little egg" (p. 1), whose tiny size is emphasised by its presence on the huge spread of the leaf, which even dominates the large face of the moon hanging behind it. The caterpillar "pops" out of the egg and begins his journey looking for food. He is completely alone with nothing but a huge smiling sun. This could connect to the developmental phase of anxiety about growing up and being alone. The "tiny" caterpillar is out on his own. His journey then takes him from Monday to Friday where he nibbles his way through five different pieces of fruit. The pages are cut away but increase in size to account for the previous day, so there is a strong sense of progression and accumulation. There is a caterpillar-sized hole through each piece of fruit, suggesting that he is just eating what he "needs", not too much and not too little.

Despite this, he is "still hungry" (p. 6), so on Saturday he eats through a whole range of food, stretching from chocolate cake to a watermelon and taking in a sausage, a pickle, some salami, and a lollipop, amongst other things in between. Again, each item of food is "one slice" or "one piece", so there is a measured and contained order to everything he eats. A narrative of "too much" is introduced because the picture shows a tiny caterpillar, dwarfed by the proportions of all this food, looking uncomfortable. The text states, "That night he had a stomach ache". The solution to this is to eat something healthy the next day. This time, it is a green leaf and "after that he felt much better" (p. 10).

On the next page, the caterpillar is no longer hungry and is no longer little, "he was a big, fat caterpillar" (p. 11). Instead of being a tiny illustration in the corner, the caterpillar suddenly becomes a huge creature that dominates the whole of the page. The shock of this is mediated by his actions. The text simply states that he built a small house around himself, which conveys a sense of agency, practicality and recognition of his needs. The text suddenly becomes dynamic and leaps into the future by narrating the process of building the cocoon, staying inside it for more than two weeks and then pushing his way out. In contrast to this, the picture becomes static and all the reader can see is the huge, brown, sealed cocoon. Time moves so fast that the sentence even crosses over to the next spread where "He was a beautiful butterfly!" (p. 13). The picture of the butterfly is beautiful, vivid, and colourful, and spreads across both the left and right pages. The caterpillar is back to his original size but remains in proportion to his beautiful wings and the effect is quite stunning to the reader.

The keyworkers can think with the non-speaking child about the difference between the beginning and the end of the story. What has happened to the caterpillar? They can think about the amount of work he had to do in providing all that he needed in order to grow and develop. They can also discuss how he felt that he could never do enough or that he might race doing too much, eating too much, until it all becomes too much to manage. Themes of greed and a feeling that needs can never be fully met can be explored and connected to the child's desire to stay safe and young in a place where he does not have to fend for himself. The book also offers the idea of progress and reaching one's full potential through hard work and modulation of feelings of wanting, wishing and greed. The caterpillar has "grown up" and transformed.

Given that part of Jake's resistance was linked to a move out of the safety of the unit it seemed pertinent to involve his family in a related task. For this, they needed lots of circles cut out of paper, all roughly the same size, divided into three piles. Each piece of paper is going to be a segment of the caterpillar, and they will all be stuck together to make a caterpillar from different time periods. One segment of the caterpillar will be when the child was very young, the second will be when he was a bit older, and the third will be at the present time. The child's siblings, friends, or family members can make this for him using art materials. Each segment of the caterpillar can be decorated differently. Some segments can be painted and decorated with glitter or sequins, and some segments need to feature things that the non-speaking child liked when he was that particular age. Others will feature places the family used to visit, people in their lives, and what happened to them. The caterpillar will be a collage of timelines for that particular age. Then the last task is to make a big butterfly for all the things the young person likes and would like in the future. This butterfly may be kept as a work in progress. It can become a space for new experiences, wishes and aims for the future.

Ankur Sharma (2010), a specialist registrar working with us, wrote a poem about a child in therapy emerging from his "hard shell". This poem can be shared to help young people to consider letting go of the safety of primitive omnipotence and allowing an adult to understand his personal narrative:

Uncurling

Tiny nine-year-old
Fingers and toes curled,
He sits opposite me, being
Grown Up Man;
"I am okay"

But then,
Dewy eyed, he fights
Lonesome thoughts
Twirling around loss of father
And, mistakes me for him; yet,
"I am all right"

Tear drops form,
Little lip pouts;
At breaking point,
So fragile.
He resists, I coax
He may cry;
I won't leave too.

A memory incited,
Too much to hold
This terrible sadness.

It drifts down his cheeks
Like tyre prints
Rolling on a snowy road
Left by
A wearied cyclist;
He cries.

Fingers and toes curled
Half, into himself,
He is now embryo.

Grown Up Man abandoned,
His spirit connects with need; and,
He tells me his story.

Dollops of tears,
A jutting lower lip
And a heart of jelly.

Snow is falling outside now;
He is uncurling,
Fragile, like a curious blossom
In winter.

Another poem or song lyric to use are the words from Adele's (Adkins, 2008) *Chasing Pavements'* song. It speaks of persistence in the face of fear of failure and of still trying and not being sure what the ending is. It is about realising and then accepting that you have and can make choices. *Chasing Pavements* suggests that responsibility does not have to be terrifying and that there are several paths from which one can choose, not just one.

Stage 9: The journey home

This chapter has specified different narratives that can be used at the individual stages of a young person's psychological development towards health. However, there is one book that we have found useful in encompassing themes relevant to the entire journey, meaning it can accompany the child as he progresses and can be a great help when he is making the transition back home. This is Maurice Sendak's *Where the Wild Things Are* (1963).

> Jake eventually began to spend longer periods of time out of the unit at home and at school. This was an extremely rocky period and he would often return back to the unit having lost weight. It was decided to have some joint sessions with the family therapist and keyworkers with the aim of Jake using their support in the sessions to help him express what might be making home difficult. Jake was able to talk about how frightening it had been to experience so many changes, leaving his home country, loss of grandmother, parents separation and brother leaving home. He did not feel he could turn to his parents, for his mother was depressed and his father felt consumed by his business school studies. He was also able to admit to a heartfelt wish that he could bring his parents back together. He also felt obliged to 'hold himself tightly together' and control his fears in order to cause as little drain on his distraught mother as possible. This admission on Jake's behalf allowed his parents to admit that they had felt very guilty about the arguments that Jake had witnessed and that they had indeed both been very wrapped up in their own distress, conflicts and grief. They tried to impress upon Jake that they would most definitely not be getting back together but that they wanted him to be able to turn to them both as parents. Sadly despite their best intentions it was apparent that there remained a lot of unresolved anger between the parents. Mother in particular seemed fragile, unsupported and in need of help for herself.
>
> Jake was not going to get his perfect story book ending but with the reality of his situation made more clear, he and his family were able to be better supported to continue to work on their relationships. What was important was that Jake had been able to shift internally so that he could make himself heard and understood by his parents, keyworkers, family therapist and individual psychotherapist. He therefore had a far greater chance of being able to allow himself to be healthy rather than clinging onto a cocoon of retreat and "not-thinking" for safety.

In *Where the Wild Things Are*, when we first meet the protagonist, Max, he is wearing a wolf suit and is making mischief of one kind or another: banging a nail into the wall, chasing his dog down the stairs. The position and tone of the text gives the impression of an omniscent narrator observing the action. In the background, a drawing of a monster hangs on the wall, and on it is written "by Max". Max is central to the story, which could be reflective of Max's centralisation of his own self. Indeed, this is affirmed by the scale used, which depicts Max taking up a large share of the drawings. This idea of the child feeling "the centre" and most important in the family can be used to think aloud with a child about how he places himself in his own family and to help him see things from different perspectives.

Max's mischief culminates in an explosive conflict between Max and his mother. The didactic voice explains 'his mother called him "WILD THING!" and Max said "I'LL EAT YOU UP!"' (p. 5). His implied 'punishment' is that he is 'sent to bed without eating anything' (p. 5). This connection between the mother, Max, and food is very interesting. It could be that food is representative of his mother's love and acceptance. He is being punished by his mother withdrawing food and love. The fact that Max threatens to eat his mother up is equally significant. Wearing a wolf suit, he seems so wild and out of control that he could destroy and consume his own mother. Then, perhaps, his mother could be perceived as holding his projected hostile feelings and for this reason he may view her as very threatening and powerful. These ideas are pertinent to a non-speaking child who has an eating disorder and could be used to explore ideas about the mouth as a link to the mother. For example, feeling like biting up and eating up mother can result in fears that food is bad, for it is filled with horrible phantasies. Likewise, both mother and her food can be experienced as bad and persecutory.

This point in the book marks a change in the teller/listener dynamic. Instead of telling the listener what is going on, the story-teller takes on the voices of both Max and his mother. We are drawn in and the sense of observer perspective is lost just as can happen in emotive interactions in real life. As the text has now become dynamic, with an interchange between Max and his mother, the picture has become static. A smaller Max stands in a disproportionately large bedroom. There are no signs of it being a child's bedroom and it is drawn in cold and dull colours. In noticing this and its similarity to Lola's story earlier, workers could think about how a world can change, feel lacking in colour and cold when one feels unloved or a lack of a loving presence. The depiction of the room could reflect Max's view of his mother, as cold, absent and lacking any recognition of the needs and nightmares of her young hurt and angry son. Indeed, Max's mother never actually appears in the book. Max's bedroom looks like an adult's bedroom, which begs the question of whether Max is allowed his own emotional space to be a vulnerable, needy child. This is an issue that can be relevant to a child who has experienced a traumatic family event, or who is stuck in difficult role-reversals in which his fragile mother or father require his support, rather than being able to support him.

At this point, there is a change from reality to a fantasy as we are told, "That very night in Max's room a forest grew" (p. 7). As the forest grows, we see Max's body language changing from a possible angry or dejected image to excitedly laughing to himself. Then he turns his back to both the teller and the listener, in a kind of monster pose. Throughout these pages, the text refers only to the forest. The storyteller could ask the listener, what do they think Max is feeling? What do they think Max is thinking? Why is the forest growing larger and larger? The latter could raise questions about how feelings can expand from hurt and anger to becoming very big and overwhelming to the self. As well as the growing forest, the frames holding the picture of the book are also expanding. By the time the forest has fully grown, the picture has taken over the entirety of the right page. This could be representative of how Max's feelings of fury are growing and his self feels very small in comparison. His excitement of feeling "a monster" is also taking over. It could also signify how his feelings are growing very big inside him as he struggles to find a way to relate to his mother. By creating "an excited monster", he creates a way to regain control and not feel so vulnerable.

Also poignant here is the fact that Max's back is turned for the first time. There can be curiousity about what it feels like to be Max and "What might Max be planning to do?" Later, there could be discussions about turning one's back on someone, what one might be feeling, why that hard back is used like a slammed door. A child in a difficult position can often say that it feels safer to turn one's hard back on help, for facing the other person represents the more risky position of opening up emotionally and being overwhelmed with painful feelings again. Subsequently, we see Max sailing a boat with his name written on it. At this point, he is looking directly at the storyteller and listener and smiling. The storyteller could again ask and think aloud to herself about her question, "What is Max thinking and feeling here?" The reader is firmly placed in Max's story, going on his imaginative journey with him, identifying with his make-believe journey. Max has been sailing for "almost over a year" (p. 15) when he meets the wild things, who seem to frighten him initially. In the early stages of admission, this can reflect a long, lonely road into withdrawal. The terror of the wild things could reflect how the non-speaking child feels that his family, the staff, everyone "out" there are bad, and the non-speaking child is the terrified victim of both external people and internal monsters found in nightmares. Max remains connected to the action pressing onward, facing horrible wild things with terrible rolling eyes and gnashing teeth. The monsters are taller than Max's boat and situated on land, while Max is still at sea. Max does not now appear scared; rather, he looks cross or slightly unimpressed. Again, in front of a non-speaking child, one could think aloud to oneself or another person about what Max is thinking or one could think about why he looks different in this picture.

Then one turns the page and Max has "tamed them with the magic trick of staring into all their yellow eyes without blinking once" (p. 17). This victory of Max over the wild things could not only reassure the child, but also exemplify that one can face horrible things and thus find the courage to have control over them in one's fantasies or imagination. By removing himself from his home and a place of conflict, Max has come to be able to control the terrible monsters. This could be used to think about the non-speaking child's retreat inward and his gradual struggle to find a way of seeing those troubling experiences "in the eye". He can thus find a way of containing his powerful emotions through seeing and lending meaning and thinking directly about them. Workers could acknowledge that Max has done his best to manage in a difficult situation. Analogies can be made to experiences and feelings of a non-speaking child. This can lead to thinking about alternative ways to manage such as through creative therapies, which enable a non-speaking child to symbolise feelings that may not have words yet and then discover ways to contain them through thinking about them.

Interestingly, the text states that the wild things "were frightened and called him the most wild thing of all... and made him king of all the wild things" (p. 20). This suggests various points of discussion. It may connect with a non-speaking child's terror in relation to the power and strength of his fury and fears. It may also open an exploration of whatever isn't safe within the family communications. There can also be discussion about the helplessness and lack of strength and power that a child may experience, either in relation to his feelings or external situations in the family or school. The sailboat journey can reflect the need to find a way of making known his sense of helplessness, the necessity of helping him own his assertive, aggressive self, and give him a sense of agency. This will enable him to use containment of emotion and relinquish his 'hard back' and omnipotent control present in his not-speaking and not-eating.

This point is reinforced later when as King of the all the wild things, Max commands his subjects to "let the wild rumpus start" (p. 22). After the rumpus, when the sun is rising, Max commands the end of the rumpus and assertively "sends the wild things off to bed without any supper" (p. 29). This echo of Max's mother's action is interesting and could be interpreted in different ways. It could be that the rumpus was cathartic and Max has expelled his wild impulses. He has learned to assertively take control of his own hostile impulses rather than being an out-of-control child. Projection of hostile feelings as a way of managing one's own difficult feelings can be thought about by staff together with a young person in relation to being either the one who has projected hostile feelings and/or the one into whom hostile feelings have been projected hostility, or both.

The idea of food being connected with love is raised again in the immediate juxtaposition between "Max the king of all wild things was lonely/and wanted to be where someone loved him best of all" (p. 30), with "Then all around from far away across the world/he smelled good things to eat" (p. 30). This smelling of good food is symbolic of Max longing for his mother and for a nurturing, loving experience. Again, this raises questions about whether love is conveyed through giving and receiving food, and about whether or not hate or anger are conveyed through taking away food or rejecting it and closing the mouth to words too. It also raises questions about the availability and reliability of that offering of food and love. Even though Max has been away for over a year, that connection is still there with his mother.

As Max returns back home and further away from the wild things, Max has ambivalent facial expressions, so the storyteller can think aloud to oneself in front of the non-speaking child about what Max is thinking and feeling. He could be ambivalent as the idea of returning evokes some difficult questions. Will Max be recognised and will he be remembered? What else will have changed? Will there be room for him when he goes back and will he be accepted? What can he do with his hurt, his hostility, his longing for his parents, his love? This can easily lead to more personal work for the child in thinking about his own return home and in considering what feelings and expectations there are about going back to home and school. How can he maintain a sense of hope, bear the difficulties he will face and manage his anxieties about change? In contrast, the book can also be used to work on themes of loss. What has Max left behind? Why does he miss his mum, and long to go back to her? Why don't the monsters want him to leave? What happens when you go away and distance yourself through hostility from the one upon whom you depend and whom you love? And where is the father in this book? It feels as though a divorced couple could be in the background of the story.

When Max returns to his bedroom, he has taken off the hood of his wolf suit, revealing the young boy underneath. The furniture in his room is now a more appropriate size for him, although there is still nothing marking it out as a child's bedroom, however, in line with the food/love connection, the fact that "he found his supper waiting for him" (p. 35) suggests reconciliation and resolution of conflict. On the very last page, the text simply states "and it was still hot" (p. 37). The use of "still" is crucial; it is the pivot upon which the central dilemma of the book hangs. It suggests that all the events took place on the same night, and so the reasoning of this must be that this was a dream or nightmare, an imaginative journey. This can help the child to think about the different journeys he has undertaken, both externally in life and internally in his dreams and nightmares. Having been let loose in his imaginative dreams or waking thoughts and having explored the wild feelings, he develops an understanding of himself and what he needs. Max realises that he has had enough and he returns back home. The idea of developing one's own internal capacity to contain and understand a kaleidoscope of different intense feelings is very important in relation to a non-speaking and non-eating child who has not been able to take this explorative journey by himself.

In contradiction to the food still being hot, the moon, which is in the last picture of the book, has become a full moon. At the beginning of the book, when Max is in his bedroom, the moon is three-quarters full. It then wanes before waxing again to become full. This can be used to represent a reality of passing time and growth. Therapeutic work could be done regarding the toleration of uncertainty about how long it will take to recover and go back home.

This story is particularly helpful in raising the fundamental and overarching question of where the wild things are; are they inside or out? This can open up thinking about the need and desire to have a "rumpus". Key work could consider what painful and conflictual events happened both externally and internally, that were internalised and distorted and now need to come "out". How can the non-speaking child let out his unthinkable feelings and phantasies? What terrible things can happen to make one so angry that one feels like a wild thing, and what are the consequences of being so angry? The child may need to consider, "Have you never been allowed or allowed yourself to feel safe enough to experience 'wild feelings'?" Again, the child needs help in differentiating "wild feelings" from "wild actions", because sometimes "wild feelings" feel like they are actions. Like Max, a child can go on a journey of self-exploration and be helped to find his own internal ways of coping, emotional regulation, and boundaries. Similar to the length of Max's one-year journey, it often takes a year for the inpatient recovery of a child who is in a *pervasive retreat from life*, which includes not talking, not walking and not eating. The child will subsequently continue in outpatient individual and family psychotherapy.

Conclusion

This chapter has introduced a way of working with narratives that can work on several levels:

First, the act of reading the picture book or sharing a poem or piece of music brings the storyteller and the non-speaking child into a shared space and potentially opens the child up to experiencing something new and mutual. Second, the non-speaking child can reflect on and relate to thoughts and feelings in specific stories as the narrator thinks aloud. Narratives can be used to model different and sometimes difficult relationships between families and their children. The particular narratives mentioned in this chapter raise specific issues that can also be helpful to think about. These are but a few examples of themes in the narratives we have described: they could be explored in much greater depth and with particular relevance to the non-speaking young person with whom one is working.

Overall, shared experiences of narratives, be they picture books, poems, drawings, dance, or music, are valid and useful forms of communicating. They link the non-speaking child's internal and external worlds, and present a non-invasive forum for connection and reflection. They are tools that offer a safe third space for exploring feelings, and in this way help the non-speaking child to begin to think more fully, to develop a safe, containing space within himself, and to form more intimate, loving connections with parents, staff, siblings, and other young people.

GLOSSARY

The following pages describe some key psychoanalytic concepts used in this book. Further exploration of psychoanalytic concepts including these terms, with relevant current references, can be located in *The New Dictionary of Kleinian Thought* edited by E. Bott Spillius, J. Milton, P. Garvey, C. Couve, and D. Steiner (2011).

Containment

This concept is based on the model of a mother as a container for the infant's projected feelings, needs, and unwanted aspects of the self. Using reverie, the mother receives the baby's projections and conveys to him the sense that his anxieties and communications are bearable and have meaning. It is through the internalising of a mindful caregiver that the infant gradually develops the capacity for mentalization. A child has a sense of containment when he believes that his feelings, though sometimes painful and frightening, are manageable and will not overwhelm or drive away the external parents (Dallos, 2006, p. 118). When a child has internalised containing parents, the child has the capacity to experience his own feelings as manageable through lending thought to them, rather than as overwhelming and requiring projection into others or the use of some other defence mechanism such as primitive omnipotence.

Countertransference

This concept refers to the whole of the therapist's feelings and unconscious reactions occurring in the encounter with the young person or the family. It is one of the most important therapeutic tools for thinking about the feelings of the young person and the family. The countertransference can provide valuable information about the unconscious feelings that are not yet in symbolic form suitable for talking to and thinking with the therapist.

Denial

The process of denial can involve disposing of limitations of the self and the importance of the people upon whom one depends. Denial can also involve idealization when bad parts of the self or other are unacknowledged leaving an idealized self or other.

Dissociation

This refers to a partial or complete disruption of the normal integration of a person's consciousness. Dissociation can be a protective response to trauma, for it allows the conscious self to distance itself from overwhelming experiences that are too much for the psyche to process.

Inner world and internal objects or figures

There is the external world with external family figures, school figures, peers and there is the internal world of internal objects or figures formed by the introjective identification with external loved and hated important figures who are distorted by one's phantasies and feelings projected onto them. The person's internal world provides the impetus for re-enactment in relation to external figures.

Internalisation/Introjection

These mechanisms involve taking in aspects, qualities, or skills of the parents and other important caregivers. Very early integration of a good breast is important for ego integration, but internalisation of the bad breast also occurs.

Introjective identification

This concept describes a process of being in a relationship with someone and taking in aspects, qualities, or skills of the person in such a way that they are gradually identified with and inform the character of an individual. Introjection of bad qualities also occurs. Introjective identification with parents and therapeutic professionals, who can metabolize and process experiences and anxiety, promotes the healthy development of the young person.

Mentalizing

This is an act of mental activity in which one imagines what other people might be thinking or feeling. It implies perceiving and interpreting behaviour as combined with intentional mental states. It involves analysing one's emotional experiences (Bateman & Fonagy, 2006, p. 2).

Omnipotence

This is a concept referring to a notion that one's thoughts have a power to protect the self from harmful anxieties. For a child using primitive omnipotence, there is a turning to his phantasies as powerful and controlling protections. The child's omnipotence is used rather than facing the reality of his persecutory fears and depending on caregivers necessary for his' emotional development.

Phantasy

"There is no impulse, no instinctual urge or response, which is not experienced as unconscious phantasy" (Isaacs, 1952, p. 83). "Unconscious phantasy is in a constant interplay with external reality, both influencing and altering the perception or interpretation of it and also being influenced by it" (S. Box, B. Copley, J. Magagna & E. Smilansky, 1994c, p. 258).

Projective identification

This process is part of normal development in psychotherapy. Through the way he is being or speaking, a person puts parts of himself into the therapist so that the therapist may feel and understand those experiences and be able to contain them, enabling them to lose their unbearable quality. The problem comes when a person loses unwanted parts of himself in the other, and then he fears he is in the presence of the therapist relating with those projected parts of himself. A person may lose awareness of good parts of himself if they are also projected into the therapist.

Re-enactment

"An essential element in this concept is replacement of recollection (or any form of mental realization) by a blindly repeating a pattern of internalized events" (Britton, 1994, p. 86)."

Regression

This is a process involving emotionally returning to an earlier stage of psychological development rather than handling an emotional crisis in an age-appropriate way.

Reparation

When the object loved is also seen to be the same object as the object hated, then some integration of the personality can occur, and there is some feeling of responsibility to repair harm done to the good object.

Splitting

This process occurs as part of normal development, but also in later life. It involves separating the gratifying experiences linked with an attuned experience with a person and keeping these good experiences separated from the persecuting, frustrating negative experiences. This leaves an idealised object and a hostile persecutory object relation until the splitting is replaced by integration of the good and bad aspects of the object.

Transference

Transference implies that there are impulses and phantasies that are aroused and made conscious during the progress of the therapy. A transference experience is part of an ongoing internal relationship to internal figures that is being re-experienced in relation to the therapist.

Working through

The process of repeating, elaborating, and amplifying interpretations. It is believed that such working through is critical for the success of therapy. Interpretations allow the person in psychotherapy to apply rational thought and conscious awareness to an emotion that previously had been hidden by defensive mechanisms in the personality. Working through can occur when a person in therapy comes up with a "thing", be it written, a piece of art, music, verbal, or some other form that was previously buried in the subconscious or unconscious mind. This "thing" is then used by the psychotherapist to say "this is an interpretation of such-and-such" event occurring in the person's internal drama and perhaps also from the person's past. This interpretation may or may not be correct. It may be suggested by the person in therapy or by the therapist. It may even be a deliberate or subconscious deliberate mis-interpretation by the person in therapy in an attempt to keep the therapist away from the root problem.

Assuming that the "thing" gives rise to a reasonably correct interpretation, using the theory of *working through*, the person in therapy will then be able to apply rational thought and conscious awareness in order to overcome the maladjustment to a current emotional situation that had previously existed because of distortions of current experiences that had occurred through projection.

REFERENCES

Acquarone, S. (2004). *Infant–Parent Psychotherapy*. London: Karnac.

Adkins, Adele, L. B. & White, E. (2008). *Chasing Pavements*. London: XL Recordings.

Allen, J. & Allen, S. (pseudonyms) (2002). How we fought for Lucy. *The Times*, 21 May.

Allen, J. G. (2003). Mentalizing. *Bulletin of the Menninger Clinic, 67*: 91–112.

Almodóvar, P. (2002). *Talk to Her* (*Hable con Ella*, original Spanish title). Sony Pictures.

Alvarez, A. (2002). Failures to link: attacks or defects, disintegration or unintegration? In: A. Briggs (Ed.), *Surviving Space: Papers on Infant Observation* (pp. 240–256). London: Karnac.

Amos, T. (1992). Crucify. From: *Little Earthquakes*, Atlantic Records.

Andrews, J., Clark, D. J. & Zinker, J. C. (1988). Accessing transgenerational themes through dreamwork. *Journal of Marital and Family Therapy, 14*(1): 15–27.

Angelou, M. (1969). *I Know Why the Caged Bird Sings*. New York: Random House.

Arlow, J. (1961). Silence and the theory of technique. *Journal of the American Psychiatric Association, 9*: 44–45.

Aron, L. (1996). Symposium on the meaning and practice of intersubjectivity in psychoanalysis: introduction. *Psychoanalytic Dialogues, 6*: 591–597.

Atwood, M. (1995). *Morning in the Burned House*. New York: Houghton Mifflin.

Baars, B., Ramsoy, T. & Laureys, S. (2003). Brain, conscious experience and the observing self. *Trends in Neurosciences, 26*: 671–675.

Baguley, I., Nicholls, J., Felmingham, K., Crooks, J., Gurka, J. & Wade, L. (1999). Dysautonomia after traumatic brain injury: a forgotten syndrome? *Journal of Neurology, Neurosurgery and Psychiatry, 67*(1): 39–43.

Balint, M. (1950). Changing therapeutic aims and techniques in psycho-analysis. *International Journal of Psychoanalysis, 31*: 117–124.

Balint, M. (1955). Friendly expanses—horrid empty spaces. *International Journal of Psychoanalysis, 36*: 225–241.

Balint, M. (1958). The three areas of the mind-theoretical considerations. *International Journal of Psychoanalysis, 39*: 328–340.

Balint, M. (1962). The theory of the parent–infant relationship—contributions to discussion. *International Journal of Psychoanalysis, 43*: 251–252.

Balint, M. (1968). *The Basic Fault: Therapeutic Aspects of Regression.* Evanston: Northwestern University Press.

Barry, L. (2009). *What It Is: Do You Wish You Could Write?* London: Jonathan Cape.

Barry, L. (2010). *Picture This: The Near-Sighted Monkey Book.* Quebec: Drawn & Quarterly.

Barzel Raveh, I. (2009). From being no-body to being somebody: on the journey back to life. The application of infant observation to work with severely traumatized brain-injured patients suffering from low levels of consciousness. Unpublished presentation to the International Infant Observation Conference, Tavistock Clinic, London.

Bateman, A. & Fonagy, P. (2004). *Psychotherapy for Borderline Personality Disorder: Mentalization-Based Treatment.* New York: Oxford University Press.

Bateman, A. & Fonagy, P. (2006). *Mentalisation-Based Treatment for Borderline Personality Disorder: A Practical Guide.* Oxford: Oxford University Press.

Bates, D. (2005). The vegetative state and the Royal College of Physicians guidance. *Neuropsychological Rehabilitation Journal, 15*(3/4): 175–183.

Bateson, G. (1972). *Steps to an Ecology of Mind: Collected Essays in Anthropology, Psychiatry, Evolution, and Epistemology.* St Albans: Paladin.

Bauby, J. D. (2004). *The Diving Bell and the Butterfly.* London: Harper Perennial.

Beckett, S. (1961). *Happy Days.* New York: Grove Press.

Benjamin, J. (1988). *The Bonds of Love.* New York: Pantheon.

Benjamin, J. (1990). An outline of intersubjectivity: the development of recognition. *Psychoanalytic Psychology, 7*: 33–46.

Benjamin, J. (1992). Recognition and destruction: an outline of intersubjectivity. In: N. Skolnick & S. Warshaw (Eds.), *Relational Perspectives in Psychoanalysis* (pp. 43–60). Hillsdale, NJ: The Analytic Press.

Beres, D. & Arlow, A. (1974). Fantasy and identification in empathy. *The Psychoanalytic Quarterly, 43*: 26–50.

Berke, J. (1989). *The Tyranny of Malice: Exploring the Dark Side of Character.* London: Simon & Schuster.

Bermudez, J. L. (1998). *The Paradox of Self-Consciousness.* Cambridge, MA: MIT Press.

Bick, E. (1968). The experience of the skin in early object relations. *International Journal of Psychoanalysis, 49*: 484–486.

Bion, W. R. (1959). Attacks on linking. *International Journal of Psychoanalysis, 40*: 308–315.

Bion, W. R. (1961). *Experiences in Groups and Other Papers.* London: Tavistock.

Bion, W. R. (1962). *Learning from Experience.* London: William Heinemann [Reprinted London: Karnac, 1984].

Bion, W. R. (1963). *The Elements of Psychoanalysis.* London: William Heinemann [Reprinted London: Karnac, 1984].

Bion, W. R. (1965). *Transformations.* London: William Heinemann [Reprinted London: Karnac, 1984].

Bion, W. R. (1967). *Second Thoughts.* London: William Heinemann [Reprinted London: Karnac, 1984].

Bloom, K. (2006). Unpublished part of preparatory manuscript for *The Embodied Self.* London: Karnac.

Blos, P. (1972). Silence: a clinical exploration. *The Psychoanalytic Quarterly, 41*: 348–363.
Bodtker, J. (1990). *Beyond Words: Interpretive Art Therapy.* Worcester: Clunie Press.
Bourne, S. (1981). *Under the Doctor: Studies in the Psychological Problems of Physiotherapists, Patients and Doctors.* England: Avebury.
Bowlby, J. (1969). *Attachment and Loss: Vol. 1 Attachment.* London and New York: Hogarth.
Bowlby, J. (1973a). *Attachment and Loss: Vol. 2: Separation: Anxiety and Anger.* New York: Basic Books.
Bowlby, J. (1973b). *Attachment and Loss. Vol. 3: Loss: Sadness and Depression.* New York: Basic Books.
Box, S. (1994a). Space for thinking in families. In: S. Box, B. Copley, J. Magagna & E. Similansky (Eds.), *Crisis at Adolescence.* Northvale, NJ, and London: Jason Aronson.
Box, S. (1994b). Engaging in the process of change with families at adolescence. In: S. Box, B. Copley, J. Magagna & E. Similansky (Eds.), *Crisis at Adolescence.* Northvale, NJ, and London: Jason Aronson.
Box, S., Copley, B., Magagna, J. & Smilansky (Eds.) (1994). *Crisis at Adolescence.* Northvale, NJ, and London: Jason Aronson.
Breuer, J. & Freud, S. (1895). *Studies in Hysteria.* James Strachey (Ed.). New York: Basic Books, 1957.
Briggs, S. (1997a). *Growth and Risk in Infancy.* London: Jessica Kingsley.
Briggs, S. (1997b). *Patterns of Containment: Relationship of Mothers and Infants Where Infants Are at Potential Risk.* London: Tavistock.
Britton, R. (1989). The missing link: parental sexuality in the Oedipus complex. In: R. Britton, M. Feldman & E. O'Shaughnessy (Eds.), *The Oedipus Complex Today: Clinical Implications* (pp. 83–101). London: Karnac, 1989.
Britton, R. (1994). Re-enactment as an unwitting professional response to family dynamics. In: S. Box, B. Copley, J. Magagna & E. Smilansky (Eds.), *Crisis at Adolescence.* Northvale, NJ, and London: Jason Aronson.
Britton, R., Feldman, M. & O'Shaughnessy, E. (1989). *The Oedipus Complex Today: Clinical Implications.* London: Karnac.
Buckholz, M. B. (1990). Using dreams in family therapy. *Journal of Family Therapy, 12*: 387–396.
Burningham, J. (1984). *Granpa.* London: Random House.
Burningham, J. (1992). *Come Away From the Water, Shirley.* London: Red Fox Random House.
Busch, R. (1978). The silent patient: issues of separation-individuation and its relationship to speech development. *International Review of Psycho-Analysis, 5*: 491–499.
Byng-Hall, J. (1980). Symptom bearer as marital distance regulator. *Family Process, 19*: 355–365.
Byng-Hall, J. (1995). *Rewriting Family Scripts.* New York: Guilford Press.
Calogeras, R. (1967). Silence as a technical parameter in psycho-analysis. *International Journal of Psychoanalysis, 48*: 536–558.
Cameron, J. (1995). *An Artist's Way: A Course in Discovering and Rediscovering Your Creative Self.* London: Pan Macmillan.
Camus, A. (1960). Create dangerously. In: A. Camus, *Resistance, Rebellion, and Death* (pp. 249–272). New York: Vintage Books.
Camus, A. (1963). *Albert Camus Notebooks, 1935–1942.* New York: Knopf.
Carle, E. (1969). *The Very Hungry Caterpillar.* New York: Putnam.
Carter, B. & McGoldrick, M. (1989). *The Changing Family Lifecycle.* Boston: Alyn & Bacon.
Case, C. (2005). *Imagining Animals: Art, Psychotherapy and Primitive States of Mind.* London: Routledge.
Cassidy, J. & Shaver, P. R. (2008). The nature of the child's ties. In: J. Cassidy & P. R. Shaver (Eds.), *Handbook of Attachment* (pp. 3–22). New York: The Guilford Press.

Child, L. (2008). *Charlie and Lola: I'm Really Ever So Not Well*. London: Puffin Books.

Chrétien de Troyes (1183). *Perceval ou le Conte du Graal*. Paris: G. F. Flammarion, 1997.

Coleridge, S. T. (1802). Dejection: an ode. In: E. H. Coleridge (Ed.), *Coleridge Poetical Works* (pp. 362–367). Oxford: Oxford University Press, 1988.

Coltart, N. (1989). Personal communication. In: J. Berke (Ed.), *The Tyranny of Malice: Exploring the Dark Side of Character*. London: Simon & Schuster.

Coltart, N. (1991). The silent patient. *Psychoanalytic Dialogues, 1*: 439–453.

Cooper, H. (2005). The sibling link. In: J. Magagna, N. L. Bakalar, H. Cooper, J. Levy, C. Norman & C. Shank (Eds.), *Intimate Transformations: Babies with their Families* (pp. 42–57). London: Karnac.

Copley, B. (2000). Family explorations. In: M. Rustin & E. Quagliata, *Assessment in Child Psychotherapy* (pp. 120–144). London: Karnac.

Cox, M. (1988). *Structuring the Therapeutic Process, Compromise with Chaos: The Therapist's Response to the Individual and the Group*. London, Bristol, Pennsylvania: Jessica Kingsley.

Da Rocha Barros, E. (2002). An essay on dreaming, psychical working out and working through. *International Journal of Psychoanalysis, 83*: 1083–1093.

Dallos, R. (2006). *Attachment Narrative Therapy*. Maidenhead: Open University Press.

Dartington, A. (1994). Where angels fear to tread: idealism, dependency, and inhibitions of thought in hospital nursing. In: A. Obholzer & V. Z. Roberts (Eds.), *The Unconscious at Work* (pp. 101–109). London and New York: Routledge.

Dartington, A. & Magagna, J. (1994). Making a space for parents. In: S. Box, B. Copley, J. Magagna & E. Smilansky (Eds.), *Crises in Adolescence*. Northvale, NJ, and London: Jason Aronson.

Daws, D. (1989). *Through the Night*. London: Free Association.

Daws, D. & Boston, M. (1981). *The Child Psychotherapist and the Problems of Young People*. London: Karnac.

Dosamantes, I. (1992). The intersubjective relationship between therapist and patient: a key to understanding denied and denigrated aspects of the patient's self. *The Arts and Psychotherapy, 19*: 359–365.

Dosamantes-Beaudry, I. (1997). Somatic experience in psychoanalysis. *Psychoanalytic Psychology, 14*: 517–530.

Dubinsky, A. (2007). Pensée et relation émotionnelle: comment le bébé se donne le temps de penser. In: A. Ciccone, D. Mellier, C. Athanassiou-Popesco, A. Carel, A. Dubinsky & A. Guedeney (Eds.), *Le bébé et le temps*. Paris: Dunod.

Dunn, J., Davies, L. C., O'Connor, T. G. & Sturgess, W. (2000). Parents' and partners' life course and family experiences: links with parent–child relationships in different family settings. *Journal of Child Psychology and Psychiatry, 41*(8): 955–968.

Eliot, T. S. (1940). East Coker: The Four Quartets. In: T. S. Eliot, *The Complete Poems and Plays* (pp. 123–129). Boston: Houghton Mifflin Harcourt, 1971.

Elmhirst, S. I. (1988). The Kleinian setting for child analysis. *International Review of Psycho-Analysis, 15*: 5–12.

Emanuel, R. (2001). A-void: an exploration of defences against sensing nothingness. *International Journal of Psycho-Analysis, 82*: 1069–1082.

Enelow, A. (1960). The silent patient. *Psychiatry, 23*: 153–158.

Epstein, N. B., Bishop, D. S. & Levin, S. (1978). McMaster model of family functioning. *Journal of Marriage and Family Counseling, 4*: 19–31.

Faimberg, H. (1988). The telescoping of generations: genealogy of certain identifications. *Contemporary Psychoanalysis, 24*: 99–117.

Fairbairn, W. R. (1952). *Psychoanalytic Studies of the Personality.* London, Henley, and Boston: Routledge & Kegan Paul.

Felmy, K. C. (1998). The icon in Orthodox theology and devotion. In: *The Art of Holy Russian Icons from Moscow, 1400–1660* (pp. 37–43). London: The Royal Academy.

Ferenczi, S. (1919). On the technique of psychoanalysis. In: *Further Contributions to the Theory and Technique of Psychoanalysis* (pp. 177–189). London: Hogarth, 1950.

Flowers, B., Keuning, D., Stoermer, M. & Vannucci, R. Jr. (2008). Human. From: *Day & Age.* Island Records.

Flynn, D. (1999). The challenges of in-patient work in a therapeutic community. In: M. Lanyado & A. Horne (Eds.), *The Handbook of Child and Adolescent Psychotherapy: Psychoanalytic Approaches* (pp. 167–181). London: Routledge.

Fonagy, P. (1991). Thinking about thinking: some clinical and theoretical considerations in the treatment of a borderline patient. *International Journal of Psychoanalysis, 72*: 639–656.

Fonagy, P. (2003). The development of psychopathology from infancy to adulthood: the mysterious unfolding of disturbance in time. *Infant Mental Health Journal, 24*(3): 212–239.

Fonagy, P., Gergely, G., Jurist, E. L. & Target, M. (2004). *Affect Regulation, Mentalization and the Development of the Self.* London: Karnac.

Fonagy, P., Steele, M., Moran, G., Steele, H. & Higgitt, A. (1993). Measuring the ghost in the nursery: an empirical study of the relation between parents' mental representations of childhood experiences and their infants' security of attachment. *American Psychoanalytic Association, 41*: 957–989.

Foulkes, S. H. (1964) *Therapeutic Group Analysis (1st American Edition).* London: George Allen & Unwin (p. 82 and p. 129)

Foukes, S. H. (1975). *Group-Analytic Psychotherapy, Method and Principles.* London and New York: Gordon and Breach.

Fraiberg, S. (1982). Pathological defences in infancy. *Psychoanalytic Quarterly, 51*: 612–635.

Fraiberg, S., Adelson, E. & Shapiro, V. (1980). Ghosts in the nursery: a psychoanalytic approach to impaired infant–mother relationships. In: S. Fraiberg (Ed.), *Clinical Studies in Infant Mental Health* (pp. 164–193). London: Tavistock.

Freeman, J., Epston, D. & Lobovits, D. (1997). *Playful Approaches to Serious Problems.* London and New York: W. W. Norton.

Freud, S. (1893). The psychotherapy of hysteria. *SE* 2 (pp. 255–305). London: Hogarth.

Freud, S. (1909b). Analysis of a phobia in a five-year-old boy. *SE 5* (pp. 5–148). London: Hogarth.

Freud, S. (1914g). Remembering, repeating and working through. Further recommendations in the technique of psychoanalysis II. *SE 12* (pp. 145–156). London: Hogarth.

Freud, S. (1920g). *Beyond the Pleasure Principle. SE 18* (pp. 7–66). London: Hogarth.

Frith, C. & Wolpert, D. (Eds.) (2004). *The Neuroscience of Social Interaction: Decoding, Imitating, and Influencing the Actions of Others.* Oxford: Oxford University Press.

Gallagher, S. (2000). Philosophical conceptions of the self: implications for cognitive science. *Trends in Cognitive Sciences, 4*(1): 14–21.

Garland, C. (1999). *Understanding Trauma: A Psychoanalytic Approach, Tavistock Clinic.* London: Duckworth.

Gersie, A. & King, N. (1989). *Storymaking in Education and Therapy.* London: Jessica Kingsley.

Giacino, J. T. & Kalmar, K. (2005). Diagnostic and prognostic guidelines for the vegetative and minimally conscious states. *Neuropsychological Rehabilitation, 15*(3/4): 166–174.

Glover, E. (1927a). Lectures on technique in psycho-analysis, part I. *International Journal of Psychoanalysis, 8*: 311–338.

Glover, E. (1927b). Lectures on technique in psycho-analysis, part III. *International Journal of Psychoanalysis, 8*: 486–520.

Graham, P. & Foreman, D. (1995). An ethical dilemma in child and adolescent psychiatry. *Psychiatric Bulletin, 19*: 84–86.

Greene, G. (2004). *The Quiet American.* London: Vintage.

Greenson, R. (1961). On the silence and sounds of the analytic hours. *Journal of the American Psychoanalytic Association, 9*: 79–84.

Hadda, J. (1991). The ontogeny of silence in an analytic case. *International Journal of Psychoanalysis, 72*: 117–130.

Hadiks, D. (1994). Non-verbal aspects of therapist attunement. *Journal of Clinical Psychology, 50*: 393–505.

Hamaguchi, P. (1995). *Childhood Speech, Language and Listening Problems.* New York: John Wiley.

Harris, M. (1970). Notes on maternal containment and good-enough mothering. *Journal of Child Psychotherapy, 4*: 35–51.

Heimann, P. (1950). On countertransference. *International Journal of Psycho-Analysis, 31*: 81–84.

Hinshelwood, R. D. (1999). Countertransference. *International Journal of Psycho-Analysis, 80*: 797–818.

Hobson, P. (2002). *The Cradle of Thought: Exploring the Origins of Thinking.* London: Macmillan.

Hodges, J., Steele, M., Hillman, S. & Henderson, K. (2003). Mental representations and defences in severely maltreated children: a story stem battery and rating system for clinical assessment and research applications. In: R. N. Emde, D. P. Wolf & D. Oppenheim (Eds.), *Revealing the Inner Worlds of Young Children: The MacArthur Stem Battery and Parent-Child Narratives* (pp. 240–267). Oxford: Oxford University Press.

Hodgson Burnett, F. (1911). *The Secret Garden.* London: Heinemann [Reprinted London: Penguin, 1951, 1994].

Hopkins, J. (1996). The dangers and deprivations of too good mothering. *Journal of Child Psychotherapy, 22*: 407–422.

Hopper, E. (1975). *Group-Analytic Psychotherapy, Method and Principles.* London and New York: Gordon and Breach.

Hopper, E. (1991). Encapsulation as a defence against the fear of annihilation. *International Journal of Psychoanalysis, 72*: 607–624.

Hopper, E. (1995). A psychoanalytical theory of drug addiction: unconscious fantasies of homosexuality, compulsions and masturbation within the context of traumatogenic processes. *International Journal of Psychoanalysis, 76*: 1121–1142.

Hopper, E. (1997). Traumatic experience in the unconscious life of groups: a fourth basic assumption. *Group Analysis, 30*: 439–470.

Hopper, E. (2003a). *The Social Unconscious: Selected Papers.* London and Philadelphia: Jessica Kingsley.

Hopper, E. (2003b). *Traumatic Experience in the Unconscious Life of Groups.* Philadelphia: Jessica Kingsley.

Houzel, D. (1999). Therapeutic application of infant observation in child psychiatry. *International Journal of Infant Observation, 2*: 42–53.

Houzel, D. (2010). Infant observation and the receptive mind. *Infant Observation, 13*(2): 119–133.

Husserl, E. (1910). Philosophy as rigorous science. Translated in: Q. Lauer (Ed.), *Phenomenology and the Crisis of Philosophy* (pp. 71–147). New York: Harper, 1965.

Isaacs, S. (1952). The nature and function of phantasy. In: M. Klein, P. Issacs, P. Heimann & J. Riviere (Eds.), *Developments in Psychoanalysis* (pp. 67–121). London: Hogarth.

Isaacs-Elmhirst, S. (1988). The Kleinian setting for child analysis. *International Review of Psychoanalysis, 15*: 5–12.

Joseph, B. (1975). The patient who is difficult to reach. In: E. Spillius (Ed.), *Melanie Klein Today: Developments in Theory and Practice, Vol. 2: Mainly Practice.* London and New York: Routledge, 1988.

Joseph, B. (1985). Transference: the total situation. *International Journal of Psycho-Analysis, 66*: 447–453.

Kabat-Zinn, J. (1990). *Full Catastrophe Living: How to Cope with Stress, Pain and Illness Using Mindfulness Meditation.* New York: Delacorte.

Kaplan, J., Saayman, G. S. & Faber, P. A. (1981). An investigation of the use of nocturnal dream reports as diagnostic indices in the assessment of family problem solving. *Journal of Family Therapy, 3*: 227–242.

Keats, J. (1820). *Ode on Melancholy.* In: G. Bullett (Ed.), *John Keats: Poems* (pp. 200–201). London: Dent, 1974.

Kerr, J. (1999). *The Tiger Who Came to Tea.* London: Harper Collins.

Khan, M. (1963). Silence as communication. *Bulletin of the Menninger Clinic, 27*: 300–317.

Killick, K. (1993). Working with psychotic processes in art therapy. *Psychoanalytical Psychotherapy, 7*(1): 25–28.

Kimmelman, M. (2004, 14 October). Looking long and hard at Morandi. *New York Times* Retrieved from http://www.nytimes.com. [last accessed August 2011].

Klein, M. (1921). The development of the child. In: *Love, Guilt and Reparation* (pp. 1–53). London: Hogarth and the Institute of Psychoanalysis, 1975.

Klein, M. (1930). The importance of symbol-formation in the development of the ego. *Love, Guilt and Reparation and Other Works 1921–45* (pp. 219–231). London: Hogarth, 1975.

Klein, M. (1931). A contribution to the theory of intellectual inhibition. In: *Contributions to Psychoanalysis 1921–1945* (Ed. E. Jones). London: Hogarth and the Institute of Psychoanalysis, 1985.

Klein, M. (1932). *Psychoanalysis of Children.* London: Hogarth and the Institute of Psychoanalysis, 1989.

Klein, M. (1935). A contribution to the psychogenesis of manic-depressive states. *The Writings of Melanie Klein, Vol. 1* (pp. 262–289). London: Hogarth.

Klein, M. (1946). Notes on some schizoid mechanisms. In: *Envy and Gratitude and Other Works 1946–1963* (pp. 1–24). London: Hogarth, 1975.

Klein, M. (1952a). The origins of transference. *International Journal of Psycho-Analysis, 33*: 433–438.

Klein, M. (1952b). Notes on some schizoid mechanisms. In: M. Klein, P. Heimann, S. Isaacs & J. Riviere (Eds.), *Developments in Psychoanalysis* (pp. 292–320). London: Hogarth, 1973.

Klein, M. (1958). On the development of mental functioning. *Envy and Gratitude and Other Works 1946–1963* (pp. 236–246). London: Hogarth, 1975.

Klein, M. (1975). *Envy and Gratitude and Other Works 1946–1963.* London: Hogarth.

Klein, S. (1980). Autistic phenomena in neurotic patients. *International Journal of Psychoanalysis, 61*: 395–402.

Kohut, H. & Wolf, E. (1978). The disorders of the self and their treatment. *International Journal of Psychoanalysis, 59*: 414–425.

Krystal, H. (1978). Trauma and affects. *Psychoanalytic Study of the Child, 33*: 81–116.

Kurtz, S. (1984). On silence. *The Psychoanalytic Review, 71*: 227–246.

Laiho, S. (2004). The psychological functions of music in adolescence. *The Nordic Journal of Music Therapy, 13*(1): 47–63.

Lask, B. (1996). Pervasive refusal syndrome. *Association for Child Psychology and Psychiatry, Occasional Papers Series, 12*: 33–35.

Lask, B. (2004). Pervasive refusal syndrome. *Advances in Psychiatric Treatment, 10*: 153–159.

Lask, B., Britten, C., Kroll, L., Magagna, J. & Tranter, M. (1991). Children with pervasive refusal. *Archives of Disease in Childhood, 66*: 866–869.

Lawrence, G. (2003). *Experiences in Social Dreaming*. London: Karnac.

Lawrence, G. (2004). *Introduction to Social Dreaming*. London: Karnac.

Leira, T. (1995). Silence and communication: nonverbal dialogue and therapeutic action. *The Scandinavian Psychoanalytic Review, 18*: 41–65.

Lennox, A. (1992). Little Bird. From: *Diva*. BMG, Columbia Records and Arista Records.

Leunig, M. (1990). *A Common Prayer*. New Blackburn, Victoria, Australia: Collins Dove.

Levy, K. (1958). Silence in the analytic session. *International Journal of Psychoanalysis, 39*: 50–58.

Liebmann, M. (2004). *Art Therapy for Groups: A Handbook of Themes and Exercises*. London: Routledge.

Liegner, E. (1974). The silent patient. *The Psychoanalytic Review, 61*: 229–245.

Likierman, M. (2001). An unsatisfied longing for an understanding without words. *Melanie Klein: Her Work in Context* (pp. 192–197). London and New York: Continuum.

Limentani, A. (1966). A re-evaluation of acting out in relation to working through. *International Journal of Psychoanalysis, 47*: 274–282.

Loewenstein, R. (1956). Some remarks on the role of speech in psycho-analytic technique. *International Journal of Psychoanalysis, 37*: 460–468.

Loewenstein, R. (1961). The silent patient: introduction. *Journal of the American Psychoanalytic Association, 9*: 2–6.

Loomie, L. (1961). Some ego considerations in the silent patient. *Journal of the American Psychoanalytic Association, 9*: 56–78.

Luepnitz, D. (1988). *The Family Interpreted*. New York: Basic Books.

MacNeice, L. (1940). Plurality. In: M. Longley (Ed.), *Selected Poems* (p. 243). London: Faber and Faber, 1966.

Magagna, J. (1993). Individual psychotherapy. In: B. Lask & R. Bryant-Waugh (Eds.), *Anorexia Nervosa and Related Eating Disorders in Childhood and Adolescence*. Hove, Sussex: Psychology Press.

Magagna, J. (1998). Psychodynamic psychotherapy in an inpatient setting. In: B. Jacobs & J. Green (Eds.), *Inpatient Psychiatric Treatment of Children and Adolescents* (pp. 124–143). London: Routledge.

Magagna, J. (2000). Families and child psychotherapy: a Kleinian perspective. In: J. Hills (Ed.), *Rescripting Family Experiences* (pp. 87–106). London: Whurr Publishers.

Magagna, J. (2002). Three years of infant observation with Mrs. Bick. In: A. Briggs (Ed.), *Surviving Space: Papers on Infant Observation*. London: Karnac.

Magagna, J., Bakalar, N.L., Cooper, H., Levy, J., Norman, C., & Shank, C. (Eds.) *Intimate Transformations: Babies with their Families*. London: Karnac.

Magagna, J. (2009). Sharing stories to identify with the non-speaking child. Unpublished excerpt.

Magagna, J. (2011). Unpublished talk, Family Explorations, given to Centro Studi Martha Harris, Venice.

Mannoni, M. (1973). *The Child, "The Illness" and Others*. Harmondsworth: Penguin Books.

McDougall, J. (1989). *Theatres of the Body: A Psychoanalytical Approach to Psychosomatic Illness*. London: Free Association.

McGowan, R. & Green, J. (1998). Pervasive refusal syndrome: a less severe variant with defined aetiology. *Clinical Child Psychology and Psychiatry, 3*: 583–590.

McKee, D. (2005). *Not Now, Bernard*. London: Andersen Press.
McNeilly, G. & Kingsley, J. (2006). *Group Analytic Art Therapy*. London: Jessica Kingsley.
Meissner, W. (2000). On analytic listening. *The Psychoanalytic Quarterly, 69*: 317–367.
Meltzer, D. (1967). *The Psychoanalytic Process*. Perth: Clunie, 1990.
Meltzer, D. (1975). Adhesive identification. *Contemporary Psychoanalysis, 11*(3): 289–310.
Meltzer, D. (1983). *Dream-Life: A Re-Examination of the Psycho-Analytical Theory and Technique*. Perth: Clunie, for the Roland Harris Trust Library, No. 12.
Meltzer, D. (1984). Personal communication.
Meltzer, D. (1992). *The Claustrum: An Investigation of Claustrophobic Phenomena*. Strathtay: Clunie.
Meltzer, D. & Harris, M. (1976). A psychoanalytical model of the child-in-the-family-in-the-community. In: A. Hahn (Ed.), *Sincerity and Other Works: Collected Papers of Donald Meltzer*. London: Karnac, 1994.
Meltzer , D., Bremner, J., Hoxter, S., Weddell, D. & Wittenberg, I. (1975). *Explorations in Autism*. Perth: Clunie.
Menzies-Lyth, I. (1959). The functioning of social systems as a defence against anxiety. In: *Containing Anxiety in Institutions: Selected Essays, Volume 1* (pp. 43–89). London: Free Association, 1988.
Menzies-Lyth, I. (1988). *Containing Anxiety in Institutions: Selected Essays, Volume 1*. London: Free Association.
Miller, J. (1989). The analysis of a nonverbal latency boy. *Bulletin of the Anna Freud Centre, 12*: 309–329.
Miller, L. (2002). Lessons from infant observation: the developing mind of the baby. *International Journal of Infant Observation, 5*(1): 21–36.
Mitrani, J. (1995). Toward an understanding of unmentalized experience. *The Psychoanalytic Quarterly, 64*, 68-112.
Moreno, J. L. (1946) *Psychodrama Vol. 1*. Beacon New York: Beacon House.
Nacht, S. (1963). The non-verbal relationship in psycho-analytic treatment. *International Journal of Psychoanalysis, 44*: 334–339.
Nacht, S. (1964). Silence as an integrative factor. *International Journal of Psychoanalysis, 45*: 299–303.
Nasar, S. (2008) *A Beautiful Mind*. New York: Simon and Schuster.
Natterson, J. (1991). *Beyond Countertransference*. Northvale, NJ: Jason Aronson.
Natterson, J. & Friedman, R. (1995). *A Primer of Clinical Intersubjectivity*. Northvale, NJ: Jason Aronson.
Nicolo, A. M. & Trapanese, G. (2005). *Quale Psicoanalisi per la Famiglia?* Milan, Italy: Franco Angeli.
North, A. & Hargreaves, D. (1999). Music and adolescent identity. *Music Education Research 1*(1): 75–92.
Nunn, K. (2001). In search of new wineskins: the phenomenology of anorexia nervosa not covered in DSM or ICD. *Clinical Child Psychology and Psychiatry, 6*: 489–503.
Nunn, K. & Thompson, S. (1996). The pervasive refusal syndrome: learned helplessness and hopelessness. *Clinical Child Psychology and Psychiatry, 1*: 121–132.
Nunn, K., Thompson, S., Moore, S., English, M., Burke, E. & Byrne, N. (1998). Managing pervasive refusal syndrome: strategies of hope. *Clinical Child Psychology and Psychiatry, 3*: 229–249.
Ogden, T. (1982). *Projective Identification and Psychotherapeutic Technique*. New York: Jason Aronson.
Ogden, T. (1986). *The Matrix of the Mind*. Northvale, NJ: Jason Aronson.
Ogden, T. (1989). *The Primitive Edge of Experience*. Northvale, NJ: Jason Aronson.

Ogden, T. (1994). *Subjects of Analysis.* Northvale, NJ: Jason Aronson.

Ogden, T. (2005). *This Art of Psychoanalysis: Dreaming Undreamt Dreams and Interrupted Cries.* London and New York: Routledge.

O'Shaughnessy, E. (1964). The absent object. *Journal of Child Psychotherapy, 1*(2): 34–43.

Oster, G. & Crone, P. (2004). *Using Drawings in Assessment and Therapy.* New York: Brunner-Routledge.

Partridge, E. (2008) Origins: A Short Etymological Dictionary of Modern English. London: Routledge.

Pasquini, P. (2007). *Tempo Lineare: Osservare, conoscere, aiutare i bambini e i genitori* (To observe, to know and to help children and their parents). Rome: Associazione Genitori e Amici del Tempo Linear—Onlus.

Patten, B. (2007). *Selected Poems.* London: Penguin.

Pepper Goldsmith, T. (2011). From symptoms to symbols: how can a creative group contribute to the transformation of deadly states of mind and the development of a capacity for mentalization in children who are psychiatric inpatients? Unpublished MA thesis, University of East London, Tavistock.

Perry, B. D., Pollard, R. A., Blakely, T. L., Baker, W. L. & Vigilante, D. (1995). Childhood trauma, the neurobiology of adaptation, and "use-dependent" development of the brain: how "states" become "traits". *Infant Mental Health Journal, 16*: 271–291.

Plato (429–547 BC). http://en.wikipedia.org/wiki/Play_therapy [last accessed August 2011].

Pullman, P. (2000). *The Amber Spyglass.* London: Scholastic.

Racker, H. (1953). The countertransference neurosis. In: *Transference and Countertransference* (pp. 105-126). Madison, CT: International Universities Press, 1968.

Rey, H. (1994). On that which the patient brings to analysis. In: J. Magagna (Ed.), *Universals of Psychoanalysis in the Treatment of Psychotic and Borderline States* (pp. 229–249). London: Free Association.

Rhode, M. (1997). Developmental and autistic aspects of vocalization. In: S. Acquarone (Ed.), *Signs of Autism in Infants* (pp. 227–236). London: Karnac, 2007.

Rhode, M. (1999). Echo or answer? The move towards ordinary speech in three children with autistic spectrum disorder. In: A. Alvarez & S. Reid (Eds.), *Autism and Personality: Findings from the Tavistock Autism Workshop* (pp. 42–79). London: Routledge.

Rhode, M. (2004). Different responses to trauma in two children with autistic spectrum disorder: the mouth as crossroads for the sense of self. *Journal of Child Psychotherapy, 30*(1): 3–20.

Rice, A. K. (1969). Individual, group and intergroup processes. *Human Relations, 22*: 565–584.

Riviere, J. (1952). The Unconscious Phantasy of an Inner World Reflected in Examples from Literature. In: M. Klein et al. *New Directions in Psycho-analysis* (pp.346-369). London: Tavistock.

Robertson, J. & Robertson, J. (1971). Young children in brief separation: a fresh look. *Psychoanalytic Study of the Child, 26*: 264–315.

Rogers, C. (1976). *Client-Centred Therapy.* London: Constable.

Rogers, R. & Hammerstein, O. (1951). Getting to know you. From: *The King and I,* Original Cast Recording. New York: Decca Records.

Romano, R. (1959). Forms of hostility in the transference. *International Journal of Psychoanalysis, 46A*: 90–106.

Ronningstam, E. (2006). Silence: cultural function and psychological transformation in psychoanalysis and psychoanalytic psychotherapy. *International Journal of Psychoanalysis, 87*: 1277–1295.

Rosenfeld, H. (1964). On the psychopathology of narcissism a clinical approach. *International Journal of Psycho-Analysis, 45*: 332–337.

Rosenfeld, H. (1971). A clinical approach to the psycho-analytic theory of life and death instincts. *International Journal of Psycho-Analysis, 52*: 169–178.

Rosenfeld, H. (1986). Personal communication.

Rosenfeld, H. (1987). *Impasse and Interpretation.* London: Tavistock.

Rustin, M. (2008). Work discussion: implications for research and policy. In: M. Rustin & J. Bradley (Eds.), *Work Discussion: Learning from Reflective Practice in Work with Children, Adolescents and Families* (pp. 267–284). London: Karnac/Tavistock Clinic Book Series.

Sabbadini, A. (1992). Listening to silence. *The Scandinavian Psychoanalytic Review, 15*: 27–36.

Saltzberger-Wittenberg, I. (1970). *Psychoanalytic Insights and Relationships.* London: Routledge, Kegan and Paul.

Saltzberger-Wittenberg, I. (1983). *The Emotional Experience of Learning and Teaching.* London: Routledge, Kegan and Paul.

Sanders, C. M. (1994). We are the stuff that dreams are made on: the use of dreams in systemic therapy. *Journal of Family Therapy, 16*: 367–381.

Sandler, P. (1997). The apprehension of psychic reality: extensions of Bion's theory of alpha-function. *International Journal of Psychoanalysis, 78*: 43–52.

Scharff, D. (2005). Infant observation augmented by the affective learning experience. In: J. Magagna, N. L. Bakalar, H. Cooper, J. Levy, C. Norman & C. Shank (Eds.), *Intimate Transformations: Babies with their Families* (pp. 198–211). London: Karnac.

Scharff, J. (1992). *Projective and Introjective Identification and the Use of the Therapist's Self.* Northvale, NJ: Jason Aronson.

Scharff, J. & Scharff, D. (2000). *Tuning the Therapeutic Instrument: Affective Learning of Psychotherapy.* Northvale, NJ: Jason Aronson.

Schon, D. (1982). *The Reflective Practitioner.* New York: Basic Books.

Schore, A. N. (2002a). Clinical implications of a psychoneurobiological model of projective identification. In: S. Alhanati (Ed.), *Primitive Mental States, Volume II: Psychobiological and Psychoanalytic Perspectives on Early Trauma and Personality Development* (pp. 1–65). London: Karnac.

Schore, A. N. (2002b). Dysregulation of the right brain: a fundamental mechanism of traumatic attachment and the psychopathogenesis of posttraumatic stress disorder. *Australian and New Zealand Journal of Psychiatry, 36*: 9–30.

Schotter, R. (2002). *Missing Rabbit.* New York: Clarion Books.

Seervai, F. (2003) *26th January and Other Poems.* Privately published poems printed in Mumbai, India: Spenta Multimedia.

Segal, H. (1957). Notes on symbol formation. *International Journal of Psycho-Analysis, 38*: 391–397.

Segal, H. (1981). *The Work of Hanna Segal: A Kleinian Approach to Clinical Practice.* London: Jason Aronson.

Segal, H. (1983). Some clinical implications of Melanie Klein's work, emergence from narcissism. *International Journal of Psycho-Analysis, 64*: 269–276.

Seligman, M. (1975). *Helplessness: On Depression, Development and Death.* San Francisco: W. H. Freeman.

Seligman, M. (1990). *Learned Optimism.* New York: Knopf.

Sendak, M. (1963). *Where the Wild Things Are.* New York: Harper.

Sharma, A. (2010). *Uncurling.* Poem published for the first time in this book.

Sherman, R. & Fredman, N. (1986). *Handbook of Structured Techniques in Marriage and Family Therapy.* New York: Brunner Mazel.

Shiel, A., Horn, S. A., Wilson, B. A., Watson, M. J., Campbell, M. J. & Meclellan, D. L. (2000). The Wessex Head Injury Matrix (WHIM) main scale: a preliminary report on a scale to assess and monitor patient recovery after severe head injury. *Clinical Rehabilitation, 14*: 408–416.

Simon, P. & Garfunkel, A. (1964). *The Sound of Silence*. Columbia Records: Catalogue number #4–43396.

Skarderud, F. (2007). Eating one's words: Part III. Mentalisation-based psychotherapy for anorexia nervosa, an outline for a treatment and training manual. *European Eating Disorders Review, 15*: 323–339.

Slochower, J. (1999). Interior experience within analytic process. *Psychoanalytic Dialogues, 9*: 789–809.

Sorenson, P. B. (2004). Primitive anxieties which interfere with attachment. *International Journal of Infant Observation, 7*(1): 46–67.

Sorenson, P. B. (2005). Transition facilitating behaviour: bridging attachment theory and British object relations. *Journal of Infant, Child and Adolescent Psychotherapy, 4*: 119–133.

Spiegel, R. (1965). Communication with depressive patients. *Contemporary Psychoanalysis, 2*: 30–34.

Spitz, R. A. (1965). *The First Year of Life*. New York: International Universities Press.

Steiner, J. (1993). *Psychic Retreats*. London: Routledge.

Stern, D. (1985). *The Interpersonal World of the Infant*. New York: Basic Books.

Stern, D. (2004). *The Present Moment*. New York: Norton.

Stolorow, R. D. & Munder Ross, J. (1978). The representational world in psychoanalytic therapy. *International Review of Psychoanalysis, 5*: 247–256.

Sunderland, M. (1997). *Drawing On Your Emotions*. Milton Keynes: Speechmark.

Symington, J. (2000). *Imprisoned Pain and Its Transformation: A Festschrift for H. Sidney Klein*. London: Karnac.

Symington, J. (2002). Mrs. Bick and infant observation. In: A. Briggs (Ed.), *Surviving Space: Papers on Infant Observation*. London: Karnac. pp. 105–117.

Symington, J. & Symington, N. (1996). *The Clinical Thinking of Wilfred Bion*. London and New York: Routledge.

Symington, N. (1983). The analyst's act of freedom as agent of therapeutic change. *International Journal of Psychoanalysis, 10*: 283–291.

Tate, A. (1993). Schooling. In: B. Lask & R. Bryant-Waugh (Eds.), *Anorexia Nervosa and Related Eating Disorders in Childhood and Adolescence*. London and New York: Routledge, 2007. pp. 313–335.

Taylor, S., Dossetor, D. R., Kilham, H. & Bernard, E. (2000). The youngest case of pervasive refusal syndrome? *Clinical Child Psychology and Psychiatry, 5*: 23–29.

Thompson, S. & Nunn, K. (1997). The pervasive refusal syndrome: the Royal Alexandra Hospital for Children experience. *Clinical Child Psychology and Psychiatry, 2*: 145–165.

Thomson, P. (1980). On the receptive function of the analyst. *International Review of Psycho-analysis, 7*: 183–205.

Trevarthen, C. (1996). *Children with Autism*. London and Philadelphia: Jessica Kingsley.

Trevarthen, C., Hubley, P. & Lock, A. (Eds.) (1978). *Secondary Intersubjectivity: Confidence, Confiding and Acts of Meaning in the First Year. Action, Gesture and Symbol: The Emergence of Language*. London: Academic Press.

Tronick, E. Z., Weinberg, M. K., Murray, L. & Cooper, P. J. (Eds.) (1997). Depressed mothers and infants: failure to form dyadic states of consciousness. In: *Postpartum Depression in Child Development* (pp. 54–81). New York: Guilford.

Tustin, F. (1980). Autistic objects. *International Review of Psychoanalysis, 7*: 27–40.

Tustin, F. (1981). *Autistic States in Children*. London and Boston: Routledge & Paul.

Tustin, F. (1986). *Autistic Barriers in Neurotic Patients*. London: Karnac.

Van Der Heide, C. (1942). Chronische schweiger in der analyse. (The chronically silent patient in analysis). *Psychoanalytic Quarterly, 11*: 444–445.

Van Der Heide, C. (1961). Blank silence and the dream screen. *Journal of the American Psychoanalytic Association, 9*: 85–90.

Waddell, M. (2002). *Inside Lives*. London: Karnac.

Waldhorn, H. (1959). The silent patient. *International Journal of Psychoanalysis, 7*: 548–560.

Warnock, M. (1976). *Imagination*. London: Faber and Faber.

Watzlawick, P., Bavelas, J. B. & Jackson, D. D. (1967). *Pragmatics of Human Communication: A Study of Interactional Patterns, Pathologies, and Paradoxes* (1st edn.). New York: Norton.

Weinberger, J. (1964). A triad of silence: silence, masochism, and depression. *International Journal of Psychoanalysis, 45*: 304–309.

Weinstein, L. (2002). Language, transference, and the developmental context in child analysis. *The Psychoanalytic Study of the Child, 57*: 355–373.

Wertman, E. (2008). Personal communication.

Whetherby, W. J. (1987). *Chariots of Fire*. New York: Dell.

Williams, G. (1997a). Double deprivation. *Internal Landscapes and Foreign Bodies: Eating Disorders and Other Pathologies*. Tavistock Series. London: Duckworth.

Williams, G. (1997b). Reflections on some dynamics of eating disorders: "no entry defenses and foreign bodies". *International Journal of Psycho-Analysis, 78*: 927–941.

Willis, S. (1999). Group analysis and eating disorders. *Group Analysis, 32*: 21–35.

Winnicott, D. W. (1949). Hate in the counter-transference. *International Journal of Psychoanalysis, 30*: 69–74.

Winnicott, D. W. (1953). Transitional objects and transitional phenomena. *International Journal of Psychoanalysis, 34*: 89–97.

Winnicott, D. W. (1958a). *Collected Papers: Through Paediatrics to Psychoanalysis*. London: Tavistock.

Winnicott, D. W. (1958b). The capacity to be alone. *International Journal of Psychoanalysis*, 39: 416–420.

Winnicott, D. W. (1960). Ego distortion and the true and false self. In: *The Maturational Process and the Facilitating Environment* (pp. 140–152). London: Hogarth Press, 1990.

Winnicott, D. W. (1962). The theory of the parent infant relationship—further remarks. *Journal of Psychoanalysis, 43*: 238–239.

Winnicott, D. W. (1988). *Babies and their Mothers*. Wokingham: Addison Wesley.

Winnicott, D. W. (1993). *Talking to Parents*. New York: Merloyd Lawrence.

Wood, D. (1999). From silent scream to shared sadness. *Group Analysis, 32*: 53–70.

Youngerman, J. (1979). The syntax of silence: electively mute therapy. *International Review of Psycho-Analysis, 6*: 283–295.

Zeligs, M. (1960). The role of transference, counter-transference, and the psycho-analytic process. *International Journal of Psychoanalysis, 41*: 407–412.

Zeligs, M. (1961). The psychology of silence: its role in the transference, countertransference and the psychoanalytic process. *Journal of the American Psychoanalytic Association, 9*: 7–43.

Zinner, J. & Shapiro, R. (1972). Projective identification as a mode of perception and behaviour in families of adolescents. *International Journal of Psycho-Analysis, 53*: 523–530.

INDEX

Printed in Great Britain
by Amazon

57508637R00226